Register Now for
to Your I

MW01492298

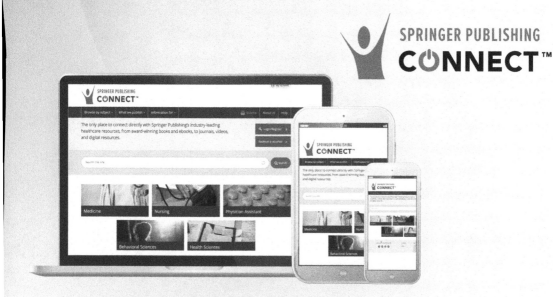

SPRINGER PUBLISHING
C⊙NNECT™

Your print purchase of *Pediatric CCRN® Certification Review* **includes online access to the contents of your book**—increasing accessibility, portability, and searchability!

Access today at:
http://connect.springerpub.com/content/book/978-0-8261-9319-3
or scan the QR code at the right with your smartphone. Log in or register, then click "Redeem a voucher" and use the code below.

> **SBRVJHT4**

Scan here for quick access.

Having trouble redeeming a voucher code?
Go to https://connect.springerpub.com/redeeming-voucher-code

If you are experiencing problems accessing the digital component of this product, please contact our customer service department at cs@springerpub.com

The online access with your print purchase is available at the publisher's discretion and may be removed at any time without notice.

Publisher's Note: New and used products purchased from third-party sellers are not guaranteed for quality, authenticity, or access to any included digital components.

Pediatric CCRN® Certification Review

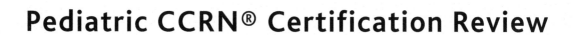

Maryann Godshall, PhD, CCRN-K, CPN, CNE, is an Associate Clinical Professor at Drexel University College of Nursing and Health Professions in Philadelphia, Pennsylvania. She obtained her BSN from Allentown College of St. Francis DeSales and her MSN as a Clinical Nurse Specialist from DeSales University. She has a post-master's degree in Nursing Education from Duquesne University, Pittsburgh, Pennsylvania. Maryann completed her PhD at Duquesne University (2014), and her research topic was "Exploring Learning of Pediatric Burn Patients through Storytelling."

Maryann has worked in Pediatrics and continues working in Pediatric Critical Care and Pediatric In-Patient Rehabilitation nursing. She has been a nurse for more than 30 years. She holds certification in pediatrics, pediatric critical care, and nursing education. She has been teaching for more than 24 years in both the university and hospital settings.

Maryann is coeditor of *The Certified Nurse Examination (CNE) Review Manual* (2022) and wrote *Fast Facts of Evidence Based Practice, Third Edition* (2020), Springer Publishing Company. She has published chapters in several books and textbooks including "Caring for the Child With a Chronic Condition and the Dying Child" and "Caring for the Child With Cancer" in *Maternal-Child Nursing Caring: Optimizing Outcomes for Mothers, Children, & Families, Second Edition* (2016); "Pediatric Nursing" in *NCLEX-RN, EXCEL* (2010), Springer Publishing Company; and in *Disaster Nursing: A Handbook for Practice* (2009); as well as many journal articles. She is a question item writer and chapter reviewer of several publications.

Other accomplishments include a Nightingale Award of Pennsylvania Nursing Scholarship. Maryann has presented locally, nationally, and internationally on a variety of pediatric, education, and critical care topics.

She is an active member in the American Association of Critical-Care Nurses, The Society of Pediatric Nursing, and Sigma Theta Tau.

Emily Warren, MSN, APRN, ACCNS-P, CCRN-K, is a pediatric Clinical Nurse Specialist (CNS) at the Johns Hopkins Hospital in Baltimore, Maryland. She obtained both her BSN and MSN from the Johns Hopkins University School of Nursing in Baltimore, Maryland.

Emily is an advanced practice nurse with 14 years of experience across the nursing care and leadership continuum. She has worked clinically as a pediatric critical care and transport nurse and currently supports nursing practice and patient care as the CNS for the four pediatric acute care units at the Johns Hopkins Hospital.

Emily is a dedicated clinician who shares her knowledge locally through mentorship and program building and is nationally recognized for her expertise across a variety of pediatric acute and critical care topics. She has and currently serves in both membership and leadership roles in nursing professional societies including the American Association of Critical-Care Nurses, the Society of Pediatric Nurses, and the National Association of Clinical Nurse Specialists.

Pediatric CCRN® Certification Review

Maryann Godshall, PhD, CCRN-K, CPN, CNE
Emily Warren, MSN, APRN, ACCNS-P, CCRN-K

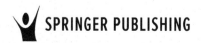

Springer Publishing Company, LLC
11 West 42nd Street, New York, NY 10036
www.springerpub.com
connect.springerpub.com/

Acquisitions Editor: Jaclyn Koshofer
Content Development Editor: Julia Curcio
Compositor: diacriTech

ISBN: 978-0-8261-9318-6
eISBN: 978-0-8261-9319-3
DOI: 10.1891/9780826193193

23 24 25 26 27 / 5 4 3 2 1

The author and the publisher of this Work have made every effort to use sources believed to be reliable to provide information that is accurate and compatible with the standards generally accepted at the time of publication. Because medical science is continually advancing, our knowledge base continues to expand. Therefore, as new information becomes available, changes in procedures become necessary. We recommend that the reader always consult current research and specific institutional policies before performing any clinical procedure or delivering any medication. The author and publisher shall not be liable for any special, consequential, or exemplary damages resulting, in whole or in part, from the readers' use of, or reliance on, the information contained in this book. The publisher has no responsibility for the persistence or accuracy of URLs for external or third-party Internet websites referred to in this publication and does not guarantee that any content on such websites is, or will remain, accurate or appropriate.

Library of Congress Control Number: 2023934384

Maryann Godshall: https://orcid.org/0000-0001-9516-0231
Emily Warren: https://orcid.org/0000-0001-8382-4766

Publisher's Note: **New and used products purchased from third-party sellers are not guaranteed for quality, authenticity, or access to any included digital components.**

Printed in the United States of America by Hatteras, Inc.

CCRN® is a registered service mark of the American Association of Critical-Care Nurses (AACN). AACN does not sponsor or endorse this resource, nor does it have a proprietary relationship with Springer Publishing.

We would like to dedicate this book to the bedside nurses in the PICU who hopefully will find this review book helpful in their pursuit of their CCRN. The work you do is beyond inspiring, and I am honored to be your peer. Thank you for all you do! We would also like to dedicate this book to the patients and families in the PICU who have taught us and continue to inspire us to learn more. It is truly an honor and privilege to have been part of your and your child's life.

Contents

Contributors

Kenya Agarwal, MSN, RN, ACCNS-P, CCRN
Children's Hospital of Philadelphia
Philadelphia, Pennsylvania

Jaclyn Campbell, DNP, APRN, CPNP-AC, CCRN
Joe DiMaggio Children's Hospital
Hollywood, Florida

Jennifer Cannon, RN, BSN, CCRN
Allentown, Pennsylvania
St. Luke's University Health Network
Bethlehem, Pennsylvania

Margaret Cates, DNP, RN, ACCNS-P, CCRN
Cardiac Intensive Care Unit
Children's Hospital of Philadelphia
Philadelphia, Pennsylvania

Julie Dunn, MSN, RN, CPN
Cardiac Intensive Care Unit
Children's Hospital of Philadelphia
Philadelphia, Pennsylvania

Erin Dwyer, MSN, APRN, ACCNS-P, CCRN
Nemours Children's Hospital
Wilmington, Delaware

Maureen Fitzgerald, EdD, MSN, CPN
Director, Academic Nursing Graduate Program
Jefferson College of Nursing
Thomas Jefferson University
Philadelphia, Pennsylvania

Kimberly Garcia, DNP, PMHNP-BC, FNP-BC, GNP-BC, NP-C, CNE, CNEcl, CARN-AP
Assistant Clinical Professor
Director, Psychiatric Nurse Practitioner Program
Drexel University
Philadelphia, Pennsylvania

Maryann Godshall, PhD, CCRN-K, CPN, CNE
Associate Professor of Nursing
College of Nursing and Health Professions
Drexel University
Philadelphia, Pennsylvania

Jennifer Highfield, DNP, APRN, CPNP-AC, CCRN
Pediatric Critical Care of South Florida
Joe DiMaggio Children's Hospital
Hollywood, Florida

David Jack, PhD, RN, CPN
Jefferson College of Nursing
Thomas Jefferson University
Philadelphia, Pennsylvania

Emily D. Johnson, MSN, CPNP-PC/AC
Charlotte R. Bloomberg Children's Center
Johns Hopkins Children's Center
Baltimore, Maryland

Lisette Kaplan, MSN, RN, CCRN
Joe DiMaggio Children's Hospital
Hollywood, Florida

Kristen Lourie, BSN, CCRN
Children's Hospital of Philadelphia
Philadelphia, Pennsylvania

Stephanie Morgenstern, MSN, APRN, ACCNS-P, CCRN
Clinical Nurse Specialist
Johns Hopkins Children's Center
Baltimore, Maryland

Rebecca Reid, MSN, RN, CCRN, CPN
Cardiac Intensive Care Unit
Children's Hospital of Philadelphia
Philadelphia, Pennsylvania

Megan Snyder, DNP, RN, ACCNS-P, CCRN
Children's Hospital of Philadelphia
Philadelphia, Pennsylvania

Molly Stetzer, MSN, RN, ACCNS-P, CWOCN, VA-BC
Children's Hospital of Philadelphia
Philadelphia, Pennsylvania

Katherine Thompson, DNP, APRN, ACCNS-P, CCRN-K
Clinical Nurse Specialist
Pediatric and Congenital Heart Center
Johns Hopkins Children's Center
Baltimore, Maryland

Angie Tsay, BSN, RN, CCRN
Johns Hopkins Hospital Children's Center
Baltimore, Maryland

Emily Warren, MSN, APRN, ACCNS-P, CCRN-K
Johns Hopkins Hospital Children's Center
Baltimore, Maryland

Reviewers

Judith Ascenzi DNP, RN, CCRN-K
Director
Pediatric Nursing Programs
Johns Hopkins Children's Center
Baltimore, Maryland

Kathryn E. Roberts, MSN, RN, CENP, CCNS, CCRN-K, FCCM
Director
Center for Nursing Excellence, Education & Innovation
Joe DiMaggio Children's Hospital
Hollywood, Florida

Foreword

The essential role of pediatric critical care nurses has never been more apparent than during the COVID-19 pandemic. Nurses are vital to the delivery of care to both pediatric patients and their families. Through education and experience, we continue to challenge ourselves as nurses to become experts in our field. This is especially so when taking care of children. Parents trust us with their most special gift: their child. We honor that trust and strive to learn to be our best for them. We guide parents through uncertain and scary times while focusing on everyone in the family unit using family-centered care.

A pediatric ICU (PICU) nurse's care is delivered with kindness, gentleness, and compassion. The nurse is the chief coordinator and navigator of care by utlizing the latest technology and treatment modalities for the most vulnerable children. Pediatric critical care nursing may be the hardest job you will ever love to do. The rewards of being part of the team that helps a fragile child slowly get stronger each day and return to their previous state of health are indescribable. To see the smile return to the face of a child who had been at the brink of death touches the soul like nothing else. We honor those bedside PICU nurses who deliver this care and do it with passion and purpose. Most PICU nurses don't want any accolades for what they do. They don't want to be a hero, they have one single purpose: to see sick children return home, to school, and back to their normal lives. PICU nurses are angels in scrubs. Thank you for what you do! It is an honor to be your peer.

This book was developed as a resource for the pediatric critical care nurse seeking to prepare them to take their certification exam to maintain their excellence in clinical practice.

Maryann Godshall and Emily Warren
PICU Nurses

Preface

Education is the passport to the future, for tomorrow belongs to those who prepare for it today.
—Malcom X

The more that you read, the more things you will know, the more that you learn, the more places you will go.
—Dr. Seuss

This book was created to be a single resource to refresh knowledge and help prepare nurses to take their pediatric CCRN® exam.

This book takes the reader through a guided, educational discussion of testable content to understand and master the pediatric CCRN® exam. We have gathered expert nurses in their fields from various hospitals to share with you their expertise and latest information available. The book is based on the blueprint provided by the American Association of Critical-Care Nurses (AACN) including testable nursing actions for the Pediatric Certified Critical Care Nurse (CCRN®) exam. It is organized by systems. Each chapter uses information, tables, figures, case studies, clinical pearls, and knowledge check questions. The reader will receive answers to those questions and rationales for the correct response and incorrect responses to support learning. After studying all the chapters, there is an additional 150-question practice exam to help prepare you for the certification exam. We wish you luck in your preparation for the pediatric CCRN® exam.

Another distinct advantage to this prep book is that when purchasing the *Pediatric CCRN® Certification Review* the learner automatically receives access to the ebook (with no expiration date). Although a full, 150-question practice exam is included at the end of the book, the ebook also offers an interactive test prep platform option for answer viewing. This feature more closely simulates taking the online exam than does a print test.

Pass Guarantee

If you use this resource to prepare for your exam and do not pass, you may return it for a refund of your full purchase price, excluding tax, shipping, and handling. To receive a refund, return your product along with a copy of your exam score report and original receipt showing purchase of new product (not used). Product must be returned and received within 180 days of the original purchase date. Refunds will be issued within 8 weeks from acceptance and approval. One offer per person and address. This offer is valid for U.S. residents only. Void where prohibited. To initiate a refund, please contact Customer Service at csexamprep@springerpub.com.

About the Pediatric CCRN® Exam

Maryann Godshall

INTRODUCTION TO THE PEDIATRIC CCRN® EXAM

The Critical Care Registered Nurse (CCRN) is a credential granted by the American Association of Critical-Care Nurses (AACN) Corporation. The pediatric CCRN® exam validates your knowledge and expertise in the care of acutely and critically ill children. More than 95,000 nurses worldwide are currently CCRN certified. Of those 95,000, more than 7,000 hold the pediatric CCRN certification. In choosing to obtain your certification, you promote continuing excellence in pediatric critical care nursing.

▶ ELIGIBILITY

LICENSING

To be eligible to take the CCRN® exam you need to have a current, unencumbered U.S. RN or APRN **license**.

PRACTICE

Candidates must meet one of the following clinical practice requirement options (AACN, 2022, p. 2):
- Practice as an RN or APRN for 1,750 hours in direct care of acutely/critically ill patients during the previous 2 years, with 875 of those hours accrued in the most recent year preceding application.
  OR
- Practice as an RN or APRN during the previous 5 years with a minimum of 2,000 hours in direct care of acutely/critically ill patients, with 144 of those hours accrued in the most recent year preceding application.

PRACTICE VERIFICATION

"The name and contact information of a professional associate must be given for verification of eligibility related to clinical practice hours. If you are selected for audit, this associate will need to verify in writing that you have met the clinical hour requirements" (AACN, 2022, p. 2).

▶ APPLICATION AND SCHEDULING

- Applicants can apply to take the exam either online or via paper application.
- There is an application fee with discounts available for groups. Employers may prepurchase exam vouchers at a further discounted rate.
- Live remote proctoring (LRP) allows you to take your exam from your own computer/desk in a quiet and private location, such as your home office. The location must be free from distractions, and your computer must meet specific compatibility requirements. Please carefully review the following information to determine if a remote proctored exam is right for you. For details, check out PSI's Remote Proctored Exam Experience video.
- The exam is available in an online or paper format.
  - Computer-based exams are administered by PSI International at over 300 testing centers across the United States and via live remote proctoring with a personal computer in a quiet, private location.

- The exam is offered year-round, Monday through Saturday.
- AACN membership is not required to take the exam.
- For more information, visit the *CCRN® Exam Handbook* online at www.aacn.org/certification /preparation-tools-and-handbooks/handbooks-and-documents.

▶ TAKING THE EXAM

- The exam is 3 hours long.
- There are 150 multiple choice questions.
  - 25 questions are pilot items being trialed for future exams and do not count toward your score.
  - 125 questions are scored.
- Your results will be determined by how many questions you get correct.
  - Some questions are more difficult than others.
  - You earn points only for the questions you answer correctly.
  - If you do not know the answer to a question, take your best guess because there is a chance of getting the answer correct.
  - If you get a minimum of 70% of the questions correct, you will receive a passing score.
- Online exam-takers receive their test results immediately upon the completion of the exam. Exam results will show on-screen, and a score report will be emailed to you within 24 hours after the completion of the exam.
- Paper exam-takers receive their test results by mail 6 to 8 weeks following the completion of the exam.
- Successful candidates will be mailed their wall certificate approximately 3 to 4 weeks after testing.
- Unsuccessful candidates are eligible for a discounted retest fee.
- For more information, visit the *CCRN® Exam Handbook* online at www.aacn.org/certification /preparation-tools-and-handbooks/handbooks-and-documents.

▶ EXAM CONTENT

COGNITIVE LEVELS OF QUESTIONS

The cognitive level of the exam items is based on a condensed version of Bloom's Taxonomy. Most of the items are written at the application and analysis levels. By testing at higher cognitive levels, it provides an indication of the candidate's critical thinking abilities when caring for acutely and critically ill patients and their families.

The AACN uses the Synergy Model, a conceptual framework that matches the skills of the practitioner to the acuity of the patient. There are no questions on the test that deal specifically with the terminology of this model but answers to specific questions in the exam based on practice utilize this model, such as questions that address the journey from novice to expert nurse.

BREAKDOWN OF THE EXAM

The following is a sample blueprint for the exam. This is a breakdown of clinical content and nursing actions. In this sample blueprint, 80% of the exam questions are on clinical judgement and 20% are on professional caring and ethical practice. The most current blueprint of the exam can be found in the *CCRN® Exam Handbook* online at www.aacn.org/certification/preparation-tools-and-handbooks /handbooks-and-documents.

SAMPLE BLUEPRINT

I. CLINICAL JUDGMENT (80%)
  A. Cardiovascular (14%)
    1. Cardiac infection and inflammatory diseases
    2. Cardiac malformations
    3. Cardiac surgery
    4. Cardiogenic shock (CS)
    5. Cardiomyopathies
    6. Cardiovascular catheterization
    7. Dysrhythmias
    8. Heart failure (HF)

      9. Hypertensive crisis
    10. Myocardial conduction system defects
    11. Obstructive shock
    12. Vascular occlusion

B. Respiratory (18%)
    1. Acute pulmonary edema
    2. Acute pulmonary embolus
    3. Acute respiratory distress syndrome (ARDS)
    4. Acute respiratory failure
    5. Acute respiratory infection
    6. Air-leak syndromes
    7. Apnea of prematurity
    8. Aspiration
    9. Chronic pulmonary conditions
    10. Congenital airway malformations
    11. Failure to wean from mechanical ventilation
    12. Pulmonary hypertension (PH)
    13. Status asthmaticus
    14. Thoracic and airway trauma
    15. Thoracic surgery

C. Endocrine/Hematology/Gastrointestinal/Renal/Integumentary (20%)
    1. Endocrine
       a. Adrenal insufficiency
       b. Diabetes insipidus (DI)
       c. Diabetic ketoacidosis (DKA)
       d. Diabetes mellitus, types 1 and 2
       e. Hyperglycemia
       f. Hypoglycemia
       g. Inborn errors of metabolism
       h. Syndrome of inappropriate secretion of antidiuretic hormone (SIADH)
    2. Hematology and Immunology
       a. Anemia
       b. Coagulopathies (e.g., immune thombocytopenic purpura [ITP], disseminated intravascular coagulation [DIC])
       c. Immune deficiencies
       d. Myelosuppression (e.g., thrombocytopenia, neutropenia)
       e. Oncologic complications
       f. Sickle cell crisis
       g. Transfusion reactions
    3. Gastrointestinal (GI)
       a. Abdominal compartment syndrome (ACS)
       b. Abdominal trauma
       c. Bowel infarction, obstruction, and perforation
       d. Gastroesophageal reflux
       e. GI hemorrhage
       f. GI surgery
       g. Liver disease and failure
       h. Malnutrition and malabsorption
       i. Necrotizing enterocolitis (NEC)
       j. Peritonitis
    4. Renal and genitourinary
       a. Acute kidney injury (AKI)
       b. Chronic kidney disease (CKD)
       c. Hemolytic uremic syndrome (HUS)
       d. Kidney transplant
       e. Life-threatening electrolyte imbalances
       f. Renal and genitourinary infections
       g. Renal and genitourinary surgery

      5. Integumentary
        a. Intravenous (IV) infiltration
        b. Pressure injury
        c. Skin failure (e.g., hypoperfusion)
        d. Wounds

D. Musculoskeletal/Neurological/Psychosocial (15%)
    1. Musculoskeletal
        a. Compartment syndrome (CS)
        b. Musculoskeletal surgery
        c. Musculoskeletal trauma
        d. Rhabdomyolysis
    2. Neurological
        a. Acute spinal cord injury
        b. Agitation
        c. Brain death
        d. Congenital neurological abnormalities
        e. Delirium
        f. Encephalopathy
        g. Head trauma
        h. Hydrocephalus
        i. Intracranial hemorrhage (ICH)
        j. Neurogenic shock
        k. Neurologic infectious disease
        l. Neuromuscular disorders
        m. Neurosurgery
        n. Pain: acute, chronic
        o. Seizure disorders
        p. Space-occupying lesions
        q. Spinal fusion
        r. Stroke
        s. Traumatic brain injury (TBI)
    3. Behavioral and Psychosocial
        a. Abuse and neglect
        b. Posttraumatic stress disorder (PTSD)
        c. Postintensive care syndrome (PICS)
        d. Self-harm
        e. Suicidal ideation and behavior

E. Multisystem (13%)
    1. Acid–base imbalance
    2. Anaphylactic shock
    3. Death and dying
    4. Healthcare-associated conditions (e.g., ventilator-association events [VAE], catheter associated urinary tract infection [CAUTI], central line associated bloodstream infection [CLABSI])
    5. Hypovolemic shock
    6. Posttransplant complications
    7. Sepsis
    8. Submersion injuries (i.e., near drowning)
    9. Hyperthermia and hypothermia
    10. Toxin and drug exposure

II. PROFESSIONAL CARING AND ETHICAL PRACTICE (20%)
  A. Advocacy/Moral Agency
  B. Caring Practices
  C. Response to Diversity
  D. Facilitation of Learning
  E. Collaboration
  F. Systems Thinking
  G. Clinical Inquiry

There are also **testable actions** that are included in the exam. They are as follows.
CLINICAL JUDGMENT

General

- Manage patients receiving:
  - continuous sedation
  - extracorporeal membrane oxygenation (ECMO)
  - nonpharmacologic interventions
  - pharmacologic interventions
  - intraprocedural and postprocedural care
  - postoperative care
  - vascular access
- Conduct physical assessment of critically ill or injured patients.
- Conduct psychosocial assessment of critically ill or injured patients.
- Evaluate diagnostic test results and laboratory values.
- Manage patients during intrahospital transport.
- Manage patients undergoing procedural sedation.
- Manage patients with temperature monitoring and regulation devices.
- Provide family-centered care.

Cardiovascular

- Manage patients requiring:
  - arterial catheterization (e.g., arterial line)
  - cardiac catheterization
  - cardioversion
  - central venous pressure (CVP) monitoring
  - defibrillation
  - epicardial pacing
  - near-infrared spectroscopy (NIRS)
  - umbilical catheterization (e.g., umbilical vein catheterization [UVC], umbilical artery catheterization [UAC])
- Manage patients with:
  - cardiac dysrhythmias
  - hemodynamic instability

Respiratory

- Manage patients requiring:
  - artificial airways (e.g., endotracheal tubes [ETT], tracheotomy)
  - assistance with airway clearance
  - chest tubes
  - high-frequency oscillatory ventilation (HFOV)
  - mechanical ventilation
  - noninvasive positive-pressure ventilation (e.g., continuous positive airway pressure [CPAP], nasal intermittent mandatory ventilation [IMV], high-flow n.cannula)
  - prone positioning
  - respiratory monitoring devices (e.g., SpO_2, SVO_2, $EtCO_2$)
  - therapeutic gases (e.g., oxygen [O_2], nitric oxide, heliox, carbon dioxide [CO_2])
  - thoracentesis

Hematology and Immunology

- Manage patients receiving:
  - plasmapheresis, exchange transfusion, or leukocyte depletion
  - transfusion

Neurological

- Conduct pain assessment of critically ill or injured patients
- Manage patients with seizure activity
- Provide end-of-life and palliative care
- Manage patients requiring:
  - neurologic monitoring devices and drains (e.g., intracranial pressure [ICP], ventricular drains, grids)
  - spinal immobilization

Integumentary
- Manage patients requiring wound prevention and/or treatment (e.g., wound vacuum assisted closures [VACs], pressure reduction surfaces, fecal management devices, IV infiltrate treatment)

Gastrointestinal
- Manage patients with inadequate nutrition and fluid intake (e.g., chewing and swallowing difficulties, alterations in hunger and thirst, inability to self-feed)
- Manage patients receiving:
  - enteral and parenteral nutrition
  - GI drains
  - intraabdominal pressure monitoring

Renal and Genitourinary
- Manage patients requiring:
  - electrolyte replacement
  - renal replacement therapies (e.g., hemodialysis, continuous renal replacement therapy [CRRT], peritoneal dialysis)

Multisystem
- Manage patients requiring progressive mobility

Behavioral and Psychosocial
- Conduct behavioral assessment of critically ill or injured patients (e.g., delirium, withdrawal)
- Manage patients requiring behavioral and mental health interventions
- Respond to behavioral emergencies (e.g., nonviolent crisis intervention, de-escalation techniques)

▶ PREPARING FOR THE EXAM

MAKE A SCHEDULE

Prepare well in advance for the exam. Timing and planning are everything! You need to make a schedule and set aside designated time to study each week even if it is just 1 hour a day. Stick to your schedule. It is easy to get distracted. Do not procrastinate!

HAVE A POSITIVE ATTITUDE

The better attitude you have toward studying, the better you will perform on the test. Don't make studying a chore. A positive attitude about studying (you are learning new information and can be excited about it) is a key factor in retaining information.

BREAK-UP MATERIAL INTO CHUNKS

Break up the content into small sections or chunks so that you are not overwhelmed. By studying smaller amounts of material, you will absorb information easier than if you tried to study a lot of material at once. Cramming for the exam is not recommended. Research has shown that cramming for tests pushes information into your short-term memory, but that same information is unavailable for long term. You want to learn this information and retain it for use in the future, not memorize and then forget. In addition, early and consistent preparation will reduce test anxiety.

ORGANIZE THE INFORMATION

Organize the information you want to study. Keep all study materials together. **You should only need this book!** Keep it with you so in the event you get unexpected down time, you can utilize it to study and review information. Review the content outline and add relevant items as needed. Using flashcards to check your facts is a great way of retaining information that may be unfamiliar to you. Underline key phrases, color code your notes, focus on visualizing a concept in your mind, and use mnemonic devices to remember items or short lists. Plan to review your notes or reread sections of content you may have found unclear.

STUDY ENVIRONMENT

This is a key area to your success. If you need silence, set up a quiet area in your home in a brightly lit space. Put away your phone, and turn off any distractors. Study when you are rested and alert; this aids in retention. Do not try to multitask. Research has consistently shown that multitasking will make your studying less effective. Consider having study groups with others who are also studying for the exam as it is helpful and good for morale. Study on your own as well but have study groups so that you can quiz each other and make sure that you truly understand concepts. When you explain concepts to others, you will understand the concept better yourself. Others might be able to explain a concept to you in a way that makes perfect sense. Utilize your peers and resources around you.

TEST TAKING TIPS

- Be sure to *read the entire question*. Do not provide an answer before you have read the entire question and all the answers. Choose your answer, then go back and read the question again to be sure what you have chosen truly answers the question being asked.
- Eliminate answers that you know are incorrect and focus on the remaining answers.
- Beware of questions that have *negatives* in them (*never, without, not*, etc.).
- Look for *key words* in questions (*always, earliest, on admission, common, best, least, immediately, initial*, etc.).
- Eliminate any answer that contain the words *always* or *never* as it will be a wrong choice.
- Identify *priority words* (which would you do first, most important, etc.).
- Identify *answers about the patients and the family* (empower, give choices, involve, etc.).
- Use a *process of elimination* (rule out answers you are sure are incorrect first).
- Identify *absolute words* (*always, never*, etc.).
- *Eliminate answers that are the same* (look for the answer that is different).
- *Identify answers that are opposite of each other*, one is usually the correct answer (increase pH or decrease pH).
- Watch out for "all of the above" answers. If you can clearly rule out one of the responses, then you have already determined that an "all of the above" response choice is not the correct answer. However, if you can identify that two responses are correct, and "all of the above" is an option, choose "all of the above." Be careful if this is a "select all that apply" question as this would not prove true in that instance.
- You should always be looking for a therapeutic response. Your initial response as the nurse is always therapeutic. For example, you must acknowledge and validate a patient's feelings. You should always acknowledge and validate before you provide information, except in the event of an emergency.
- Know who or what is the actual focus of the question. Is it a friend, family, or a significant other instead of the patient? A lot of information in the question may be there to purposely distract you. Ask yourself, "What is the question really asking me?"
- **When in doubt and you don't know the answer:** Remember Maslow's hierarchy of needs and the ABCs (airway, breathing, and circulation). When these goals are met, safety is the priority. After safety comes psychological needs. Learning takes place only if the learner (patient) is motivated to learn.
- Oftentimes the longest option (the answer with most words or explanation) is the correct answer.
- Order matters. If a question asks the order of an event, pay close attention to words that indicate sequencing (*first, before, later, next*).
- If you really can't decide which choice is best, and you can't come back to it, make an educated guess.

ANSWER PRACTICE QUESTIONS

There are many sources of practice questions. This book provides some questions in each chapter along with a comprehensive exam at the back of the book. When quizzing yourself, look at the questions you got wrong to determine why it is the wrong answer. The questions in this book will provide rationale for correct and incorrect answers. If you are unclear of the content, go to the content review section of each chapter or seek alternate resources. Pay attention to questions where you made an educated guess at the answer. This is a sign you may not have a solid understanding of that content. In addition, pay attention to questions that you found difficult and took a lot of time to answer even if you got them correct. This might signify you may not have a solid understanding of the content or concept. As with your initial RN exam, the more questions the better, provided that you are utilizing quality questions. You can find additional questions on the AACN website.

REVIEW CLASSES

There are many vendors that offer 1- or 2-day review classes. This can be "live" in person or in an online or virtual format. Some have found this beneficial and others have not. If you find yourself undisciplined with your study schedule, review classes may benefit you. These offerings can be recorded and you can listen to them anytime. It is up to you and how you learn best.

THE DAY OF THE EXAM

Get everything you will need for the exam together the night before. Be sure to get a good night's sleep. Cramming until the early morning hours is not helpful. Do not overconsume coffee or any other stimulant like green tea. The day of the exam, arrive early. You don't want to feel rushed. Plan for traffic issues. Eat a light breakfast or a nutritious snack, not a snack full of sugar. Use the bathroom before the exam. Relax and control test anxiety. It is normal to feel anxious about taking the exam. Anxiety is a natural way our body responds to any stress. Some anxiety is helpful and increases awareness, whereas uncontrolled anxiety will impede your ability to think critically. Some strategies that might be used to reduce test anxiety are:

- Schedule the exam during a time that is less stressful for you in your life.
- Before starting the exam, breathe. Take a few cleansing breaths to allow oxygen to flow to your brain. Visualize. Close your eyes and imagine yourself sitting by the ocean or at your favorite place. Then slowly open your eyes and begin.
- Talk yourself up during the exam, for example, "I got this." Put positive energy out in the universe for your success.
- Stop negative thoughts like "what if" and second guessing. Don't make up reasons why an answer could be correct. Take the questions and answers as they are written.
- Practice yoga or meditation while studying or the morning of the exam.

THE EXAM ITSELF

- What if you get stuck on a question? Try not to take too long on one question. If you don't know the answer, skip it, and move on to questions you do know and can readily answer, then go back to the more difficult ones later.
- Correlate the test questions to something you have seen in your clinical practice.
- Take each question as it comes. When you move on to the next question, forget the previous question. Focus only on the question you are answering.
- If you find yourself becoming anxious, go back to closing your eyes and breathing for a moment.
  Preparation for the exam is key. If you are not successful on your initial attempt, you can take the exam again. Good luck!

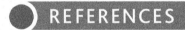 REFERENCES

American Association of Critical-Care Nurses. (2022, October). *CCRN exam handbook*. https://www.aacn.org /~/media/aacn-website/certification/get-certified/handbooks/ccrnexamhandbook.pdf

Cardiovascular System Review

Margaret Cates, Julie Dunn, and Rebecca Reid

When thinking about pediatric cardiac defects and disorders, nurses can become easily overwhelmed. Establishing a strong understanding of normal anatomy and physiology of the heart and general principles related to cardiac output (CO) will support your understanding and ability to critically think through the patient's diagnosis, treatment, and management.

In order to understand what is abnormal, knowing what is normal is necessary. In the normal heart anatomy, unoxygenated blood returns to the heart through the superior vena cava (SVC) and the inferior vena cava (IVC) into the right atrium (RA), which is where unoxygenated blood from the heart returns via the coronary sinus. Unoxygenated blood leaves the RA via the tricuspid valve and enters the right ventricle (RV). The blood then enters the pulmonary artery (PA), through the pulmonary valve (PV) and the two branch (into the left and right) PAs to the lungs to be oxygenated. In the lungs, an exchange of gases occurs between oxygen (O_2) and carbon dioxide (CO_2). The four pulmonary veins return the now oxygenated blood to the left atrium (LA) of the heart, through the mitral valve (MV) and into the left ventricle (LV). Blood exits this chamber into the ascending aorta and the aortic valve (AV). The blood then may fall backward in diastole into the aortic cusps and enters the coronary arteries to feed the heart oxygenated blood. The majority of the blood continues upward and through the innominate artery, the left common carotid artery, the left subclavian artery, and then down through the descending thoracic aorta (Figure 2.1).

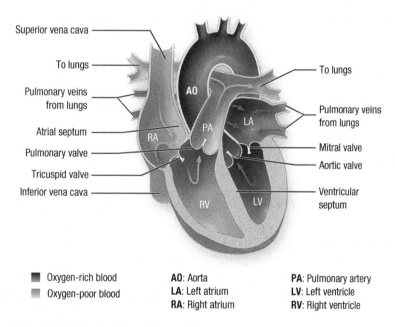

Figure 2.1 Normal cardiac anatomy
Source: Copyright 2014, Children's Hospital of Philadelphia. Reprinted with permission.

Important concepts of the cardiovascular system include:

- **CO** is comprised of stroke volume (SV) and heart rate (HR): **CO = SV × HR**. **SV** is the amount of blood ejected from the heart with each contraction. **HR** is the number of times the heart beats per minute. Good CO is demonstrated by good peripheral perfusion. CO is influenced by preload, afterload, compliance, and contractility (Figure 2.2).

- **Preload** is the amount of blood returned to the heart from the pulmonary and systemic circulations at the end of diastole. **Afterload** is the workload that the ventricles must overcome to pump blood to the lungs or body; the workload is the pulmonary (PVR) or systemic vascular resistance (SVR).
- **Compliance** is the ability of the heart to stretch and fill during diastole. Good compliance is demonstrated by a ventricle that fills without a large increase in ventricular pressure. Poor compliance may be referred to as a "stiff heart" where small increases in ventricular preload significantly increase ventricular pressures.
- **Contractility** is the ability of the heart muscle to shorten or shrink with enough force to eject blood from the ventricle to the lungs and body. Contractility is estimated by echocardiography and directly measured by cardiac catheterization.

Understanding the impact that clinical conditions, like metabolic acidosis and hypoxemia, and interventions, like O_2, fluid, and medication administration, have on preload, afterload, compliance, and contractility are essential to the management of the critically ill infant or child with cardiac disease.

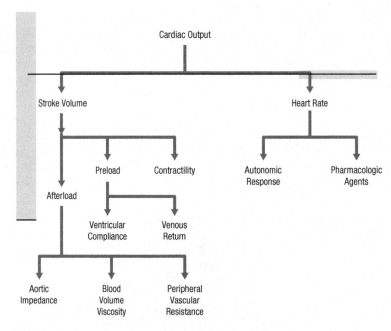

Figure 2.2 Cardiac output (CO)

▶ CARDIAC MALFORMATIONS

Congenital heart disease (CHD) is the most common birth defect affecting about 1% of all births in the United States (CDC, 2022a). One in four infants born with CHD will have critical CHD, which requires intervention in the first year of life. The exact cause of CHD is unknown but is attributed to both environmental and genetic factors. Prematurity, chromosomal abnormalities, and extracardiac birth defects increase morbidity and mortality risk. Early diagnosis is associated with improved outcomes. Prenatal diagnosis through routine ultrasound and fetal echocardiogram has increased over recent years. However, not all CHD is diagnosed prenatally. As such, all 50 states screen for critical CHD prior to discharge from the birth hospital. Screening takes place with the use of the right upper extremity and a lower extremity pulse-oximetry reading. If there is a difference between the two readings or oxygen saturation levels are low, the baby is referred for cardiology consultation and echocardiogram to rule out CHD.

FETAL AND TRANSITIONAL CIRCULATION

During embryological development, the heart develops between the 3rd and 8th week of pregnancy, complete with fetal circulation delivering oxygenated blood to the fetus and removing CO_2. Fetal circulation is distinctly different from post-fetal circulation, with aspects of fetal circulation playing a key role in the management of the neonate born with critical CHD. Key differences include:

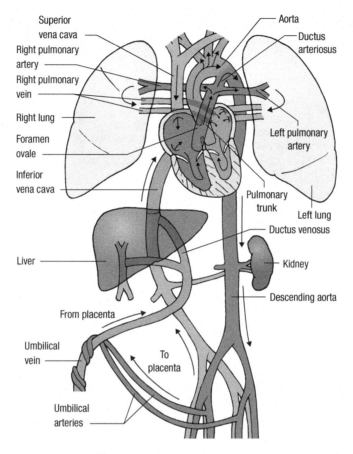

Figure 2.3 Fetal circulation

Source: Hoffman, J., Thompson-Bowie, N., & Jnah, A. (2019). *Fetal and neonatal physiology for the advanced practice nurse.* Springer Publishing Company.

- gas exchange occurs via the placenta instead of the lungs
- presence of intracardiac shunts (foramen ovale, ductus arteriosus, ductus venosus)
- high pulmonary vascular resistance (PVR)
- low SVR
- low CO (Figure 2.3)

The foramen ovale is an opening between the RA and LA of the heart. The ductus arteriosus is a blood vessel that connects the PA to the aorta. The ductus venosus is a blood vessel that connects oxygen rich blood from the placenta to the IVC.

Transitional circulation begins as the umbilical cord is clamped and circulation is separated from the placenta coupled with extrauterine respiration. During transitional circulation:

- Gas exchange transitions to the lungs once separate from the placenta.
- PVR drops considerably in the first 12 to 24 hours of life and continues to fall to normal levels around 6 to 8 weeks of age.
- SVR and CO increases.
- Functional closure of intracardiac shunts occurs by 24 to 72 hours of life.

CONGENITAL HEART DISEASE CLASSIFICATION

CHD is broadly classified into two types: **acyanotic** and **cyanotic** (Figure 2.4).

Acyanotic CHD is further divided into two types:
- increased pulmonary blood flow
- outflow obstruction

When a patient has acyanotic CHD, there may be a right to left shunt with oxygenated blood being delivered to the systemic circulation.

Cyanotic CHD is further divided into two types:

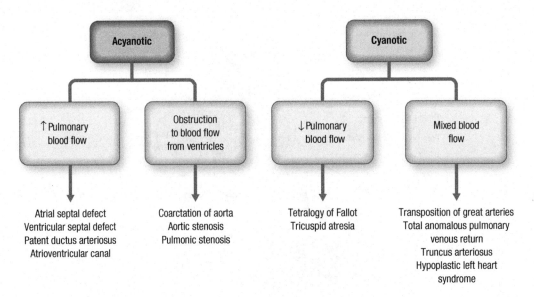

Figure 2.4 Classification of acyanotic and cyanotic congenital heart disease (CHD)

- decreased pulmonary blood flow
- mixed blood flow

With cyanotic CHD, there is the presence of a right to left shunt, which results in deoxygenated blood being delivered to the systemic circulation. This results in O_2 saturation levels below the normal level.

Clinicians should include CHD in their differential diagnosis, in the setting of a murmur and cyanosis, cyanosis that worsens with crying, a failed hyperoxia test—meaning saturations do not improve with administration of 100% oxygen, significant weight loss, poor feeding with tachypnea, infant that presents as potentially septic, discordant upper and lower extremity pulses, and presence of a genetic syndrome. CHD is associated with the following genetic syndrome:

- Trisomy 21: Down syndrome
- Trisomy 18: Edwards syndrome
- Turner syndrome
- Williams syndrome
- DiGeorge syndrome
- Noonan syndrome

▶ ACYANOTIC CONGENITAL HEART DISEASE

INCREASED PULMONARY BLOOD FLOW

The hallmark of CHD with increased pulmonary blood flow is the presence of a *left to right shunt*, where blood shunts from the high-pressure left side of the heart to the low-pressure right side of the heart. This increased blood flow through the pulmonary circulation results in signs and symptoms of congestive heart failure (HF). Examples of CHD with increased pulmonary blood flow include:

- **patent ductus arteriosus** (**PDA**; Figure 2.5 and Table 2.1)
- **atrial septal defect** (**ASD**; Figure 2.6 and Table 2.2)
- **ventricular septal defect** (**VSD**; Figure 2.7 and Table 2.3)
- **atrioventricular canal defect** (**AVC**; Figure 2.8 and Table 2.4)

Table 2.1 Patent Ductus Arteriosus (PDA)

Anatomy and Physiology	■ Ductus arteriosus does not close after birth ■ Left to right shunt from aorta to PA ■ Increased incidence in preterm infants ■ More common in females than males

(continued)

Table 2.1 Patent Ductus Arteriosus (PDA) (*continued*)

Signs and Symptoms	Presentation is determined by the size and length of the PDA ■ Tachycardia ■ Tachypnea ■ Widened pulse pressure ■ Systolic murmur at left upper sternal border ■ Hyperdynamic precordium ■ Cardiomegaly and increased pulmonary markings on CXR
Treatment	Pharmacologic management ■ COX inhibitor—indomethacin, ibuprofen, and less commonly acetaminophen Surgical management ■ Division and/or ligation via left thoracotomy Cardiac catheterization management ■ Coil or occlusion device ■ Minimally invasive ■ Expertise required
Nursing Implications	Surgical complications ■ Damage to recurrent laryngeal or phrenic nerve ■ Chylothorax ■ Bleeding ■ Infection ■ Ligation of PA or aorta ■ Rupture of ductus or aorta Cardiac catheterization complications ■ Device migration ■ Thrombosis from vascular access ■ Infection ■ Arrhythmias ■ Hemolysis ■ Damage to PA, ductus arteriosus or aorta

AO, aorta; COX, cyclooxygenase; CXR, chest x-ray; PA, pulmonary artery; PDA, patent ductus arteriosus.

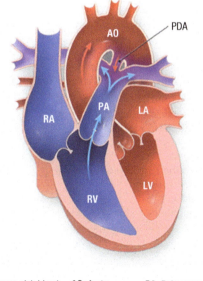

● Oxygen-rich blood   **AO**: Aorta   **PA**: Pulmonary artery
● Oxygen-poor blood   **LA**: Left atrium   **LV**: Left ventricle
● Mixed blood   **RA**: Right atrium   **RV**: Right ventricle

Figure 2.5 Patent ductus arteriosus (PDA)
Source: Copyright 2014, Children's Hospital of Philadelphia.
Reprinted with permission.

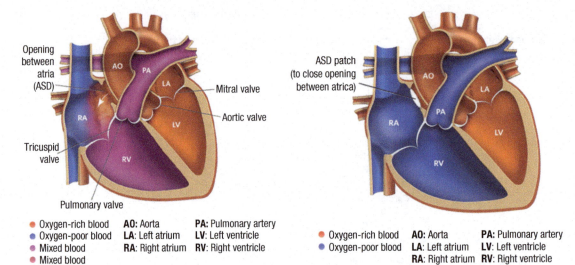

Figure 2.6 A. Atrial septal defect (ASD)

Figure 2.6 B. Surgical repair
Source: A,B: Copyright 2014, Children's Hospital of Philadelphia. Reprinted with permission.

Table 2.2 Atrial Septal Defect (ASD)

Anatomy and Physiology	▨ Opening between RA and LA ▨ Left to right shunt from LA to RA ▨ Greater than 3 mm ASD; less than 3 mm patent foramen ovale
Signs and Symptoms	▨ Tachypnea ▨ Tachycardia ▨ Systolic ejection murmur at left upper sternal border ▨ Cardiomegaly and increased pulmonary markings on CXR
Treatment	Surgical management ▨ Patch closure with pericardium or prosthetic material; primary closure with suture for small defects ▨ CPB Cardiac catheterization management ▨ Occlusion device deployed under fluoroscopy ▨ Antiplatelet therapy with aspirin for 6–12 months
Nursing Implications	Surgical complications ▨ First-degree heart block ▨ Atrial arrhythmias ▨ Pericardial effusions Cardiac catheterization complications ▨ Atrial arrhythmias ▨ Heart block ▨ Thrombosis from vascular access ▨ Device migration

ASD, atrial septal defect; CPB, cardiopulmonary bypass; CXR, chest x-ray; LA, left atrium; RA, right atrium.

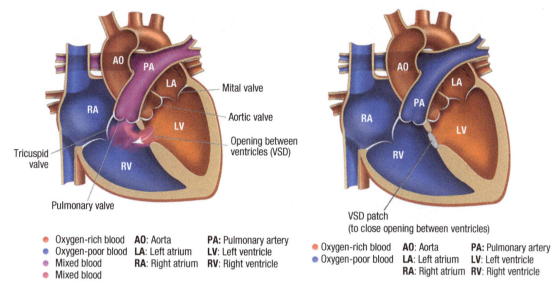

Figure 2.7 A. Ventricular septal defect (VSD)

Figure 2.7 B. Surgical repair
Source: A,B: Copyright 2014, Children's Hospital of Philadelphia. Reprinted with permission.

Table 2.3 Ventricular Septal Defect (VSD)

Anatomy and Physiology	■ Opening between RV and LV ■ Left to right shunt from LV to RV ■ Muscular VSDs often close spontaneously
Signs and Symptoms	■ CHF symptoms around 6 to 8 weeks of life with PVR falls to normal levels—increasing left to right shunt and pulmonary over circulation. ■ Tachypnea ■ Tachycardia ■ Diaphoresis ■ Poor feeding
Treatment	Surgical management ■ Patch closure with prosthetic (Dacron or Gortex) material; primary closure with suture for small defects. ■ CPB Cardiac catheterization management ■ Occlusion device may be appropriate for muscular VSDs that do not spontaneously close
Nursing Implications	Surgical complications ■ Heart block due to injury of AV node or electrical conduction system ■ Residual VSD ■ RV dysfunction from ventriculostomy Cardiac catheterization complications ■ Arrhythmias ■ Thrombosis from vascular access ■ Device migration

AV, aortic valve; CHF, congestive heart failure; CPB cardiopulmonary bypass; LV, left ventrical; PVR, pulmonary vascular resistance; RV, right ventricle; VSD, ventricular septal defect.

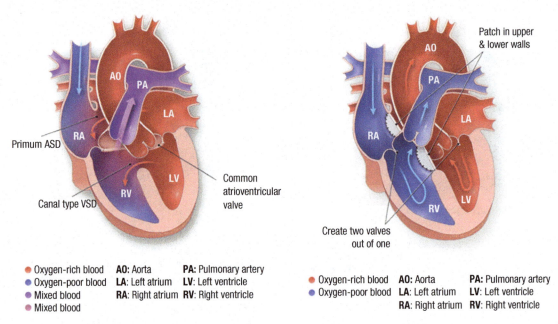

Figure 2.8 A. Atrioventricular canal defect (AVC)

Figure 2.8 B. Surgical repair
Source: A,B: Copyright 2014, Children's Hospital of Philadelphia. Reprinted with permission.

Table 2.4 Atrioventricular Canal Defect (AVC)

Anatomy and Physiology	■ Endocardial cushion defect is comprised of the ASD and VSD along with abnormal development of the tricuspid and MVs ■ Complex left to right shunting across the atrial and ventricular septum ■ Types: complete or incomplete and balanced or unbalanced ■ Complete AVC requires intervention in the first 6 months of life ■ Associated with Trisomy 21 or Down syndrome
Signs and Symptoms	■ Tachycardia ■ Tachypnea ■ Diaphoresis ■ FTT ■ Systolic ejection murmur at left upper sternal border ■ Lack of CHF symptoms should raise suspicion for PH
Treatment	■ Surgical repair involves one or two patch closure of the ASD and VSD and repair of the AV valve
Nursing Implications	■ Postoperative complications include AV valve regurgitation, AV valve stenosis. ■ Afterload reduction key to reduce stress on AV valve ■ Monitor for PH with CVP or RA; treat with 100% oxygen or inhaled nitric oxide ■ Arrhythmias ■ Heart block

ASD, atrial septal defect; AV, aortic valve; AVC, atrioventricular canal defect; CHF, congestive heart failure; CVP, central venous pressure; FTT, failure to thrive; MV, mitral valve; PH, pulmonary hypertension; RA, right atrium; VSD, ventricular septal defect.

Prolonged exposure to increased pulmonary blood flow can have detrimental effects on the pulmonary vasculature, ultimately resulting in pulmonary hypertension (PH). Careful observation, preoperative management with diuretics, and timely intervention are essential to prevent such long-term complications.

OUTFLOW OBSTRUCTION

Characterized by ventricular outflow tract obstruction, patients with this type of CHD will present with hypertension proximal to the area of obstruction and decreased perfusion distal to the area of obstruction. Examples include:

- **pulmonary stenosis** (Figure 2.9)
- **aortic stenosis** (Figure 2.10)
- **coarctation of the aorta** (**CoA**; Figure 2.11 and Table 2.5)

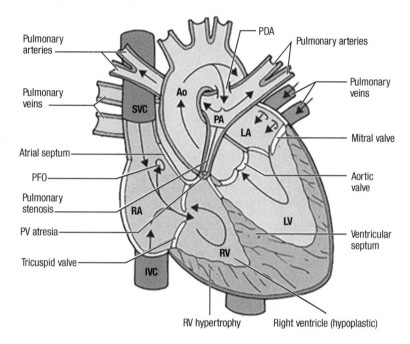

Figure 2.9 Pulmonary stenosis

Source: Hoffman, J., Thompson-Bowie, N., & Jnah, A. (2019). *Fetal and neonatal physiology for the advanced practice nurse.* Springer Publishing Company.

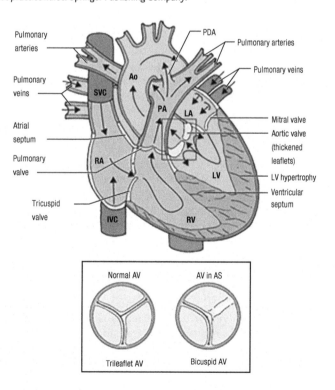

Figure 2.10 Aortic stenosis

Source: Hoffman, J., Thompson-Bowie, N., & Jnah, A. (2019). *Fetal and neonatal physiology for the advanced practice nurse.* Springer Publishing Company.

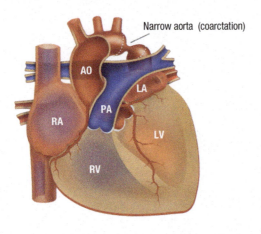

Narrow aorta (coarctation)

- ● Oxygen-rich blood
- ● Oxygen-poor blood

AO: Aorta
LA: Left atrium
RA: Right atrium

PA: Pulmonary artery
LV: Left ventricle
RV: Right ventricle

- ● Oxygen-rich blood
- ● Oxygen-poor blood

AO: Aorta
LA: Left atrium
RA: Right atrium

PA: Pulmonary artery
LV: Left ventricle
RV: Right ventricle

Figure 2.11 A. Coarctation of the aorta (CoA)

Figure 2.11 B. Surgical repair
Source: A,B: Copyright 2014, Children's Hospital of Philadelphia. Reprinted with permission.

Table 2.5 Coarctation of the Aorta (CoA)

Anatomy and Physiology	▪ Commonly discrete narrowing of the aorta at the area of the ductus arteriosus ▪ Critical CoA is ductal dependent; presents in the neonatal period and requires PGE_1 infusion for initial stabilization
Signs and Symptoms	▪ Upper extremity BP > lower extremity BP ▪ LV dysfunction ▪ Bounding upper extremity pulses ▪ Weak, thready to absent femoral or lower extremity pulses ▪ Systolic ejection murmur ▪ Thrill at suprasternal notch
Treatment	▪ CoA that presents in infancy will be repaired surgically due to risk of re-coarctation. Presentation later in childhood repair via balloon angioplasty in cardiac catheterization may be appropriate Surgical management ▪ End-to-end anastomosis or patch aortoplasty techniques via thoracotomy or median sternotomy ▪ Left subclavian flap method no longer approach of choice due to impacts of ligation of left subclavian artery—decreased perfusion, BP and limb growth
Nursing Implications	▪ Postoperative complications include hypertension (expected 24–48 hours after repair), mesenteric arteritis, bowel ischemia, bleeding, and thoracotomy associated with recurrent laryngeal or phrenic nerve damage and chylothorax ▪ Re-coarctation is common, but subsequent intervention is often via cardiac catheterization

AO, aorta; BP, blood pressure; CoA, coarctation of aorta; LV, left ventricle; PGE_1, prostaglandin.

Undiagnosed outflow obstruction CHD may present as obstructive shock. The neonate that presents in obstructive shock following ductus arteriosus closure with CoA requires timely administration of prostaglandin (PGE_1) infusion. This infusion aims to reopen the ductus arteriosus providing improved systemic CO until surgical intervention can occur. The typical infusion dose of PGE_1 infusion is 0.01 to 0.4 mcg/kg/min. The side effects are dose dependent, and infusion should be decreased as appropriate to maintain ductal patency while minimizing side effects. Side effects of PGE_1 include: apnea, flushing, hypotension, and fever.

> **Clinical Pearl**
>
> *Infants requiring PGE₁ infusion should be monitored closely for apnea. Physical stimulation, nasal cannula with 21% FiO₂, and IV caffeine may be needed to mitigate PGE₁ related apnea. If these interventions are not successful, intubation and mechanical ventilation may be required.*

Pulmonary and aortic stenosis are defined as narrowing above, at, or below the PV or AV, respectively. The most common approach to intervention is balloon valvuloplasty via cardiac catheterization, and in more extreme cases, surgical intervention or replacement of the valve may be indicated.

▶ CYANOTIC CONGENITAL HEART DISEASE

DECREASED PULMONARY BLOOD FLOW

CHDs with decreased pulmonary blood flow are characterized by an obstruction on the right side of the heart that results in a right to left shunt and cyanosis. Examples of cyanotic CHD with decreased pulmonary blow flow include:
- **tricuspid atresia** (Figure 2.12)
- **Tetralogy of Fallot** (**TOF**; Figure 2.13 and Table 2.6)

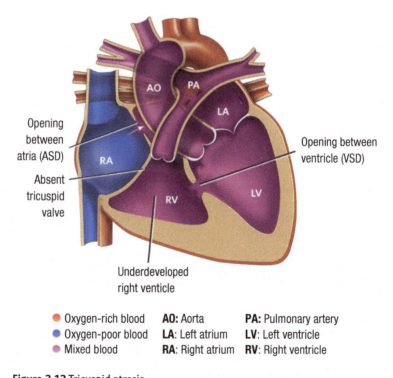

Figure 2.12 Tricuspid atresia
Source: Copyright 2014, Children's Hospital of Philadelphia. Reprinted with permission.

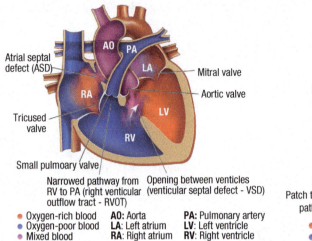

Figure 2.13 A. Tetralogy of Fallot (TOF)

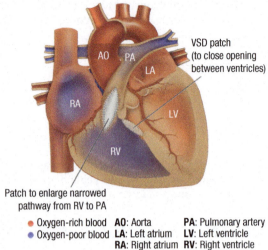

Figure 2.13 B. Surgical repair
Source: A,B: Copyright 2014, Children's Hospital of Philadelphia. Reprinted with permission.

Table 2.6 Tetralogy of Fallot (TOF)

Anatomy and Physiology	▪ Most common cyanotic CHD ▪ Comprised of four defects: narrow RV outflow tract, VSD, overriding aorta, and RV hypertrophy ▪ Degree of cyanosis
Signs and Symptoms	▪ Cyanosis ▪ Tachypnea ▪ Dyspnea ▪ Poor weight gain
Treatment	Neonatal intervention ▪ Full neonatal surgical repair not common; aorto-pulmonary shunt may be indicated ▪ Cardiac catheterization interventions to increase pulmonary blood flow until full repair may be necessary. May include PDA stent, pulmonary valvuloplasty, RV outflow tract stent Surgical repair ▪ Typically, between 2 and 6 months of age ▪ Includes VSD closure, resection of RV outflow tract obstruction with transannular patch May also include pulmonary valvuloplasty and pulmonary arterioplasty ▪ CPB
Nursing Implications	Hypercyanotic or Tet spells ▪ Episodic increase in RV outflow tract obstruction and decrease in pulmonary blood flow ▪ Increased cyanosis and decreased oxygen saturations ▪ Typically occurs between 2 and 4 months of age ▪ Interventions aim to decrease PVR (100% oxygen, morphine, treat acidosis with sodium bicarbonate, beta-blockers) and increase SVR (knee-chest position, fluid bolus, blood, phenylephrine) ▪ Surgery should be schedule following first hypercyanotic spell Postoperative complications ▪ Low CO syndrome, RV dysfunction with poor compliance ▪ Arrhythmias—JET ▪ Endocarditis risk requires subacute bacterial endocarditis prophylaxis

CHD, congenital heart disease; CO, cardiac output; CPB, cardiopulmonary bypass; JET, junctional ectopic tachycardia; PDA, patent ductus arteriosus; PVR, pulmonary vascular resistance; RV, right ventricle; SVR, systemic vascular resistance; VSD, ventricular septal defect.

TRICUSPID ATRESIA

Tricuspid atresia is defined as agenesis of the tricuspid valve resulting in no communication between the RA and RV. It requires additional defects, like ASD or VSD, for survival. Initial stabilization may require use of a PGE_1 infusion. Treatment will require single ventricle palliation with need for neonatal intervention dependent on the specific substrate of the defect.

MIXED BLOOD FLOW

Cyanotic CHD with mixed blood flow is comprised of more complex defects where the direction of blood flow can be both right to left and left to right. These defects are critical CHD and typically considered incompatible with life without intervention. Examples of cyanotic CHD with mixed blood flow includes:

- **transposition of the great arteries** (**TGA**; Figure 2.14 and Table 2.7)
- **total anomalous PV return** (Figures 2.15 and 2.16 and Table 2.8)
- **truncus arteriosus** (Figure 2.17 and Table 2.9)
- **hypoplastic left heart syndrome** (**HLHS**; Figure 2.18 and Table 2.10)

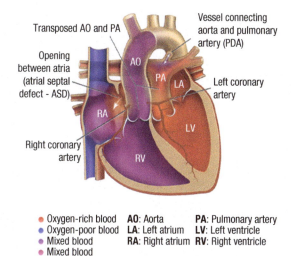

- ● Oxygen-rich blood   **AO**: Aorta   **PA**: Pulmonary artery
- ● Oxygen-poor blood   **LA**: Left atrium   **LV**: Left ventricle
- ● Mixed blood   **RA**: Right atrium   **RV**: Right ventricle
- ● Mixed blood

Figure 2.14 A. Transposition of the great arteries (TGA)

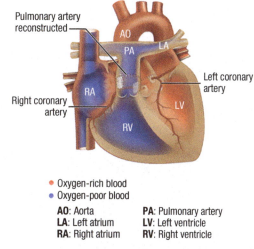

- ● Oxygen-rich blood
- ● Oxygen-poor blood

  AO: Aorta   **PA**: Pulmonary artery
  LA: Left atrium   **LV**: Left ventricle
  RA: Right atrium   **RV**: Right ventricle

Figure 2.14 B. Arterial switch operation
Source: A,B: Copyright 2014, Children's Hospital of Philadelphia. Reprinted with permission.

Table 2.7 Transposition of the Great Arteries (TGA)

Anatomy and Physiology	■ Parallel circulation with aorta arising from the RV and PA arising from the LV Communication between circulations is essential (ASD, VSD, or PDA) ■ PGE_1 infusion to maintain ductal patency after birth ■ Target preductal oxygen saturations above 80% ■ Anticipate need for mechanical ventilation and correction of metabolic acidosis
Signs and Symptoms	■ Cyanosis ■ Tachycardia ■ Tachypnea ■ Metabolic acidosis
Treatment	■ Balloon atrial septostomy via cardiac catheterization may be indicated for restrictive ASD and/or persistent hypoxemia ■ Surgical intervention with arterial switch operation in the first week of life
Nursing Implications	■ Postoperative complications include bleeding, coronary insufficiency, LCOS, arrhythmias

ASD, atrial septal defect; LCOS, low cardiac output syndrome; LV, left ventricle; PA, pulmonary artery; PDA, patent ductus arteriosus; PGE_1, prostaglandin; RV, right ventricle; VSD, ventricular septal defect.

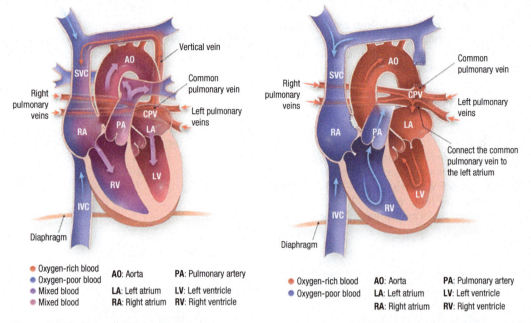

Figure 2.15 A. Supracardiac total anomalous pulmonary venous return (TAPVR)

Figure 2.15 B. Surgical repair
Source: A,B: Copyright 2014, Children's Hospital of Philadelphia. Reprinted with permission.

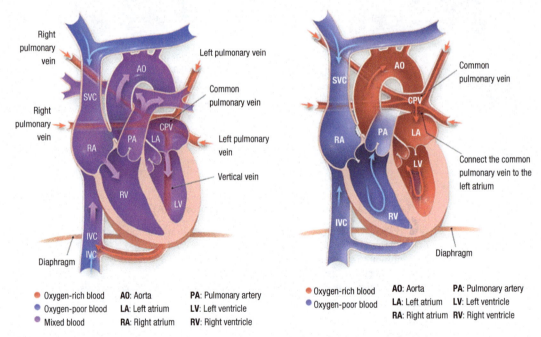

Figure 2.16 A. Infradiaphragmatic total anomalous pulmonary venous return (TAPVR)

Figure 2.16 B. Surgical repair
Source: A,B: Copyright 2014, Children's Hospital of Philadelphia. Reprinted with permission.

Table 2.8 Total Anomalous Pulmonary Venous Return (TAPVR)

Anatomy and Physiology	▪ Pulmonary veins do not return to the LA as normal ▪ Four types: supracardiac, cardiac, infradiaphragmatic, and mixed ▪ Obstructed TAPVR is considered a medical emergency requiring immediate surgical intervention. Infradiaphragmatic is the type most likely to be obstructed
Signs and Symptoms	▪ Tachypnea ▪ Increased work of breathing ▪ Cyanosis ▪ "Snowman" cardiac silhouette on CXR ▪ Obstructed TAPVR will present with cyanosis, respiratory distress, metabolic acidosis, and CS
Treatment	▪ Requires surgical intervention with CPB cardioplegia, and possible DHCA ▪ Specifics of surgical repair depend on the type of TAPVR
Nursing Implications	▪ Postoperative complications include LCOS and bleeding ▪ Potential for elevated PVR and pulmonary hypertensive crisis—anticipate need for 100% oxygen, inhaled nitric oxide, sedation with or without neuromuscular blockade

CPB, cardiopulmonary bypass; CS, cardiogenic shock; DHCA, deep hypothermic cardiac arrest; LA, left atrium; LCOS, low cardiac output syndrome; PVR, pulmonary vascular resistance; TAPVR, total anomalous pulmonary venous return.

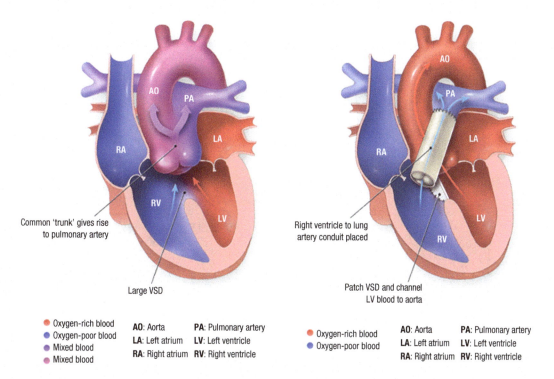

Common 'trunk' gives rise to pulmonary artery

Large VSD

● Oxygen-rich blood
● Oxygen-poor blood
● Mixed blood
● Mixed blood

AO: Aorta **PA**: Pulmonary artery
LA: Left atrium **LV**: Left ventricle
RA: Right atrium **RV**: Right ventricle

Right ventricle to lung artery conduit placed

Patch VSD and channel LV blood to aorta

● Oxygen-rich blood
● Oxygen-poor blood

AO: Aorta **PA**: Pulmonary artery
LA: Left atrium **LV**: Left ventricle
RA: Right atrium **RV**: Right ventricle

Figure 2.17 A. Truncus arteriosus

Figure 2.17 B. Rastelli operation
Source: A,B: Copyright 2014, Children's Hospital of Philadelphia. Reprinted with permission.

Table 2.9 Truncus Arteriosus

Anatomy and Physiology	▦ Single arterial trunk and valve that arises from both the RV and LV and a VSD ▦ Classified into four types based on how the pulmonary arteries branch off of the single arterial trunk ▦ Associated with DiGeorge Syndrome

Signs and Symptoms	▦ Presentation will depend on balance of pulmonary and systemic circulation.
	▦ Immediately after birth, PVR is high, resulting in less pulmonary blood flood and right to left shunting of blood and cyanosis.
	▦ As PVR falls in the first 12–24 hours of life, pulmonary blood flow increases leading to pulmonary over circulation and decreased systemic blood flow
	  ● Assess for CHF—tachypnea, tachycardia, etc.
	  ● Assess for decreased systemic blood flow—decreased urine output, necrotizing enterocolitis.
	  ● May present similarly to neonatal sepsis

Treatment	▦ Requires neonatal surgical intervention with CPB cardioplegia, and possible DHCA ▦ Rastelli operation with VSD closure; requires reoperation in the future for conduit revisions as the patient grows
Nursing Implications	▦ Postoperative complications include LCOS, ischemia, bleeding, arrhythmias, truncal valve insufficiency, and residual VSD ▦ Potential for elevated PVR and pulmonary hypertensive crisis—anticipate need for 100% oxygen, inhaled nitric oxide, sedation with or without neuromuscular blockade

CHF, congestive heart failure; CPB, cardiopulmonary bypass; DHCA, deep hypothermic cardiac arrest; LCOS, low cardiac output syndrome; LV, left ventrical; PVR, pulmonary vascular resistance; RV, right ventrical; VSD, ventricular septal defect.

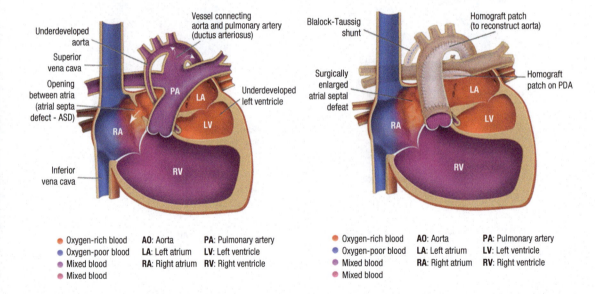

Figure 2.18 A. Hypoplastic left heart syndrome (HLHS)

Figure 2.18 B. Palliation stage 1 (*continued*)

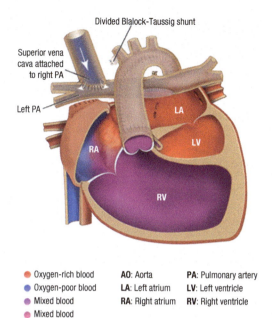

Figure 2.18 C. Palliation stage 2

- Oxygen-rich blood
- Oxygen-poor blood
- Mixed blood
- Mixed blood

AO: Aorta   **PA**: Pulmonary artery
LA: Left atrium   **LV**: Left ventricle
RA: Right atrium   **RV**: Right ventricle

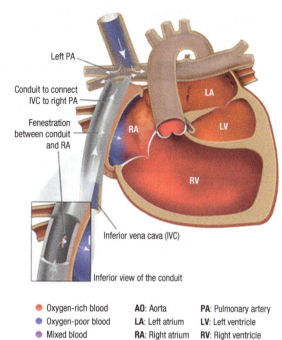

- Oxygen-rich blood
- Oxygen-poor blood
- Mixed blood

AO: Aorta   **PA**: Pulmonary artery
LA: Left atrium   **LV**: Left ventricle
RA: Right atrium   **RV**: Right ventricle

Figure 2.18 D. Palliation stage 3
Source: A,B,C,D: Copyright 2014, Children's Hospital of Philadelphia. Reprinted with permission.

Table 2.10 Hypoplastic Left Heart Syndrome (HLHS)

Anatomy and Physiology	■ Underdevelopment of the left sided heart structures; either stenosis or atresia of the mitral or AV that results in hypoplasia of the LV and ascending aorta and ASD. The underdeveloped left side of the heart does not support systemic blood flow and oxygen delivery to the body ■ Ductal dependent heart disease. Prenatal diagnosis allows for initiation of PGE_1 infusion to maintain systemic blood flow and oxygen delivery. Postnatal diagnosis will present with cardiogenic and obstructive shock as ductus arteriosus closes
Signs and Symptoms	Postnatal presentation ■ Tachypnea ■ Increased work of breathing ■ Cyanosis, pale, mottled ■ Irritability ■ Poor feeding Restrictive ASD—does not allow for systemic and pulmonary venous return to mix ■ Profound cyanosis and hypoxemia ■ Left atrial hypertension and pulmonary edema
Treatment	HLHS with restrictive ASD ■ Balloon atrial septostomy Staged single ventricle palliation—intervention does not result in normal biventricular anatomy ■ Norwood with aortopulmonary or Sano shunt in neonatal period with CPB cardioplegia, and DHCA ■ Bidirectional Glenn to route the SVC to the PA. May require cardiopulmonary bypass ■ Extracardiac Fenestrated Fontan to route the IVC to the PA completing single ventricle circulation with CPB
Nursing Implications	■ Preoperative management includes balancing pulmonary and systemic perfusion, assessing for metabolic acidosis, limited oxygen delivery to prevent pulmonary over circulation, promote parental bonding, provide enteral and parenteral nutrition. ■ Norwood postoperative complications: LCOS, hypoxemia, shunt thrombosis/obstruction, residual arch obstruction, ventricular dysfunction, AV valve regurgitation neurologic injury, NEC, and poor growth

(continued)

Table 2.10 Hypoplastic Left Heart Syndrome (HLHS) (*continued*)

	▪ Bidirectional Glenn postoperative complications: avoid positive pressure ventilation to improve passive return of blood through SVC to PA, SVC syndrome, pleural effusion, hypoxemia due to elevated PVR, and arrhythmia requiring pacemaker ▪ Extracardiac Fenestrated Fontan postoperative complications: avoid positive pressure ventilation to improve passive return of blood through the PA, LCOS, arrhythmias (atrial fibrillation and atrial flutter), ventricular dysfunction, AV valve insufficiency, bleeding, protein losing enteropathy, plastic bronchitis, VTE, kidney and liver dysfunction, neurodevelopmental and behavioral health problems

ASD, atrial septal defect; AV, aortic valve; CPB, cardiopulmonary bypass; DHCA, deep hypothermic cardiac arrest; HLHS, hypoplastic left heart syndrome; IVC, inferior vena cava; LCOS, low cardiac output syndrome; LV, left ventrical; NEC, necrotizing enterocolitis; PA, pulmonary artery; PGE₁, prostaglandin; PVR, pulmonary vascular resistance; SVC, superior vena cava; VTE, venous thromboembolism.

The field of pediatric CHD continues to advance, and outcomes improve with more adults today living with CHD than children. This patient population requires specialized care from early diagnosis, preoperative planning, and intervention, to postoperative management and lifelong follow up for complex CHD. Long-term outcomes are complicated by neurodevelopment, behavioral, and mental health problems that are the focus of much research to support patients with complex CHD to thrive into adulthood.

▶ CARDIAC SURGERY

Outcomes for children with congenital and acquired heart disease continue to improve with advancements in cardiothoracic surgery. Cardiac surgery is often classified as closed-heart surgery or open-heart surgery, which requires the use of cardiopulmonary bypass (CPB). Since the invention of CPB in the 1950s, the technology has been adapted and improved to better support the complex needs of the neonate, infant, and child requiring cardiac surgery.

CLOSED-HEART SURGERY

Closed-heart surgery refers to surgery that does not require the use of the CPB machine. A thoracotomy is the typical incision for this type of surgery but may also require a median sternotomy incision (MSI). A thoracotomy incision is made on the side of the chest between two ribs, where there are more nerves and muscle compared to the sternum making this incision more painful than an MSI. Examples of closed-heart surgeries include:
▪ coarctation repair
▪ patent ductus arteriosus ligation
▪ vascular ring repair
▪ aortopulmonary shunts
▪ some interventions on the PA, like PA banding

OPEN-HEART SURGERY

Open-heart surgery refers to surgery that requires the use of the CPB machine. This approach is utilized to take over the function of the heart and lungs to deliver oxygenated blood to the body while providing a bloodless and often still field for the surgeon to operate. This type of surgery requires an MSI and a partial thymectomy to access the heart. The heart is enclosed in a sac called the pericardium that will be cut open to allow access for the surgeon to cannulate for the CPB machine.

There are different techniques to cannulate, but the general principles include placing venous cannula(s) in the superior and inferior vena cava or RA to drain blood from the heart to the CPB machine where it is oxygenated and returned to the patient through an aortic cannula. This empties the heart and provides a bloodless field for the surgical team.

Cardioplegia, a high potassium concentrated solution, is administered once a patient is on CPB to stop the heart and create a still field for the surgical team. Not all surgeries require cardioplegia. The patient's temperature is regulated by the CPB machine and the targeted temperature management depends on the surgical repair being performed (Table 2.11).

Table 2.11 Cardiopulmonary Bypass Machine Temperature Regulation

Temperature Management	Goal
Normothermic conditions	34°C–37°C
Mild hypothermic conditions	28°C–34°C
Moderate hypothermic conditions	24°C–28°C
Deep hypothermic conditions	15°C–24°C

Hypothermia is leveraged to decrease metabolic demands during surgery, providing myocardial protection. Complex surgeries require increased hypothermic conditions including the use of deep hypothermic cardiac arrest (DHCA).

In addition to deep hypothermic conditions, with DHCA, the bypass cannulas are removed and delivery of oxygenated blood to the patient stops during that time. The risk of neurologic and end-organ dysfunction increases with the length of DHCA. The surgical team strategizes to minimize DHCA time as much as possible. While there is not a clear "safe" time limit for DHCA, studies suggest that times less than 30 to 40 minutes poses less risk than longer times (Das et al., 2021). Once the surgical repair is completed, the patient is rewarmed to normothermic conditions and weaned from the CPB machine. During this time, modified ultrafiltration (MUF) takes place to hemoconcentrate the blood returned to the patient decreasing volume overload, inflammatory response, blood product need, and improving coagulation and lung function. Additionally, a transesophageal and/or transthoracic echo may be performed to evaluate the surgical repair and vasoactive infusions will be initiated and titrated to support optimal cardiac function. If the heart function is unable to support weaning from the CPB machine following an adequate surgical repair, extracorporeal membrane oxygenation (ECMO) may be considered to support cardiac and pulmonary function.

Common surgeries that require CPB include:
- ASD or VSD closures
- AVC repair
- arterial switch operation for TGA
- TOF repair
- other surgical repairs of complex congenital heart defects

NURSING IMPLICATIONS AND TREATMENT

Pediatric critical care nurses play an essential role in the management of neonatal, infant, and pediatric cardiac surgical patients to optimize outcomes. Knowledge of the surgical repair, general principles of cardiac surgery, including CPB, detailed physical assessment, and integration of physiologic and laboratory data supports the nurse and critical care team to respond to the individualized needs of this patient population and intervene prior to clinical deterioration. Collaboration with the critical care team is essential for optimal and efficient postoperative management.

Patients are at risk for infection, bleeding, low CO, and neurologic and end-organ injury following surgery. Infection risk is mitigated with preoperative bathing and infection preventing practices and perioperative antibiotic prophylaxis. Bleeding is monitored closely postoperatively with less than 3 mL/kg/hr and thinning and lightening color of output being a reassuring sign; greater than 5 mL/kg/hr is concerning for surgical bleeding and the surgeon should be notified. Chest tubes are utilized to monitor bleeding and may be placed in the mediastinal, pleural, or pericardial space based on the specific needs of the patient. Chest tube output is monitored closely postoperatively with less than 3 ml/kg/hr and thinning and lightening color of output being a reassuring sign; greater than 5 ml/kg/hr is concerning for surgical bleeding and the surgeon should be notified. An abrupt stop in chest tube output is concerning for occlusion and risk for cardiac tamponade related to blood collecting around the heart.

Clinical Pearl

Signs and symptoms of tamponade include tachycardia, narrowed pulse pressure, pulsus paradoxus, elevated central venous pressure (CVP) and RA pressure, and muffled heart sounds.

LOW CARDIAC OUTPUT SYNDROME

Approximately 25% of patients will experience low cardiac output syndrome (LCOS) following cardiac surgery requiring CPB with peak impacts 6 to 18 hours after bypass (Chandler & Kirsch, 2016). LCOS is defined by decreased CO caused by myocardial dysfunction, increased PVR and SVR that results in an imbalance in oxygen delivery and oxygen consumption, anaerobic metabolism, and lactic acidosis. Risks for LCOS include prolonged CPB times, DHCA, myocardial ischemia, ventricular dysfunction, complex surgery, and significant residual lesions. The nurse anticipates the following physical exam findings with LCOS:

- cool, mottled extremities
- delayed capillary refill time (CRT)
- decreased pulses and narrowed pulse pressure
- tachycardia
- altered level of consciousness (LOC)
- decreased blood pressure (BP) is a late sign

There are supportive strategies leveraged by the critical care team to support patients through LCOS postoperative, which include:

- **optimizing preload** with judicious use of volume resuscitation, assessing for improved CO response with decreased HR and increased arterial BP
- **supporting systolic function** with the use of inotropic infusions such as dopamine, dobutamine, and epinephrine
- **afterload reduction** through the use of the phosphodiesterase inhibitor, milrinone, by decreasing PVR and SVR and providing inotropic support; inhaled nitric oxide, nitroprusside, nitroglycerin, and nicardipine may also be utilized.
- **increased intrathoracic pressure** using positive pressure ventilation, which decreases SVR and supports systolic function
- **mechanical circulatory support (MCS),** like ECMO, may be required in the setting of LCOS refractory to medical management

INVASIVE HEMODYNAMIC MONITORING

Catheters placed into an artery, vein, or directly into the heart or great vessels and connected to fluid-filled transducers provide continuous waveform and numerical displays of hemodynamic data like arterial BP, central venous pressure (CVP), right atrial, left atrial, PA pressures, and pulmonary artery occlusive pressures also know as a "wedge" pressure (Figures 2.19 and 2.20, Table 2.12).

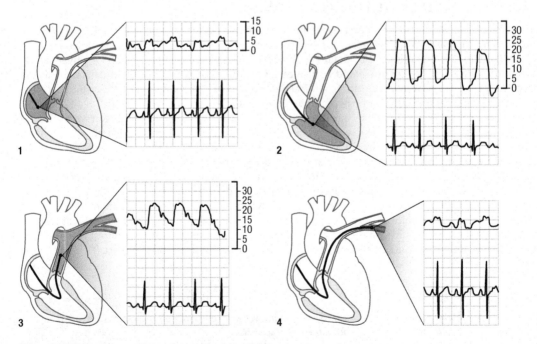

Figure 2.19 Comparison of wave forms of a PA catheter
Source: Slota, M. C. (2019). *AACN core curriculum for pediatric high acuity, progressive, and critical care nursing.* Springer Publishing Company.

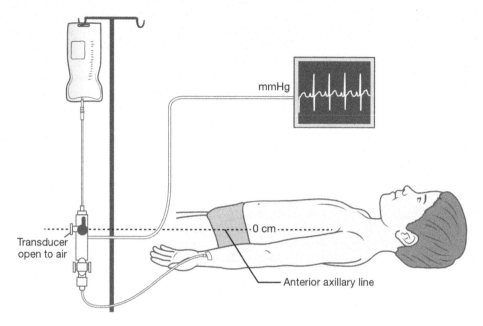

Figure 2.20 Diagram of position of phlebostatic axis
Source: Slota, M. C. (2019). *AACN core curriculum for pediatric high acuity, progressive, and critical care nursing.*
Springer Publishing Company.

Table 2.12 Invasive Hemodynamic Monitoring

	Catheter Location	Normal Values	Indication
Arterial	Radial, ulnar, femoral, dorsalis pedis, posterior tibial arteries; less commonly, axillary or mammary arteries or aorta; umbilical artery in neonates	Dependent on age	BP monitoring: assess pulse pressure (widened or narrowed), pulsus alternans (LV failure), pulsus paradoxus during inspiration (pericardial effusion, hypovolemia)
CVP	Internal jugular, SVC, femoral vein	0–5 mmHg	Measure of preload/venous return and end diastolic RV function; blood sampling for mixed venous O_2 saturations
RA	Right atrium		
LA	Left atrium	4–12 mmHg	Measure of preload to left side of the heart and end diastolic LV function
PA	Pulmonary artery	~1/4–1/3 systemic BP; mean 5–15 mmHg	Assess for PH management of CS and LV failure; blood sampling for mixed venous O_2 saturations
PAOP	PA catheter advanced to a pulmonary arterial branch and balloon inflated	4–12 mmHg	Surrogate of LA pressure

BP, blood pressure; CS, cardiogenic shock; CVP, central venous pressure; LA, left atrium; LV, left ventricle; PA, pulmonary artery; PAOP, pulmonary artery occlusive pressure; PH, pulmonary hypertension; RA, right atrium; SVC, superior vena cava.

Hemodynamic monitoring catheters must be positioned correctly and calibrated at the phlebostatic axis for accurate measurement. Each catheter location has a unique waveform that should be monitored by the pediatric critical care nurse for indications of changes in CO.

NONINVASIVE MONITORING

In addition to invasive monitoring, many methods of noninvasive monitoring are performed follow cardiac surgery, like:

■ EKG
■ noninvasive blood pressure measurement (NIBP)
■ pulse oximetry
■ near-infrared spectroscopy (NIRS) with multisite measurement to assess for changes in CO
■ echocardiogram

▶ CARDIOGENIC SHOCK

Cardiogenic shock (CS) is defined as a low CO state in which ineffective CO cannot meet the metabolic demands of body tissues due to myocardial dysfunction. This high-acuity state is characterized by low CO, end-organ hypoperfusion, tissue hypoxia, systemic hypotension, and elevated ventricular filling pressures. CS brings substantial risk for morbidity and mortality in children.

The common causes of CS are:

■ CHD
■ arrhythmias
■ heart infections
■ cardiomyopathy
■ postoperative period following cardiac surgery

Diagnosis is confirmed with established myocardial dysfunction, when other probable causes of hypotension have been excluded (Kar, 2015). Myocardial dysfunction may be secondary to acidosis, ischemia, myocardial inflammation, drugs, and toxins.

The major compensatory response to improve systemic perfusion in CS is *tachycardia.* As the myocardial pump begins to fail, there is a rise in ventricular diastolic pressures, resulting in increased wall stress and myocardial oxygen requirement. The decrease in CO and systemic perfusion causes anaerobic metabolism, resulting in lactic acid formation. This triggers sympathetic stimulation to increase cardiac contractility and renal fluid retention. The body's compensatory responses can be counterproductive and lead to further deterioration of the critically ill child.

Clinical signs of further deterioration include:

■ hypotension
■ oliguria
■ cold extremities
■ altered LOC
■ cyanosis

These deteriorating clinical signs may persist even after attempts to correct arrhythmias, hypoxia, acidosis, and hypovolemia have been made. Physical examination findings include tachycardia, reduced capillary refill, diaphoresis, hepatomegaly, edema, dyspnea, jugular vein distension, tachypnea, crepitation, decreased urine output, gallop heart sounds, precordial heave, irritability, feeding difficulties, and failure to thrive (FTT).

Mortality is reduced with early recognition and management. The management focuses on improving CO and function to restore oxygen delivery to the tissues and minimize myocardial oxygen demand. The treatment management is compiled of a combination of cardiorespiratory therapies (e.g., mechanical ventilation, sedation, and maintaining normothermia), vasoactive medications (e.g., epinephrine, dopamine), and subsequent anatomic cardiac defects correction. Treatment with MCS such as ECMO or a ventricular assist device (VAD) may be considered in relation to hemodynamic instability and serve as a bridge to recovery, surgery, or transplant.

With treatment of other forms of shock, fluid resuscitation can improve a patient's status. However, in CS fluid boluses can result in *fluid overload* and *pulmonary edema* and *should be used with caution.* It is recommended to administer fluid boluses in smaller aliquots of 5 to 10 mL/kg.

ECMO is an important treatment modality utilized in pediatric refractory CS.

Clinical scenarios requiring ECMO as a treatment modality:

■ LCOS after cardiac surgery
■ cardiac arrest from severe myocardial dysfunction, which resulted in CS
■ decompensated cardiomyopathy
■ acute fulminant myocarditis

▶ OBSTRUCTIVE SHOCK

Decreased CO caused by physical impairment of blood flow out of the heart is classified as obstructive shock. This obstruction results in increased afterload. The causes of obstructive shock include:

- cardiac tamponade
- tension pneumothorax
- pulmonary or aortic stenosis
- CoA
- pulmonary embolism (PE)
- thrombus

Presentation may mimic hypovolemic shock; however, physical exam will reveal systemic venous congestion in obstructive shock. Timely identification of the obstruction and interventions to alleviate it are imperative to effective management and patient survival (Table 2.13).

Table 2.13 Obstructive Shock

Cause of Obstructive Shock	Presentation	Intervention
Cardiac tamponade	■ Muffled heart sounds ■ Poor perfusion ■ Pulsus paradoxus ■ Jugular vein distention	Pericardiocentesis
Tension pneumothorax	■ Asymmetric breath sounds ■ Tracheal deviation	Needle decompression or chest tube placement
CoA	■ Upper extremity BP higher than lower ■ Thready to absent lower extremity pulses ■ Bounding upper extremity pulses	Neonatal presentation—initial stabilization with PGE$_1$ infusion for ductal patency, followed by surgical intervention
PE	■ Chest pain ■ Tachypnea ■ Dyspnea ■ Hypoxia	Antithrombotic therapy, thrombectomy, and supportive care as needed

BP, blood pressure; CoA, coarctation of the aorta; PE, pulmonary embolism; PGE$_1$, prostaglandin.

Clinical Pearl

Hypertension is defined as a BP greater than the 95th percentile in children less than 13 years of age and greater than 140/90 mmHg in children greater than 13 years of age on three separate readings.

▶ HYPERTENSIVE CRISIS

Hypertension in children is often due to secondary causes like renal disease and neurological causes. Hypertension is defined as a BP greater than the 95th percentile in children less than 13 years of age and greater than 140/90mmHg in children greater than 13 years of age on three repeat readings. In the setting of primary hypertension, initial presentation as a hypertensive crisis is rare (Upsal & Halbach, 2020). Hypertensive crisis is a life-threatening acute increase in BP resulting in end-organ damage or even death. *Encephalopathy* is the most common presentation in children due to cerebral edema caused by elevated BP (Upsal & Halbach, 2020). Presentation may include decreased LOC (lethargy or coma) and/or seizures. In addition to end-organ damage to the brain, other areas of damage include:

- **eyes**: papilledema, retinal hemorrhage, exudates
- **heart**: HF
- **kidneys**: renal insufficiency

NURSING IMPLICATIONS AND TREATMENT

Management of hypertensive crisis includes intravenous antihypertensive medications like:

- hydralazine
- nicardipine

- esmolol
- nitroprusside
- labetalol

In patients with increased intracranial pressure, BP must be lowered slowly to reduce further end-organ damage. Initial stabilization may also include maintaining airway, breathing and circulation depending on the clinical presentation. Accurate BP measurement is essential; initially noninvasive measurement with the appropriate size cuff will be utilized, but continuous, ongoing monitoring should be obtained with an arterial line. Underlying causes of the hypertensive crisis may influence additional treatment interventions, like pain management or anxiolysis.

▶ CARDIAC CATHETERIZATION

Minimally invasive diagnostic and/or interventional procedure where percutaneously placed catheter(s) are guided via fluoroscopy into the heart. Common access sites in infants and children include the femoral artery and/or vein, subclavian vein, and jugular vein. Angiography is utilized to define anatomy, perform pressure and oxygen saturation measurements and evaluate the following (Table 2.14):

- CO
- Cardiac index (CI); normal is 2.5 to 4 L/min/m².
- pulmonary flow (Qp)
- systemic flow (Qs)
- The ratio of Qp to Qs (Qp: Qs); normal is 1:1,
- PVR; normal is 1 to 3 Woods units/m²,
- SVR 20 units/m²

Table 2.14 Cardiac Catheterization

Measurement	Calculation
CO	SV × HR
CI	CO/BSA in m²; normal is 2.5–4 L/min/m²
SV	(CO/HR) × 1000
Qp	VO²/PV saturation − PA saturation
Qs	VO²/aortic saturation − mixed venous saturation
PVR	(mean PA pressure − mean LA pressure)/Qp
SVR	(mean Ao pressure − mean RA pressure)/ Qs
Qp: Qs	(Ao − SVC)/(PV − PA)

Ao, aorta; BSA, body surface area; CI, cardiac index; CO, cardiac output; HR, heart rate; LA, left atrium; PA, pulmonary artery; PV, pulmonary valve; PVR, pulmonary vascular resistance; Qp, pulmonary flow; Qs, systemic flow; RA, right atrium; SV, stroke volume; SVC, superior vena cava; SVR, systemic vascular resistance; Vo², oxygen consumption

Diagnostic data evaluate previous cardiac surgical and catheterization interventions and proposed surgical or catheterization interventions. Interventions performed by cardiac catheterizations include:

- balloon valvuloplasty and dilation of vessels to relieve stenosis
- placement of coils and/or devices to close septal defects or occlude vessels
- placement of stents and valves
- balloon atrial septostomy
- endomyocardial biopsy
- electrophysiology (EP) studies to manage arrhythmias

There are also hybrid approaches with the simultaneous use of cardiac catheterization and cardiac surgical intervention to care for complex physiology, like the high-risk infant born with HLHS (Alphonso et al., 2020). Complications of cardiac catheterization include:

- adverse reaction to contrast
- arrhythmias or heart block
- air embolization
- blood loss
- hypotension
- infection
- myocardial infarction

- venous or arterial thrombosis
- perforation
- radiation exposure
- death (rarely)

Cardiac catheterization provides the most accurate hemodynamic data and minimally invasive options to address cardiac anomalies.

NURSING IMPLICATIONS AND TREATMENT

Nursing considerations following cardiac catheterization include **maintaining hemostasis** and **monitoring for complications** with detailed physical assessment and monitoring. Patients will be required to lay supine, also called flat time, following removal of catheters used for the procedure and the length of the flat time will depend on the vessels accessed and center specific guidelines and closure method. Nursing assessment should include a **comprehensive cardiovascular assessment** with a focus on access site and neurovascular assessments. The access site should be assessed for bleeding and hematoma; there is typically a pressure dressing in place immediately following the procedure limiting visual assessment to some degree. The neurovascular assessment is based on cardiac catheterization access site. For example, a patient that received right femoral vein and artery access, neurovascular assessment of the pulses, capillary refill, color, and temperature of the right leg are essential. If unable to palpate, obtain a Doppler ultrasound, or any other concerning neurovascular assessment finding, the nurse should be concerned about a thrombus and should notify the provider for additional evaluation. Postcardiac catheterization thrombus will be treated with antithrombotic medication based on the severity and location of the thrombus, such as heparin, enoxaparin, and tissue-type plasminogen activator (tPA).

▶ VASCULAR OCCLUSION

Venous thromboembolism (VTE) is less common in infants and children compared to adults; however, it is seen in hospitalized infants and children. Virchow's triad is recognized as factors necessary to develop VTE and is comprised of **endothelial blood vessel injury**, **venous stasis**, and **hypercoagulability**. Risk factors for VTE in pediatrics include:

- trauma
- vascular injury
- central venous catheters (CVC)
- immobility
- age risk increased in infancy and again in adolescence (Albisetti & Chan, 2022)
- estrogen-containing contraceptives

Underlying disease that increases risk for VTE includes:

- inherited thrombophilia—Factor V Leiden, Prothrombin mutation, Antithrombin, Protein C and Protein S deficiency (Albisetti & Chan, 2022)
- infection
- malignancy
- CHD

Common types of VTE include:

- deep vein thrombosis (DVT)—most commonly in the lower extremities, unless associated with CVC
- PE—rare in children, and less likely to be hemodynamically significant (Albisetti & Chan, 2022)
- superior vena cava syndrome (SVCS)

Presentation and diagnosis of VTE is determined by the location of the thrombus (Table 2.15).

Table 2.15 Venous Thromboembolism (VTE)

VTE Location	Clinical Presentation	Diagnosis
DVT	- Pain - Swelling - Redness - Warmth - Asymptomatic	- Ultrasound with Doppler - Angiography - Venogram

(continued)

Table 2.15 Venous Thromboembolism (VTE) *(continued)*

VTE Location	Clinical Presentation	Diagnosis
SVCS	■ Facial swelling ■ Cough ■ Dyspnea ■ Jugular vein distention ■ Edema—nipple line and above (head, neck, and arms)	■ Clinical exam ■ CXR ■ CT scan

CXR, chest x-ray; DVT, deep vein thrombosis; SVCS, superior vena cava syndrome; VTE, venous thromboembolism.

NURSING IMPLICATIONS AND TREATMENT

Management of VTE focuses first on prevention with the use of compression stockings, sequential compression devices, prophylactic enoxaparin, routine repositioning, and optimizing mobility based on the patient's clinical status. In the setting of a VTE, treatment shifts to therapeutic anticoagulation—typically with enoxaparin, ongoing observation, supportive care, and, if indicated, thrombectomy.

CARDIAC INFECTION AND INFLAMMATORY DISEASES: ACQUIRED CARDIOVASCULAR DISORDERS

Acquired cardiovascular disorders include disease processes or abnormalities that develop after birth. It can occur in children treated for congenital heart defects or it can be detected in the otherwise normal heart. They may develop from the following:
■ autoimmune response
■ infection
■ familial tendencies
■ environmental factors

Rare cases of myocarditis and pericarditis with associated chest pain and high troponin levels have been reported to the Vaccine Adverse Event Reporting System following inoculation with the COVID-19 vaccine. The majority of adolescents and young adults have a rapid recovery of symptoms with a mild clinical course after suspected myocarditis related to the COVID-19 vaccine.

According to the Centers for Disease Control and Prevention (CDC; 2022b), cases of myocarditis have occurred in the following:
■ post mRNA COVID-19 vaccination (Pfizer-BioNTech or Moderna)
■ more often in male adolescent and young adults after the second dose
■ onset most often occurs within a week of vaccination

The CDC continues to recommend the COVID-19 vaccine to curb the pandemic. The benefit of the COVID-19 vaccine with the known risks of contracting the COVID-19 illness and possible severe complications outweigh the rare risk of temporary myocarditis and pericarditis associated with the COVID-19 vaccine.

Clinical Pearl

There are three layers of heart: the epicardium, myocardium, and endocardium.
■ *epicardium: the outer layer of the heart*
■ *myocardium: the middle layer of the heart*
■ *endocardium: the inner layer of the heart*

▶ MYOCARDITIS

Myocarditis is an inflammation and necrosis of the heart muscle (myocardium) associated with impaired systolic ventricular function. The common etiology of myocarditis is infectious, with a virus being the most prevalent cause. Noninfectious causes include medications, autoimmunity, hypersensitivity reactions, and toxins. Myocarditis may have spontaneous recovery or sustain irreversible myocardial injury.

Currently, *diagnosis through cardiac catheterization with direct tissue examination remains the gold standard in myocarditis*. However, given the invasive nature of endomyocardial biopsy, the diagnostic focus is shifting to cardiac magnetic resonance (CMR) imaging with the incorporation of clinical findings and laboratory data (Law et al., 2021). Electrocardiography, echocardiography, and chest x-ray (CXR) demonstrate the variable findings associated with myocarditis.

SIGNS AND SYMPTOMS

Myocarditis signs and symptoms may include:

- fatigue
- chest pain
- syncope
- shortness of breath
- cough
- heart murmur
- nausea and vomiting
- abdominal pain
- edema
- diminished pulses
- fever
- palpitation
- arrhythmias
- dyspnea
- tachypnea
- gallop
- diarrhea
- hepatomegaly
- cyanosis

Clinical presentation may range from mild symptoms to HF and, in more severe cases, life-threatening arrhythmias or CS.

Patients with **acute myocarditis** typically present with:

- recent HF symptoms
- a poorly functioning ventricle that may show dilation
- viral symptoms in the preceding weeks

Patients with **chronic persistent myocarditis** present with cardiac symptoms such as chest pain and often display preserved systolic function.

Chronic myocarditis patients have histologic evidence of persistent myocardial inflammation. Patients with fulminant myocarditis present in CS and may require inotropes or MCS. Tachyarrhythmias are common in fulminant myocarditis. Atrial or ventricular arrhythmias may be associated with a poor early outcome, and antiarrhythmic therapy should be initiated. Standard treatment methods focus on **supportive therapy to allow the heart to recover**. Anticipatory care in children is crucial and monitoring in an intensive care unit may be necessary for initial management and treatment. Initial treatment with bedrest is important and supportive care is similar to treatment methods utilized in other scenarios of acute HF. Oral HF therapy is used once the patient is beyond the acute stage of illness and continues to display signs of HF or persistent systolic dysfunction.

Additional supportive care with **milrinone for inotropy** (squeeze of the heart) may be initiated as first-line therapy. **Dopamine and epinephrine** are inotropes with vasopressor properties that are reserved for patients with hypotension and CS since they have more chronotropic (increased HR) and arrhythmogenic potential. The treatment modalities of **intravenous immunoglobulin (IVIG), corticosteroids,** and use of **antiviral therapy** if a viral infection is found remain center and practitioner specific.

Acute myocarditis can progress rapidly to hemodynamic compromise requiring the use of MCS with either ECMO or a VAD. Many patients have a complete recovery. However, patients with an acute episode of myocarditis who recover but develop severe chronic HF or those who require long-term MCS may require heart transplantation. When hemodynamic compromise is suspected in the patient trajectory, transferring to a center that provides pediatric MCS with ECMO and transplantation should be considered.

▶ PERICARDITIS

Pericarditis results from inflammation of the pericardium, which is a double-walled, thin membrane or sac-like structure surrounding the outer surface of the heart. The pericardium protects, lubricates, and supports the function of the heart. The pericardium anchors the heart to the mediastinum to keep it in place within the chest cavity, and it has two layers (fibrous and serous) with a fluid-filled pericardial cavity between the two layers.

The etiology of pericarditis is often idiopathic; however, it can be attributed to several factors including:

■ infections (viral, fungal, bacterial, parasitic)
■ medications
■ heart surgery
■ heart attack
■ other medical conditions (e.g., autoimmune and trauma)

SIGNS AND SYMPTOMS

The common clinical presentation includes:

■ pericardial friction rub
■ muffled heart sounds
■ tachycardia
■ tachypnea
■ fever
■ pain

Pericardial pain presents mostly in the chest and in some patients, radiates to the shoulder, neck, back, and abdomen.

NURSING IMPLICATIONS AND TREATMENT

LABS AND DIAGNOSTICS

■ CXR
■ echocardiogram

Clinical findings on chest radiography may reveal cardiomegaly, and echocardiograms may show pericardial effusions or suspected tamponade physiology.

TREATMENT AND MANAGEMENT

Cardiac tamponade requires emergency treatment within an ICU setting, as the excessive pericardial fluid leads to increased intrapericardial pressure, which impairs the heart ability to fill and decreases CO. Pericardiocentesis is a procedure utilized to remove the pericardial fluid drainage, and in some cases of symptomatic acute pericarditis, it may be indicated to restore optimal intracardiac hemodynamics. Surgical therapy with a pericardiotomy is performed when the appropriate clinical response is not achieved by percutaneous drainage.

First line treatment includes **nonsteroidal anti-inflammatory drugs (NSAIDs)** to treat pain and inflammation, and in some patients, colchicine has been used to control persistent inflammation. Depending on the etiology, they may need antibiotics or antifungal medications.

COMPLICATIONS

Acute pericarditis may have complications that include cardiac tamponade, constrictive pericarditis, and recurrent pericarditis. Acute pericarditis may last a few weeks and resolve with rest or simple treatment therapies. Recurrent pericarditis may be due to inadequate treatment or an immune mediated process, but in some recurrent cases the etiology remains unknown. In severe cases, pericarditis may lead to constrictive pericarditis and cardiac tamponade. Constrictive pericarditis results from acute or chronic inflammation leading to a thickened pericardium, which impairs the ventricular filling of the heart.

▶ ENDOCARDITIS

Infective endocarditis (IE) is an infection of the inner surface of the heart or the heart valves (endocardium). It is caused by a microorganism traveling in the bloodstream (e.g., bacteremia), which lodges onto abnormal heart valves or structural heart abnormalities. IE may occur after invasive surgeries including cardiac procedures, especially when synthetic material is utilized such as with valves, genitourinary tract, and gastrointestinal (GI) surgeries. IE may also occur from long-term indwelling catheters or exposure to bacteremia from dental practices such as teeth brushing or dental procedures.

In IE, microorganisms can grow and form vegetations, platelet thrombi, and fibrin deposits within the endocardium. The infection can invade adjacent tissue, including the aortic and MV, causing further complications as the lesions may break off and embolize elsewhere in the body, most significantly in the kidney, spleen, or central nervous system (CNS). Extracardiac manifestations of IE such as Osler nodes, Janeway spots, splinter hemorrhages, splenomegaly, and petechiae on the oral mucous membranes are less common in children than adults. Other nonspecific symptoms are prolonged low-grade fevers, malaise, weight loss, diaphoresis, rigors, arthralgias, myalgias, and HF symptoms.

NURSING IMPLICATIONS AND TREATMENT

LABS AND DIAGNOSTICS

A definitive diagnosis is obtained with a **blood culture** to identify the causative agent. The most common causative agents are *Staphylococcus aureus* and *Streptococcus viridans*.

TREATMENT AND MANAGEMENT

The treatment requires a prolonged course of parenteral drug therapy, which includes the administration of intravenous high-dose antibiotics for at least 2 weeks and often for 4 to 8 weeks to eradicate the infecting microorganism. Periodic blood cultures are obtained to evaluate the response to antibiotic therapy. Echocardiograms are completed to assess valve damage, vegetation, and ventricular function. In some cases, cardiac surgery is needed to repair or replace damaged valves.

The American Heart Association (AHA) emphasizes the importance of maintaining good oral hygiene to decrease the risk of developing IE. According to the AHA, only high-risk patients that are included in the AHA guidelines (e.g., prosthetic heart valve or previous diagnosis of IE) should receive prophylactic antibiotic therapy one hour before a specific dental procedure (e.g., gingival tissue manipulation or oral mucosal perforation).

▶ KAWASAKI DISEASE

Clinical Pearl
Kawasaki disease (KD) is an acute illness that causes inflammation of the blood vessels (vasculitis), and the most significant complication is the development of coronary artery abnormalities that can lead to the formation of aneurysms.

KD, also known as mucocutaneous lymph node syndrome, is an acute systemic vasculitis (inflammation of the blood vessels) that primarily affects young children and infants. KD is the leading cause of acquired heart disease in developed countries with the highest risk in children of Asian descent. The etiology of KD remains unknown. Uncomplicated KD is self-limiting and resolves in 6 to 8 weeks; however, 20% to 25% of children develop cardiac sequelae without treatment. Timely diagnosis with treatment is pertinent in preventing cardiac complications. KD involves widespread inflammation in the small and medium size blood vessels and the most significant complication in KD is the development of coronary artery abnormalities that can lead to the formation of aneurysms.

SIGNS AND SYMPTOMS

KD clinical manifestations may be divided into acute, subacute, and convalescent phases (see Table 2.16).

Table 2.16 Clinical Manifestations of Kawasaki Disease

Acute Phase	Subacute Phase	Convalescent Phase
High fever unresponsive to antipyretics and antibiotics Nonpurulent conjunctivitis Pharyngeal mucosal inflammation with red, cracked lips, strawberry tongue Rash Edematous hands and feet Erythematous palms and & soles Cervical lymphadenopathy Irritability and inconsolability Abdominal pain Vomiting and diarrhea Pyuria Cardiac manifestations may include myocarditis, MR decreased LV function, pericardial effusion, and coronary artery enlargement	Resolution of fever and acute manifestations Thrombocytosis Periungual desquamation (around the nail) Irritability persists Temporary arthritis Cardiac manifestations may include damaged coronary vessels continuing to stretch or dilate	Clinical manifestations resolved Temporary arthritis Phase ends with resolution of elevated inflammatory markers—CRP, ESR Cardiac complications may include damaged coronary vessels continuing to stretch or dilate

CRP, C-reactive protein; ESR, erythrocyte sedimentation rate; LV, left ventricle; MR, mitral regurgitation.

NURSING IMPLICATIONS AND TREATMENT

LABS AND DIAGNOSTICS

There is not a specific test for diagnosis. Diagnosis is based on clinical manifestations and associated laboratory results that support the diagnosis (Box 2.1). Laboratory findings may include:

- **elevated cardiac biomarkers (troponin)**
- **elevated natriuretic peptides (brain natriuretic peptide [BNP] and N-terminal pro-BNP [NT-proBNP])**
- anemia
- leukocytosis
- thrombocytosis
- transient elevation of liver enzymes
- decreased albumin
- elevated CRP
- erythrocyte sedimentation rate (ESR)

Box 2.1 Diagnosis of Kawasaki Disease

The case definition of KD (also referred to as typical or classic KD) is based on the clinical presentation of a fever lasting 5 days or more, and the presence of at least four of the following five clinical manifestations:
- bilateral conjunctivitis without exudate
- rash; erythema multiforme-like or maculopapular, diffuse erythroderma
- cervical lymphadenopathy (at least 1.5 cm in diameter), usually unilateral
- erythema and edematous hands and feet
- oral mucosal changes

TREATMENT AND MANAGEMENT

The standard treatment of KD includes:

- high-dose intravenous immune globulin (IVIG)
- oral acetylsalicylic acid (ASA; aspirin) therapy

Administration of IVIG has been shown to reduce the duration of fever and decrease the formation of coronary aneurysms, especially if administered within the first 10 days of the illness.

▶ MULTISYSTEM INFLAMMATORY SYNDROME IN CHILDREN

The coronavirus disease 2019 (COVID-19) is caused by severe acute respiratory syndrome coronavirus 2 (SARS-CoV-2) infection resulting in a global pandemic. Most children infected with SARS-CoV-2 are asymptomatic or have mild disease symptoms. A rare but severe complication associated with the SARS-CoV-2 infection is multisystem inflammatory syndrome in children (MIS-C).

SIGNS AND SYMPTOMS

Patients with MIS-C have a variety of symptoms including:
- fever
- abdominal pain
- GI symptoms
- rash
- oral mucosal changes
- nonpurulent conjunctivitis
- headache
- changes in the LOC

MIS-C may cause coronary artery dilation, acute myocardial dysfunction, pericardial effusion, myocarditis, arrhythmias, or conduction abnormalities.

NURSING IMPLICATIONS AND TREATMENT

LABS AND DIAGNOSTICS

Laboratory findings in MIS-C associated with ICU admission and shock include:
- elevated BNP
- D-dimer
- troponin
- CRP
- ferritin
- decreased lymphocyte
- decreased platelet counts

TREATMENT AND MANAGEMENT

Treatment of MIS-C continues to evolve and includes **supportive care** and the use of immune-modifying medications such as **intravenous immunoglobulin** (**IVIG**; Atles et al., 2022). Supportive treatment includes management of HF symptoms in some patients and the patients presenting in vasoplegic shock often require care in ICUs for administration of vasoactive and inotrope medications.

MIS-C patients may require respiratory support with the use of noninvasive or mechanical ventilation and in severe cases, some patients will require ECMO. Management of MIS-C may include antiplatelet and anticoagulation therapy for the risk of thrombotic events with some patients.

▶ HEART FAILURE

Blood entering the heart needs to move through the heart with forward flow for adequate CO. When altering events prevent this from happening, HF is likely. Therefore, HF is a symptom of a disease. Arrhythmias, muscle overgrowth or weakness, obstruction, and too much space or not enough space can all affect the process for oxygenated blood to perfuse the coronary arteries, the brain, and the body. Without enough CO, the human body will fail, and death can occur.

The principle of blood flowing toward the path of least resistance is ever present. The coronary arteries sit just above the AV and require the closure of the AV to pull oxygenated blood in for adequate cardiac function. If the blood cannot go the normal path, it backs up. When blood backs up, the heart cannot keep expending the necessary energy to keep the body performing at a peak level, presenting as fatigue or decreased feeding abilities/appetite.

As the body recognizes that it is not receiving enough oxygen when the blood is not able to easily travel, the renin-angiotensin-aldosterone system kicks in to increase preload. This causes retention of salt and water, increasing contractility with the stretching of the heart muscle. Over time, a failing heart will not be able increase contractility to accommodate this volume and more congestive HF symptoms will occur, such as pulmonary and systemic congestion, hepatomegaly, and edema. As the heart fails, the vessels after the heart will constrict to keep BP elevated to maintain adequate perfusion. The patient's HR will increase to improve CO, but this causes an increase in myocardial oxygen demand. Cyclic adenosine monophosphate (cAMP) is released to increase myocardial contractility from more calcium uptake. This higher calcium level can predispose patients to arrhythmias from transient electrical depolarizations. HF is a vicious cycle.

SIGNS AND SYMPTOMS

LEFT HEART FAILURE

The blood backing up from the LV creates mitral regurgitation (MR), which increases the size of the LA. If the blood volume here is too great, it backs up into the lungs. Signs and symptoms include:

- crackles/rales
- pleural effusions
- pulmonary edema
- tachypnea
- pulmonary congestion

The sympathetic stimulation will present as increased HR, decreased peripheral pulses with poor perfusion evidenced by cool and mottled skin and diaphoresis.

RIGHT HEART FAILURE

The right side of the heart is not able to pump into the lungs due to either high PA pressures or PVR, obstruction from pulmonary stenosis or pulmonary atresia, leading to signs of congestive HF. In children this can present as:

- hepatomegaly
- peripheral edema
- ascites

Arrhythmias may occur due to atrial stretch, increased blood volume in the RA, affecting the conduction pathway, or due to ischemia in the coronary arteries.

NURSING IMPLICATIONS AND TREATMENT

Left-sided HF can lead to right-sided HF. The right heart has to compensate for what the left heart is not able to do. Chronically elevated left sided pressures create high PVR. The right heart has had to pump against high PVR, and the RV remodeled in an inadequate way. Often after a left ventricular assist device (LVAD) is placed, the right heart is put to the test. After the left side is offloaded by having a machine do the work of the LV, the right heart that was used to working harder no longer has that force to pump against. Often compensatory vasoactive mediators cause PH, and it may take some time and medications to decrease the pulmonary pressure. For the LVAD to work, it requires preload to the left side from the blood volume from the lungs. After an LVAD is placed, the patient may require blood products and volume, which can cause the deconditioned RV to have tricuspid regurgitation, with decreased contractility against an increased afterload (Fida et al., 2015). The patient will be placed on iNO (inhaled nitric oxide) and milrinone to help the right side easily pump out. The need for optimized forward flow is high to prevent right sided HF. Keeping the CVP in a postoperative LVAD patient below 15 is the goal. There are many times that a right ventricular assist device (RVAD) will need to be placed, making the patient a bi-VAD.

When using VAD therapy, the patient will often be on an afterload reducer like **nicardipine** or **nitroprusside** to optimize the BP and maintain a mean arterial pressure (MAP) between tightly controlled levels. VADs are preload dependent and afterload sensitive. There needs to be enough blood volume for the VAD to work, and the heart needs to be able to send the blood out without too much difficulty.

A patient with a VAD may or may not have a palpable pulse. Two factors that determine this are the level of native heart function and if the VAD is a continuous flow, nonpulsatile system. A Doppler BP can be obtained by tightening a BP cuff on the arm and using the Doppler to listen for the radial pulse returning after the pressure is slowly released. The MAP should be at the ordered level to maintain tight control, considering preload and afterload.

Clinical Pearl

Heart failure: When a part of the heart isn't functioning as it should, due to poor muscular tone, conduction issues, or blood pathway problems, the heart will fail. There are signs to look for which will indicate which part of the heart is having trouble. Left HF leads to right HF.

CARDIOMYOPATHIES

When thinking about cardiomyopathies, *the heart muscle is where the problem lies*. There are a few different types, which can occur alongside other congenital heart defects. This section will address cardiomyopathies not related to defects. The goal of treatment is to try and "remodel" the heart muscle with medications, preventing fulminant HF (see Figure 2.21). Through decreasing oxygen demand and the work for the heart with the use of medications, symptom relief can improve the quality of life for this patient. These patients may live at home on continuous infusions such as milrinone to allow the heart to work less hard and on enteral feeds to maintain enough caloric intake for the body. Often these patients will start being worked up for transplant.

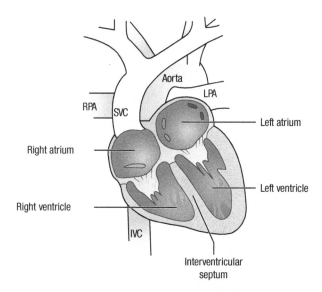

Figure 2.21 Normal heart
Source: Copyright 2018, Children's Hospital of Philadelphia. Reprinted with permission.

▶ HYPERTROPHIC CARDIOMYOPATHY

Hypertrophic cardiomyopathy (HCM) is an autosomal dominant gene mutation and is the most common genetic cardiac disorder, found in 1:500 of the general population. It is characterized by an overgrowth of the left ventricular heart muscle, especially near the septum (Figure 2.22). The LV is not dilated, though the chamber is filled with excessive muscular tissue. This can restrict the outflow of blood from the ventricle, leading to diastolic dysfunction. Diastolic dysfunction can be thought of as a stiffened chamber that restricts the ability of the heart to fill. This can lead to poor blood flow or perfusion for the coronary arteries and to the brain and body. When the LV does not have adequate blood volume, perfusion is compromised, which may lead to ventricular arrhythmias and sudden death. Left ventricular outflow tract obstruction (LVOTO) occurs when so much tissue compromises the filling of the left side of the heart and prevents blood from leaving. This can lead to MV dysfunction as the path of least resistance leads to backflow into the LA and then the pulmonary veins and lungs.

SIGNS AND SYMPTOMS

Often asymptomatic, family history of sudden cardiac deaths, syncope, chest pain, exertional dyspnea, exercise intolerance. Presenting symptom may be sudden cardiac death from LVOTO. When blood is not able to leave the heart and perfuse the coronaries, ischemia occurs. If enough blood volume does not supply the brain, syncope will occur.

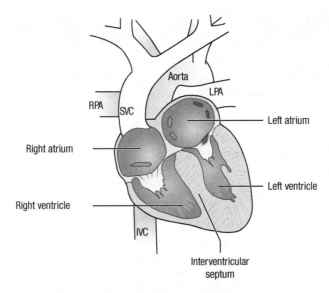

Figure 2.22 Hypertrophic cardiomyopathy (HCM)
Source: Copyright 2018, Children's Hospital of Philadelphia. Reprinted with permission.

NURSING IMPLICATIONS AND TREATMENT

ASSESSMENT

Often first found at a well-child visit with the practitioner hearing a murmur, which leads to further tests.

LABS AND DIAGNOSTICS

- **Abnormal EKG** found more than 75% of the time shows left ventricular hypertrophy, abnormal QRS axis. Holter may be ordered to look at the bigger picture—arrhythmias may occur most during exercise.
- **Echocardiograms** show thickened LV without LV dilation, diastolic dysfunction, and possible LVOTO.
- **Exercise stress test** may show an abnormal BP response: BP decreased.

TREATMENT AND MANAGEMENT

- **Avoid tachycardia:** Avoid athletic activities that raise HR, dehydration, inotropes.
- **beta-blockers** to slow rate and optimize ventricular filling
- cautious use of **diuretics** due to limiting preload
- **antiarrhythmics and/or implantable cardioverter-defibrillator (ICD)** placement due to risk of sudden death
- **surgical myomectomy** when unresponsive to medical treatments
- **heart transplantation**

HCM prevents blood from filling the LV and ejecting well, compromising oxygenated blood flow to the coronaries leading to ischemia. Increased ventricular filling time using beta-blockers and automatic implantable cardioverter-defibrillator (AICD) implantation are useful therapies to help prevent sudden death. It is the most common cause of sudden death in young adults and athletes.

▶ DILATED CARDIOMYOPATHY

LV dilation with systolic dysfunction (impaired contractility) are the presenting characteristics of dilated cardiomyopathy (DCM; Figure 2.23). A change in the preload should change the contractility, but in DCM this does not happen. It is the most common cardiomyopathy in children. DCM can occur from many different causes such as a genetic mutation, familial, mitochondrial disease, metabolic disease, systemic myopathy or neuromuscular disease, post myocarditis, or even peripartum. The heart chamber becomes enlarged as the heart muscle becomes weaker with poor contraction. The walls of the heart do not become thicker because the heart muscle is not able to grow as it could in a normal heart.

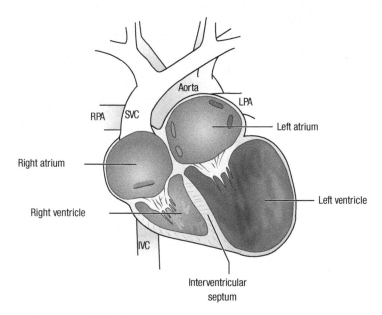

Figure 2.23 Dilated cardiomyopathy (DCM)
Source: Copyright 2018, Children's Hospital of Philadelphia. Reprinted with permission.

SIGNS AND SYMPTOMS

DCM is characterized by a large LV and muscle weakness. This cardiomyopathy allows blood to sit in the LV or regurgitate back through the MV, dilating the LA and forward flow is impaired. With DCM, the presentation can be mild to severe. In infants, feeding intolerance or poor growth may be noted. There could be respiratory symptoms, poor perfusion to the GI system, fatigue, exercise intolerance. Some children may compensate well for a time and have few symptoms. Remember in infants, HR is more compensatory than SV per Frank Starling's law. As DCM becomes more symptomatic, the signs of HF become more prominent including with signs of respiratory distress, congestive HF and GI symptoms due to poor perfusion. There is also a high risk of stroke as blood can sit in the ventricle, having time to clot before being ejected.

NURSING IMPLICATIONS AND TREATMENT

ASSESSMENT

Findings include:
- tachycardia
- tachypnea
- increased work of breathing
- loss of appetite or poor weight gain
- exercise intolerance
  May have:
- peripheral edema
- cool extremities
- delayed capillary refill

LABS AND DIAGNOSTICS

- **CXR** reflects pulmonary edema, pleural effusions, hepatomegaly.
- **Echocardiograms** show depressed systolic function, an enlarged LV.
- **EKG** may show a tachyarrhythmia, flat inverted T waves, atrial enlargement.
- **BNP** is helpful to trend when assessing the degree of HF or improvement.
- **Liver enzymes** assess degree of hepatic involvement.

TREATMENT AND MANAGEMENT

- **Inotrope** support helps contractility, diuresis to decrease blood volume (preload), which helps in remodeling the LV and allows a decrease in the amount of blood that the heart will have to pump.
- **Milrinone** and **angiotensin-converting enzyme (ACE) inhibitors** or other **afterload reducers** will allow the heart to pump blood out easier, improving forward flow.
- **Anticoagulation** reduces the risk of clots if function is several depressed, such as an ejection fraction of less than 20%.
- **Mechanical ventilation** used for LV afterload reduction and to reduce metabolic demand.
- **MCS** used via ECMO or other VAD therapies, when worsening of CHF symptoms, decreased left ventricular systolic function with progression to diastolic dysfunction, increased MR. Heart transplant considered with decompensated HF.

▶ MUSCULAR DYSTROPHY

Muscular dystrophy is a known risk for later development (late teens), most often with DCM. Screening begins every year starting at age 6, then annually after age 10. Treatment includes ACE inhibitors and even a VAD as a destination therapy.

▶ RESTRICTIVE CARDIOMYOPATHY

Less than 5% of cardiomyopathies are restrictive cardiomyopathies (RCMs), which has the poorest prognosis. RCM is often from an abnormality in the sarcomere contractility protein gene, with 25% having a family history of cardiomyopathy (Figure 2.24). This can also be idiopathic from metabolic disorders, with only a 20% survival rate at 5 years from diagnosis and 66% to 100% need heart transplants by age 6 (Callow & Scheffer, 2019). RCM is characterized by diastolic dysfunction (stiffened chamber) of either or both ventricles, decreased LV compliance and relaxation with impaired filling, leading to increased left ventricular end diastolic pressure (LVEDPP) and LA enlargement from the backflow of blood through the MV. Systolic function is not impaired.

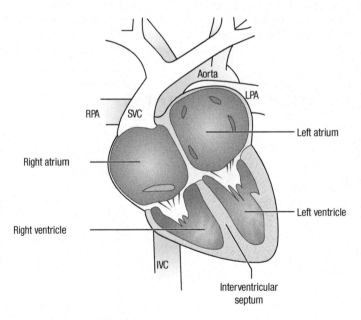

Figure 2.24 Restrictive cardiomyopathy
Source: Copyright 2018, Children's Hospital of Philadelphia. Reprinted with permission.

SIGNS AND SYMPTOMS

RCM presents with exercise intolerance, difficulty breathing, chest pain, FTT, ascites, edema, recurrent respiratory infections, chronic congestion, and fatigue.

NURSING IMPLICATIONS AND TREATMENT

ASSESSMENT

Findings include:
- lyspnea
- syncope
- Aascites
- FTT
- arrhythmias
- PVR

LABS AND DIAGNOSTICS

- **EKG:** atrial enlargement, ST/T wave abnormalities, Holter to assess for further arrhythmias
- **Echocardiogram shows bi-atrial enlargement:** "Mickey Mouse" ears, abnormal diastolic filling and dysfunction with normal systolic function. Elevated PA pressures
- **labs:** BNP, liver enzymes
- **Cardiac catheterization** measures filling pressures and pulmonary arterial pressure (PAP).

TREATMENT AND MANAGEMENT

- **Avoid tachycardia.**
- Ensure **adequate preload** to optimize diastolic filling, avoid fluid overload.
- **anticoagulation, ICD**
- **Optimize growth** and promote **stable hemodynamics.**
- **heart transplantation**

> ### Clinical Pearl
>
> *Cardiomyopathies: to differentiate the main types think about DCM (dilated) as big, HCM (hypertrophic) as bad since sudden death can occur with HCM, and RCM (restrictive) as ugly since heart transplantation is the best treatment option.*

▶ LYMPHATIC DISORDERS (CARDIAC SURGERY RISK)

The lymphatic system is responsible for cleaning out fluids that leak out of the blood vessels. The thoracic duct moves the fluids back into the circulatory system. When a patient has had cardiac surgery that involves a thoracotomy, the thoracic duct may be nicked, leading to chylous drainage from a pleural chest tube placed in the operating room. Prior to this chest tube being pulled, thoracotomy patients should drink fatty liquids, like milk, to check for this common surgical risk. If a white, milk-like substance is found in the chest tube, it is sent to the lab for a cell count, as the *white fluid is indicative of chyle*. The patient will need to be on a fat-free diet for about 6 weeks. Fat molecules that typically would seep through the lymphatic system will no longer be present, allowing the duct to heal.

Another cause of increased lymphatic drainage is with single ventricle surgeries causing a change in intrathoracic pressures. Higher pressures within the chest make it harder for fluids to be brought back into the lymphatic vessels. This can cause pleural effusions within the lungs. The abdomen has increased risk of ascites and protein losing enteropathies (PLE) due to abnormalities in lymphatic flow.

Another lymphatic condition common to cardiac children is plastic bronchitis. Lymph can ooze into the patient's airway, drying into caulk-like formations that are shaped like the bronchioles. This "cast" is made from fluid that has leaked out of the lymphatic vessels, which are known to transport white blood cells (WBCs) and protein, into the patient's airway lined with mucus. These casts can become stuck in a patient's airway, causing asphyxiation. In this emergency situation, a bronchoscopy needs to be done at the bedside to pull the cast out. This needs to be done quickly, as depending on the position of the cast, air may not be able to enter the body effectively. Inhaled tPA is an effective treatment for these patients.

NURSING IMPLICATIONS AND TREATMENT

ASSESSMENT

- **chylothorax:** presence of milk-like substance in chest tube after patient drinks a fatty liquid
- **increased lymphatic production:** ascites, generalized edema, abdominal distention
- **plastic bronchitis:** difficulty breathing, choking on cast, airway emergency

LABS AND DIAGNOSTICS

- **chest tube drainage cell count:** triglyceride level greater than 150, indicating the presence of chyle
- serum: **low albumin <3**
- **CXR:** pleural effusions, ascites, edema
- **bronchoscopy:** visualization of casts

TREATMENT AND MANAGEMENT

- **Chylous effusions:** fat-free diet for about 6 weeks: an infant can have skimmed breast milk, Vivonex, Portagen, or Tolerex; a child above 3 years of age can eat fat-free foods and drink Boost, Breeze, or Carnation Breakfast Essentials.
- increased **respiratory support** with increased fluid in chest and/or abdomen
- drainage of accumulating fluid with a **chest tube**
- **diuretics**
- Assess for difficulty breathing from fluid in the chest should the lymphatic vessel not heal once the 6 weeks have passed.
- **lymphatic embolization**—thoracic duct coiling, gluing
- **inhaled tPA** for plastic bronchitis

ARRHYTHMIAS AND MYOCARDIAL CONDUCTION SYSTEM DEFECTS

Conduction of the heart involves a shift of energy, which causes the heart to move in a specific pattern that allows for effective CO to occur. In the normal heart, the sinoatrial (SA) node is where conduction begins. The electrical message is sent to the atrioventricular (AV) node and down to the ventricles via the bundle of His, to the bundle branches, and then through the Purkinje fibers (Figure 2.25). For effective CO to occur, the electrical activity should travel down this pathway at a normal rate.

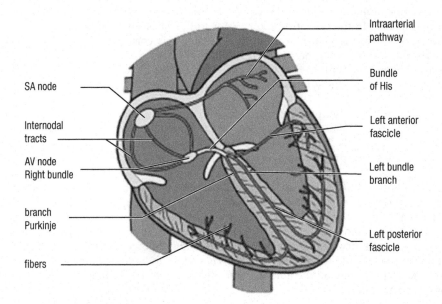

Figure 2.25 The cardiac conduction system

Source: Hoffman, J., Thompson-Bowie, N., & Jnah, A. (2019). *Fetal and neonatal physiology for the advanced practice nurse.* Springer Publishing Company.

To visualize conduction, the EKG is performed. Each part of the normal conduction cycle is defined using letters from the alphabet, "PQRST" with the occasional "U" wave. The "P" wave is when the atria contract, or atrial depolarization. "QRS" is when the ventricles contract (depolarization), and "T" is ventricular repolarization (Figure 2.26; see Figure 2.27 for normal sinus rhythm.).

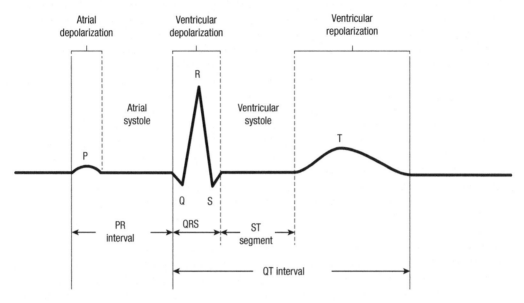

Figure 2.26 Ventricular repolarization

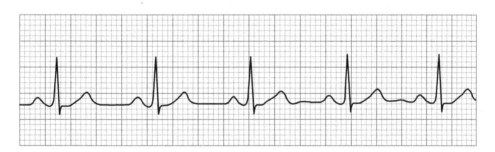

Figure 2.27 Normal sinus rhythm

Each part of the conduction cycle has a function that correlates with moving the heart muscle in a manner that pushes blood from one chamber to the next, into the lungs, filling the coronaries, sending the blood out to the body. If this does not happen in the pattern of regular, strong contractions, abnormal problems can occur. Some problems include clot formation if the blood is not able to move out of a chamber, or when the majority of the blood may not leave a chamber, this can eventually cause dilation or backflow. If the HR is too high, blood will not fill the chamber and only small amounts will be sent to the body, compromising perfusion.

The electrical activity flowing through the heart causes the muscles to contract in a rhythmic way. This "conduction" moves blood into the next location necessary for adequate CO. When assessing a rhythm, always look at rate, regular or irregular, P wave for every QRS, narrow or wide QRS complex. Congenital alterations, familial history, rare infections, or postcardiac surgery conduction disorder can lead to poor perfusion or even life-threatening arrhythmias. Over time, conduction disturbances can cause cardiomyopathies due to poor emptying of the heart chambers.

Whatever rhythm is on the monitor, the first thing the nurse should do is assess. Look at the patient. Are they conscious? Are they mentating? Do they have a pulse? Is it strong? What is the BP? Based on this first step, the second step can range from checking electrolytes to starting CPR.

▶ LONG QT SYNDROME

One in 2,500 people are found to have this conduction disorder. It is often caused by an inherited faulty gene but can also be triggered later in life from medications like antibiotics, antipsychotics, or anti-arrhythmics. Sodium ion channels in the heart are blocked, causing a delay in the T wave. The T wave on the EKG is when ventricular repolarization occurs, which is the time the cells are recharging for the next cycle. The r-on-t phenomenon is an attempt for ventricular depolarization while in the repolarization phase is underway, this can trigger ventricular tachycardia (VT) presenting as Torsade's de pointes. This can be a self-limiting arrhythmia presenting as fainting or seizures, or sudden cardiac death if it deteriorates into ventricular fibrillation.

SIGNS AND SYMPTOMS

- fainting
- seizures
- history of cardiac arrest

NURSING IMPLICATIONS AND TREATMENT

ASSESSMENT

Patients are well-appearing unless in arrhythmia.

LABS AND DIAGNOSTICS

- genetic screening if familial disposition
- EKG
- exercise stress test
- Holter

TREATMENT AND MANAGEMENT

- Patient should avoid strenuous exercise.
- Beta-blockers, such as nadolol (Corgard), decrease risk in arrhythmias arising from stress.
- ICD placement for those at high risk
- Potassium supplementation can be used to lower excitability threshold.

▶ WOLFF-PARKINSON-WHITE SYNDROME

In Wolff-Parkinson-White Syndrome (WPW), a short circuit is created when the heart develops in the womb. A strand of heart muscle in the atria becomes an extra electrical path. This tissue is unusual as it is muscle and not made up of the automaticity cells that are in the normal conduction pathway. Supraventricular tachycardia (SVT) frequency is quite variable in WPW and can happen daily or even just a few times per year. Triggers can be strenuous exercise, too much caffeine or alcohol, or completely random. When an impulse travels down this short circuit, it can either follow the normal conduction path or go around in a circular pattern causing the heart to beat very quickly. When this happens, it is called a reentrant tachycardia or SVT. One in 1,000 people are found to have WPW, though reentrant arrhythmias occur in 50% of these. The biggest issue is when the heart rhythm degenerates into atrial fibrillation with a fast ventricular response or decompensates into ventricular fibrillation.

SIGNS AND SYMPTOMS

- history of fainting
- feeling palpitations or racing in the chest

NURSING IMPLICATIONS AND TREATMENT

ASSESSMENT

- asymptomatic unless in SVT
- **if symptomatic:**
  - will palpate/auscultate a fast pulse
  - dizziness

- chest pain
- fainting
- shortness of breath
- feeling anxiety

LABS AND DIAGNOSTICS

- EKG or Holter shows regular rhythm.
- short PR interval
- wide QRS
- **presence of delta wave:** a "slurred upstroke" of the QRS: slight angle into the complex noted on V6
- occasional SVT
- exercise stress test when old enough to assess for risk of sudden cardiac death
- Holter

TREATMENT AND MANAGEMENT

- **Vagal maneuvers:** Teach patient to blow through a straw or syringe opening, bear down, cough, elicit diving reflex by putting bag of ice on the face of an infant
- medications
  - **beta-blockers daily:** slows electrical impulses in the heart
  - **Adenosine** in the hospital—blocks abnormal electrical signals. Brief asystole while heart resets. Often used in stable SVT. **Very** short half-life (<10 seconds): MUST give via rapid IV push with saline flush after.
- **Cardioversion:** restores heartbeat to normal rhythm. Used in unstable SVT. Can be painful, remember to give sedation/pain medication prior.
- ablation to prevent recurrence of symptoms destroys the abnormal pathway through heat or freezing in a cardiac catheterization with electrophysiology presence
- Teach patient to seek treatment for chest pain lasting more than 15 minutes or if heartbeat doesn't go back to normal within a few minutes.

▶ ECTOPIC ATRIAL TACHYCARDIA

Ectopic atrial tachycardia (EAT) is noted for abnormal automaticity with a gradual onset and resolution, differing from SVT's sudden HR increase and decrease. Over time, this can lead to HF when EAT goes unrecognized. Because of the abnormal automaticity, this rhythm can be irregular with frequent premature atrial contractions (PACs), there can be an exaggerated response to exercise, and EAT can appear quite variable on EKG. Treatment with antiarrhythmics, beta-blockers, digoxin, and esmolol are options, with calcium channel blockers being used in older children. Ablation can also be performed for EAT in the cardiac catheterization lab.

Clinical Pearl

Digoxin has a narrow therapeutic range and toxicity is a risk with this cardiac glycoside. Nurses caring for patients receiving digoxin should be familiar with signs and symptoms of toxicity, which include nausea, vomiting, hypotension, bradycardia, and visual changes including blurred vision and yellow halos. The antidote for digoxin toxicity is digoxin immune fab.

▶ JUNCTIONAL ECTOPIC TACHYCARDIA

Junctional ectopic tachycardia (JET) is most commonly found after surgical heart repairs, though very rarely has been noted to be congenital in nature. This abnormal rhythm originates in the AV node and is attributed to ischemia and injury to the conduction tissue during surgery. This rhythm can be regular or irregular, has a gradual onset and resolution, and has rate variability (Figure 2.28). Decreased CO with hypotension occurs when the heart is not able to fill due to a fast HR. When JET is found in postoperative patients, it is usually self-limiting and will spontaneously resolve within a week of surgery. Treatment consists of correcting electrolytes, starting medications such as antiarrhythmics including amiodarone, beta-blockers to slow the heart down and most importantly keeping the patient cool. JET often occurs in a postoperative TOF patient that is too warm following surgery. Another treatment option in these patients is using dexmedetomidine, which is known for lowering HR in patients.

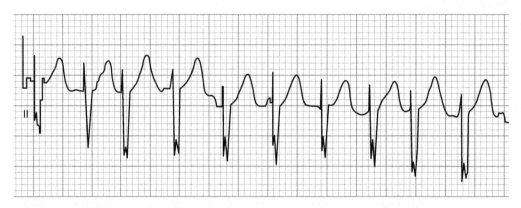

Figure 2.28 Junctional esctopic tachycardia (JET)

HEART BLOCK

When thinking about heart blocks (Figure 2.29), consider where the problem is. The lower the baseline HR the lower the block is: AV blocks have a slower HR than a first-degree block. The block prevents electrical signals from completing their route effectively, altering the conduction cycle. This can occur from damage to the heart muscle such as in postoperative patients, can be a congenital defect, or can even happen from an infection. Some conduction defects are more serious than others. The most serious may require implantation of a permanent pacemaker.

FIRST-DEGREE HEART BLOCK

This block is measured from the PR interval, so the PR interval is prolonged (>0.20 seconds). The delay is in the conduction through the AV node. The P wave is present for first-degree block. This is not usually a symptomatic disorder, unless the rate is too slow to maintain good CO.

SECOND-DEGREE HEART BLOCK

There are two types of second-degree blocks: Mobitz I (also known as Wenckebach) and Mobitz II. To remember how to differentiate, there is a rhyme that is known: "Longer, longer, longer drop, now I know it's Wenckebach. If that p keeps marching through, then you know it's Mobitz 2." Second-degree type 1 AV block aka Wenckebach (Mobitz I) is often thought of as a 2:1 (or 3:1) block depending on how many P waves there are for every conducted QRS. The PR interval gradually increases until a QRS complex is dropped. This usually occurs in a regular pattern; an example is every 4th QRS is dropped second-degree, type 2, AV block. With Mobitz II, the PR interval does not change. Some P waves aren't able to send the message down the line to continue the conduction of the QRS. There may be multiple P waves with no QRS, meaning no ventricular contraction. The P waves are regular, but the QRS is variable. Hemodynamic stability depends on the ventricular rate in this block.

THIRD-DEGREE HEART BLOCK AKA COMPLETE HEART BLOCK

In this block, the atria and ventricles do not communicate. The P waves are regular and the QRS complex is regular, but there is no relationship between each other. The atria and ventricles don't communicate with each other and do their own thing. There is complete atria and ventricular dissociation. When conduction begins at the ventricle level, the HR will be very low.

First-degree AV block

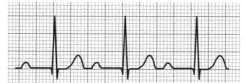

Second-degree AV block Type 1 (Mobitz 1 or Wenchebach)

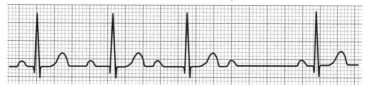

Second-degree AV block Type 2 (Mobitz II)

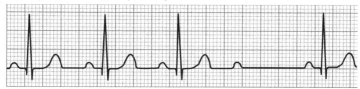

Second-degree AV block (2:1 block)

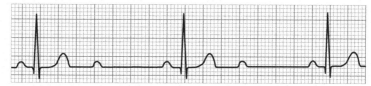

Third-degree AV block with junctional escape

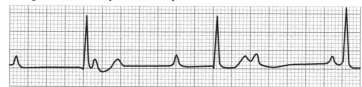

Figure 2.29 Types of AV heart blocks.
Source: Npatchett—CC BY-SA 4.0.

JUNCTIONAL HEART BLOCK

A junctional rhythm is characterized by the absence of a P wave. The conduction originates from the AV node and the rate would be slower than with first degree. The loss of the atrial kick can contribute to some hypotension and possible CO concerns.

SIGNS AND SYMPTOMS

- dizziness or fainting
- fistory of congenital heart surgery
- congenital heart block
- poor CO

NURSING IMPLICATIONS AND TREATMENT

ASSESSMENT

- must be determined if the patient is on medications that can cause a block: calcium channel blockers, dexmedetomidine, beta-blockers, digoxin, antiarrhythmics
- must be determined if the patient is stable

LABS AND DIAGNOSTICS

- EKG or Holter
- echocardiogram: assesses how the heart is functioning with block
- exercise stress test

TREATMENT AND MANAGEMENT

- Stop medication that may be causing block.
- transvenous pacing
- permanent pacing if condition does not resolve within 7 to 10 days

▶ NEONATAL HEART BLOCK

When a woman with Lupus is pregnant, one concern is that her baby will be born with autoimmune congenital heart block. Weekly monitoring should begin between 16 and 24 weeks. There is a reduced risk when hydroxychloroquine is initiated early in the pregnancy (De Carolis et al., 2020). The neonate will present in utero with second- or third-degree heart block. If the intrinsic rate is high enough to generate adequate CO the rhythm may be watched closely in the postnatal period, but most often these patients need pacing initiated quickly.

▶ LYME DISEASE HEART BLOCK

Lyme carditis presents after cardiac "invasion" of untreated Lyme (Chaudhry et al., 2017). Tissue damage in the heart occurs from inflammation as the immune system kicks in to destroy bacteria. EKG/telemetry can reveal quite variable conduction delays with the majority being a mild heart block that self resolves. Occasionally, these patients present in second- or third-degree heart block with dizziness and fatigue, shortness of breath, and chest pain. The rhythm can devolve further as treatment begins. The patient with inadequate CO due to a low ventricular rate will need emergent transcutaneous or transvenous pacing. Isoproterenol (Isuprel) can also be used temporarily. Often after antibiotics are administered, the patient's heart will heal, and the conduction disturbance will resolve in about 2 weeks. Rarely is a permanent pacemaker necessary, but it is an option should the resolution take longer than anticipated.

▶ ST SEGMENT ELEVATION

When the heart muscle is unable to access oxygenated blood, ischemic changes are evident on the EKG in the form of ST segment elevation, sometimes referred to as "tombstones" depending on the amount of ischemia. This can occur from torsion post-surgical repair, often associated with TGAs from the arterial switch operation. The surgery involves removing the coronary arteries from the aorta and sewing them onto the PA (which becomes the neoaorta). The surgeons assess in the operating room if the heart is able to receive adequate oxygenated blood before closing the chest, but there are times when ST elevation isn't evident until after the patient returns to the ICU. ST segment elevation may also occur from an anomalous left coronary artery from the pulmonary artery (ALCAPA) found within weeks to a few months after birth when the baby presents in fulminant HF. When the heart has received unoxygenated blood from the coronary artery, damage to the muscle arises and the heart fails. Coronary artery embolisms also can cause ST segment elevation due to blockage from plaque, fat, or a blood clot, which is especially more common in adults.

SIGNS AND SYMPTOMS

- irritability and chest pain
- poor feeding/eating
- diaphoresis especially with feeding
- circumoral cyanosis
- tachypnea
- tachycardia
- feeling tired
- poor appetite
- nausea/vomiting
- anxiety

NURSING IMPLICATIONS AND TREATMENT

ASSESSMENT

The nurse must determine if the patient is stable. This condition can be an emergency, as this is myocardial ischemia: time = muscle death. Adequate resources should be available. The healthcare team should prepare for the patient to travel to the cath lab and be alert for worsening status.

LABS AND DIAGNOSTICS

- echocardiogram to assess coronary artery
- 12 lead EKG to assess degree of elevation, greater than 2 mm concerning
- elevated troponin level
- computed tomography angiography (CTA) to assess blood flow in heart

TREATMENT AND MANAGEMENT

- catheterization lab for emergent stent placement
- operating room if unable to place stent

▶ COMMON ARRHYTHMIAS SEEN IN A CARDIAC ICU

PREMATURE ATRIAL CONTRACTIONS

PACs are very common, can be a single PAC, or can present as bigeminal PACs—one PAC every other beat. A patient with PACs is typically asymptomatic. Check for perfusion: pulses, cap refill, BP. Check electrolytes. Notify frontline practitioner (Figure 2.30).

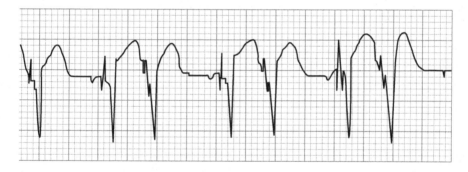

Figure 2.30 Premature atrial contractions (PACs)

PREMATURE VENTRICULAR CONTRACTIONS

Premature ventricular contractions (PVCs) can be single or more frequent. PVCs are common, especially with low K^+. Bigeminal PVCs can be multi-focal-upright or upside down. Can lead to VT. Check and correct electrolytes. Notify frontline practitioner if frequent or bigeminal. The heart is feeling irritable (Figure 2.31).

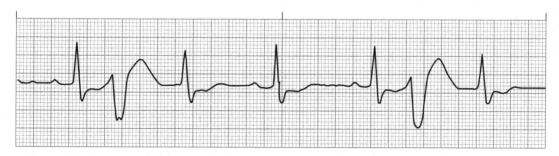

Figure 2.31 Premature ventricular contractions (PVCs). A wide QRS complex that is not preceded by a P wave. PVCs alternating with every other beat is called bigeminy and PVCs every third beat is called trigeminy.

SUPRAVENTRICULAR TACHYCARDIA

Supraventricular tachycardia (SVT) is common in postoperative children with WPW. Reentrant tachycardia—sudden onset and can have a sudden resolution. High HR—usually >220 in infants, >170 in older kids. Watch for that sudden onset, which is usually the biggest clue that it is SVT and not a different arrhythmia. Assess if stable or unstable. Hypotension and poor mentation determine stability. Adenosine will be given for stable SVT, dose doubled with second administration—always remember very short half-life. Cardioversion 0.5 to 2 joules per kilogram for unstable (Figure 2.32).

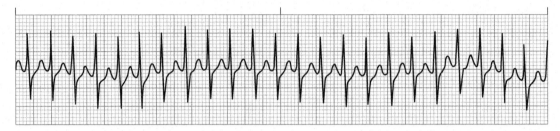

Figure 2.32 Supraventricular tachycardia (SVT). No discernable P waves, narrow complex, rate >180 beats per minute for child or >220 beats per minutes for infant.
Source: Children's Hospital of Philadelphia

Clinical Pearl

Synchronized cardioversion is done when the patient has a pulse rate. You need to synchronize (learn) the heart rhythm, so the charge is delivered on the "R" wave of the QRS complex. If energy delivered any other time, you could cause a more serious rhythm change. Defibrillation can be done at any time because there typically isn't a pulse. Defibrillation is done for V-fib and pulseless V-tach.

VENTRICULAR TACHYCARDIA (VT: **Figure 2.33***):* Can initially be "stable" but may deteriorate quickly. Notify frontline practitioner. Check for a pulse. Call a code if no pulse and begin CPR. Cardioversion will be done for VT with a pulse, defibrillation for VT without a pulse: 2 to 4 joules per kilogram.

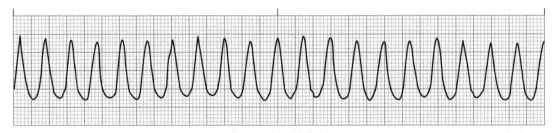

Figure 2.33 Ventricular tachycardia (VT). Rapid rate and regular with wide QRS complexes.

VENTRICULAR FIBRILLATION (Vfib or VF: **Figure 2.34***):* The heart cannot pump blood out and the patient is in cardiac arrest. No pulse, no contraction, call a code and begin CPR. Defibrillation is necessary to get the heart out of this lethal rhythm. An automated external defibrillator (AED) can be used if not in an ICU. These are now widely available since recognition that AEDs save lives.

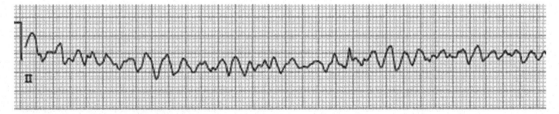

Figure 2.34 Ventricular fibrillation (Vfib or VF)
Source: Children's Hospital of Philadelphia.

ATRIAL FLUTTER (**Figure 2.35**): A short circuit in the atria cause a fast rhythm in a regular, sawtooth pattern. This can cause symptoms of palpitations, shortness of breath, dizziness. Increased risk of stroke and HF. Decreased CO due to decreased heart filling time. More common in children after surgery involving the atrial conduction path. An EKG will be ordered when notifying the frontline provider. Treatment consists of antiarrhythmics and possibly ablation.

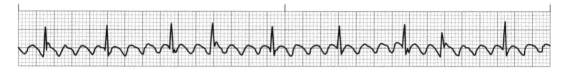

Figure 2.35 Atrial flutter. Sawtooth appearance, fast atrial rate (300 bpm), normal QRS complex. Rare in infants and children and may occur after cardiac surgery involving the atria.

ATRIAL FIBRILLATION (Afib; **Figure 2.36***):* Fast and chaotic, irregular atrial rhythm that can occur with cardiomyopathy, WPW, or postcardiac surgery in children. Very rarely associated to a child without any comorbidities. An EKG will be ordered after notifying the frontline practitioner. The AV node blocks most of the impulses, creating a more stable rhythm. The risk of clots is higher with this and decreased CO is likely. Antiarrhythmics, anticoagulation, and ablation of the AV node with permanent pacemaker placement may be used to treat this. For unstable Afib, cardioversion is used to reset the rhythm.

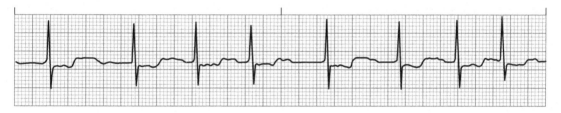

Figure 2.36 Atrial fibrillation. Regularly irregular, no correlation between P waves and WRS, rate can be normal or rapid, multiple excited cardiac cells in atrium firing simultaneously and only one enters the ventricle, which then contracts
Source: Children's Hospital of Philadelphia.

BUNDLE BRANCH BLOCK (BBB; **Figure 2.37***):* Most often a benign condition, with a slight delay in conduction through the bundle branches. An EKG can determine if it is a left or a right BBB. Left BBB can be more significant than right BBB. This appears as "bunny ears" on the QRS.

A.   **B.**

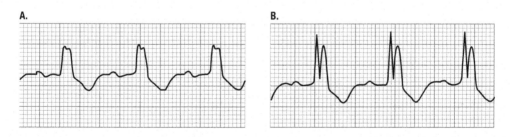

Figure 2.37 A bundle branch block widened QRS, ST, and T wave displacement opposite to the deflection of the QRS complex. Either right or left bundle branch blocks. Right BBB has a "bunny ear" appearance.

VAGAL INDUCED BRADYCARDIA: When suctioning, placing a nasogastric tube or intubating, or even an orally intubated patient that is too awake, there are times when the rhythm will quickly slow down. This can lead to arrest if the noxious stimulus is not removed. During intubation, atropine is given in neonates and infants to increase the HR proactively to prevent severe bradycardia.

SIGNS AND SYMPTOMS OF COMMON ARRHYTHMIAS

Possible poor perfusion.

NURSING IMPLICATIONS AND TREATMENT

ASSESSMENT

- observation of patient
- observation of rhythm
- assessment of CO
- decreased urine output
- weak or absent peripheral pulses
- lengthened CRT
- decreased or acutely altered mentation and LOC

LABS AND DIAGNOSTICS

- serum electrolytes, specifically K^+
- EKG

TREATMENT AND MANAGEMENT

- Immediately provide airway management, oxygen, and CPR according to the American Heart Association Pediatric Life Support Guidelines for pediatric cardiac arrest algorithms for patients with signs and symptoms of cardiopulmonary compromise (hypotension, acutely altered mental status, loss of pulse).
- Give supplemental K^+ if on diuretic therapy.
- **Correct reversible causes:** hypoxia, acidosis.
- Establish rate and rhythm control through pacing.
- medications:
  - **bradyarrhythmias:** atropine, epinephrine, isuprel
  - **tachyarrhythmias:** antiarrhythmics, adenosine, beta-blockers

Clinical Pearl

Arrhythmias: Is the patient stable or unstable? This is defined by adequate BP, consciousness, perfusion, chest pain, urine output, and if a long-term conduction issue, how is their heart being affected? To identify the rhythm on a monitor, assess for rate, regularity, P wave for every QRS, narrow or wide QRS. Cardioversion is for unstable patients with a pulse, defibrillation for no pulse. With pulseless electrical activity (PEA), all that can be done is assess and treat the cause and continue good CPR and the administration of IV epinephrine.

▶ PACEMAKERS

A machine that can generate electrical impulses to the heart to begin the conduction cycle of depolarization and contraction of the chambers. Indications for pacing include:

- heart block secondary to surgery
- congenital complete heart block
- bradyarrhythmias
- long QT
- neurocardiogenic syncope

Pacing can occur for the atria, ventricles, or both. Lead wires are most often bipolar in current state, functioning as both ground and active. A rate is set on this machine to create optimized CO. Electricity is sent through the wires to obtain "capture," or cause a contraction of the heart. This is measured by the output of the current.

Clinical Pearl

Pacer SPIKES on the electrocardiography indicates pacing:
- ***atrial** pacing—sharp spike before the P wave*
- ***ventricular** pacing—sharp spike is before the QRS*
- ***AV sequential** pacing (both atria and ventricles—sharp spikes before the P wave and QRS)*

- **Temporary pacing (aka transthoracic):** Leads/electrodes attach to a cable connected to the pacemaker/defibrillator.
- **Transcutaneous (external):** Noninvasive, electrodes are placed on the skin. Electrode pads placed on the front and the back of the patient to deliver stimulation to the heart through the chest wall. This requires much higher energy levels to obtain capture. Pacing in this method can be painful and sedation is recommended. This method is the least reliable form of pacing and requires the pads to be removed for CXRs and frequent changing of the pads during active pacing to maintain capture. Leads attached to the defibrillator are required along with the pads when using this method.
  Transvenous: Electrode tip placed via a sheath in a large vein, sitting in the RA and RV—typically femoral, right internal jugular, or left subclavian. This can be placed quickly at the bedside—good for patients that are born with congenital heart block, or when in heart block from myocarditis or Lyme carditis.
- **Epicardial:** Wires placed in the operating room directly to the RA, RV, or both during open heart surgery. Often placed when surgeon working in areas that may disturb the conduction pathway: AVC, VSD, TOF repair. It's easier to place a lead in the operating room and remove several days later when the patient is stable.
- **Permanent pacing:** Implanted into the chest, with leads attached to the heart muscle. Smaller patients <12 kg may require epicardial leads placed through a thoracotomy or sternotomy. Transvenous leads can be used for patients >12 kg. The generator is usually placed in the abdominal wall or above the heart in a surgically placed pocket. Battery voltage needs to be checked regularly, with a surgical plan as the battery end-of-life becomes apparent. Leads can fracture, more often epicardial, causing loss of capture and quickly declining CO. See Figure 2.38 for loss of pacemaker capture, Figure 2.39 for undersensing, Figure 2.40 for oversensing, and Figure 2.41 for noncapture.

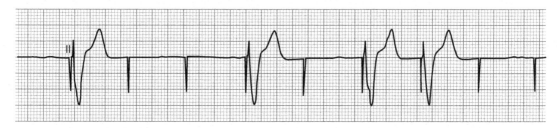

Figure 2.38 Loss of pacemaker capture

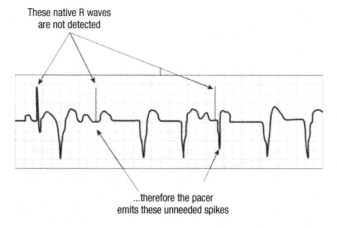

Figure 2.39 Undersensing. Device fails to detect existing cardiac depolarizations and therefore competes with the native rhythm.
Source: Slota, M. C. (2019). *AACN core curriculum for pediatric high acuity, progressive, and critical care nursing.* Springer Publishing Company.

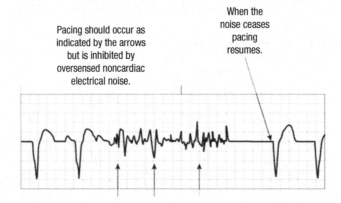

Figure 2.40 Oversensing
Source: Slota, M. C. (2019). *AACN core curriculum for pediatric high acuity, progressive, and critical care nursing.* Springer Publishing Company.

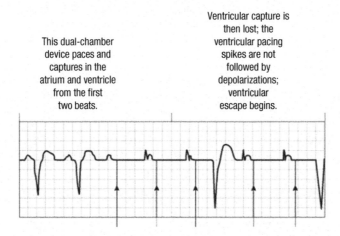

Figure 2.41 Noncapture. Device emits stimuli that fail to depolarize the myocardium.
Source: Slota, M. C. (2019). *AACN core curriculum for pediatric high acuity, progressive, and critical care nursing.* Springer Publishing Company.

PACEMAKER SETTINGS

Mode: Consider what is needed to obtain the best CO. If the patient needs a higher rate and the atria and ventricles are communicating, atrial single chamber pacing (AAI) may be best. If the patient is in a complete heart block, ventricle single chamber pacing (VVI) might be the best option (Table 2.17).

Rate: HR is set on the pacemaker and can be used to overdrive pace when patient is in a tachyarrhythmia.

AV interval: equivalent to PR interval

Capture threshold (Milliamps, mA): How much energy is required to take over the conduction of the heart. Internal pacing is generally between 5 to 10 mA, with the mA set 5 higher to maintain capture. Transthoracic pacing has to go through the chest wall and requires mA generally above 40. Capture is evident when a pacer spike is followed by a contraction, either a P wave or a QRS, depending on the mode.

Sensing threshold (Millivolts, mV): When the heart is able to maintain good conduction, the pacemaker should allow this to happen. This can be controlled by lowering the mV threshold to increase pacer sensitivity and raising the mV to decrease the sensitivity.

Table 2.17 Pacemaker Modes

Mode	Activity	Indication
AAI—atrial demand	Paces and senses atrium, inhibits pacing if adequate activity sensed	Sinus bradycardia, provides atrial kick if AV conduction system intact
VVI—ventricular demand	Paces and senses ventricle, inhibits pacing if adequate activity sensed	AV dissociation, allows CO but without atrial kick
DDD—AV sequential (dual chamber) pacing	Paces and senses atrium and ventricle, Paces if inadequate activity sensed	Heart blocks, provides atrial kick

AAI, atrial single chamber pacing; AV, atria and ventricles; DDD, dual chamber pacing; CO, cardiac output; VVI, ventricle single chamber pacing.

▶ COMMON CARDIAC MEDICATIONS

See Table 2.18 for a summary of common cardiac medications.

Table 2.18 Common Cardiac Medications

Category	Common Names	Actions Simplified	Common Side Effects
Vasoactive/ Inotrope	**Epinephrine** (alpha and beta1 and beta2) **Dopamine** (alpha) **Dobutamine** (beta1) **Isoproterenol** (alpha and beta2) **Norepinephrine** (alpha and beta) **Vasopressin** (alpha effects)	Improves CO through Adrenergic effects: alpha—vasoconstrict blood vessels to increase BP beta1—increase contractility, increase AV conduction, increase HR increase in coronary blood flow beta2—arterial vasodilation fast onset of action—1–10 minutes, short half-life	Arrhythmias, tachycardia, headache, palpitations Increased myocardial oxygen demand with epinephrine and isoproterenol Decreases diastolic BP Tissue necrosis from infiltrated peripheral administration Watch for hypertension with patients on MAOIs or SSRIs Watch peripheral tissue perfusion for higher dosages, including GI perfusion
Anti-hypertensives	**Nitroglycerine** **Nitroprusside** **Labetalol** **Clonidine** **Hydralazine** **Nicardipine**	Vasodilator on peripheral veins and arteries Decreases cardiac oxygen demand by decreasing preload and afterload— decrease in PVR	Hypotension due to relative hypovolemia, bradycardia
Anti-coagulation/ Anti-platelet	**Heparin** **Argatroban**—for patients with HIT **Bivalirudin** **Enoxaparin** **Warfarin** **Apixaban** **Aspirin** **Clopidogrel** **Dipyridamole**	Systemic anticoagulation or prevention of platelet aggregation—used to prevent clot formation in ventricular dysfunction Used for mechanical devices, shunts, coronary stenosis or coronary injury	Bleeding, thrombocytopenia, bruising

(continued)

Table 2.18 Common Cardiac Medications (*continued*)

Category	Common Names	Actions Simplified	Common Side Effects
ACE inhibitors	Enalapril Captopril	Renin-angiotensin antagonist: arterial and venous dilation, afterload reduction	Hypotension, cough
Phosphodiesterase Inhibitors	Milrinone	Improve cardiac contractility and CO without interaction of the alpha and beta receptors—does not increase HR Afterload-reducer decreases pulmonary and SVR Works within a few minutes, half-life few hours Used in ventricular failure, low CO syndrome, congestive HF, PH	Hypotension, atrial and ventricular ectopy
Diuretics	Furosemide Bumetanide Chlorothiazide	Treats fluid overload, edema, pulmonary edema, HF, hypertension, hyperkalemia	Hypokalemia, hyponatremia, hypovolemia
Beta-blockers	Propranolol, Esmolol, Nadolol Sotalol Atenolol	Beta-adrenergic blockers slow the HR down, decreases AV node conduction Reduces myocardial irritability, reduces force of contraction helps widen veins and arteries to improve blood flow	Hypotension, bradycardia, hypoglycemia, dyspnea Esmolol: irregular heart rhythm, HF
Anti-arrhythmic	Amiodarone Flecainide Procainamide Mexiletine Lidocaine	Increases threshold for electrical stimulation, decreases excitability of cardiac muscle-Amiodarone decreases AV conduction Onset effects noted within a few minutes of continuous administration	Hypotension, bradycardia, heart block Monitor electrocardiography, watch ectopy Long term issues with Amiodarone—monitor closely—hepatic, thyroid, pulmonary, and ocular changes
Calcium Channel Blocker	Verapamil Diltiazem Nifedipine	Dilates peripheral arteries, decreased peripheral vascular resistance Helps with fast/irregular heartbeat by blocking influx of calcium during cardiac depolarization Increase supply of blood to the heart	Hypotension Rarely used in neonates or infants (exception with nicardipine—a calcium channel blocker used postsurgically for afterload reduction—often with coarctation repairs)

(*continued*)

Table 2.18 Common Cardiac Medications (*continued*)

Category	Common Names	Actions Simplified	Common Side Effects
MISCELLANEOUS	Adenosine	Slows conduction through AV node, converts SVT to NSR	Extremely short half-life, will not work if not given very fast
	Atropine	Anticholinergic, blocks vagal stimulation of the heart, treats sinus bradycardia, given for intubation if concerned about vagal bradycardia	Asystole, tachycardia
	Digoxin	Improves contractility, antiarrhythmic, slows HR, improves filling	Bradycardia; monitor apical HR before administering, frequent lab draws significant risk for toxicity
	PGE$_1$	Vasodilation with relaxation of smooth muscles—used for maintaining PDA—duct dependent congenital defects	Apnea common side effect especially at higher doses, fever, flushing, hypotension
	Spironolactone	Mild diuretic, but used in HF to help "remodel" and improve myocardial function	Electrolyte imbalances

ACE, angiotensin-converting enzyme; AV, atrioventricular; BP, blood pressure; CO, cardiac output; GI, gastrointestinal; HF, heart failure; HIT, heparin-induced-thrombocytopenia; HR, heart rate; MAOI, monoamine oxidase inhibitors; NSR, normal sinus rhythm; PDA, patent ductus arteriosus; PGE1, prostaglandin E1; PVR, PH, pulmonary hypertension; pulmonary vascular resistance; SSRI, selective serotonin reuptake inhibitor; SVT, supraventricular tachycardia.

CASE STUDY 1

An 8-year-old patient is admitted to the cardiac ICU with an acute episode of chest pain and nausea followed by syncope while at school. The patient has no past medical history but was positive for adenovirus 5 days ago. Chest radiograph reveals cardiomegaly. Her suspected diagnosis is acute viral myocarditis.

Initial Vital Signs:
- Temp: 38°C, oral 100.4°F
- Heart rate (HR): 150
- Respiratory rate (RR): 24
- Blood pressure (BP): 88/42
- Mean BP: 58

Physical Exam
- General: calm
- Neurologic: drowsy, responds to stimuli
- Cardiac: S1, S2, + gallop, +1 pulses throughout, and cap refill <3 seconds. Pale, cool hands and feet
- Respiratory: Lungs coarse bilaterally. Tachypnea with mild subcostal retractions at rest.
- Gastrointestinal (GI): Hepatomegaly with liver edge 3 cm below costal margin and tender to palpation. Active bowel sounds.

1. Which laboratory values would it be useful to obtain during the nurse's assessment? (Select all that apply.)
   A. White blood cell (WBC), erythrocyte sedimentation rate (ESR), C-reactive protein (CRP)
   B. Brain natriuretic peptide (BNP), Troponin, creatinine kinase MB (CKMB)
   C. Basic metabolic profile (BMP), liver function tests (LFTs)
   D. 25-hydroxyvitamin D, iron

2. Which additional studies will the provider likely order? (Select all that apply.)
   A. Biopsy
   B. Electrocardiography
   C. Echocardiography
   D. MRI
   E. CT

3. Which of the following initial treatment options do you anticipate the provider ordering?
   A. Initiation of bed rest
   B. Placement of a Foley
   C. Obtaining blood cultures
   D. Administration of intravenous (IV) milrinone

The nurse is preparing to complete another set of vital signs 2 hours later when the patient's cardiac monitor suddenly alarms and reveals a wide-complex ventricular tachycardia (VT). The patient is lethargic and has palpable +1 carotid and femoral pulses.

Vital Signs:
- Heart rate (HR): 188
- Respiratory rate (RR): 10
- Blood pressure (BP): 68/38
- Mean BP: 50

(See answers next page.)

ANSWERS TO CASE STUDY QUESTIONS

1. A) White blood cell (WBC), erythrocyte sedimentation rate (ESR), C-reactive protein (CRP); B) Brain natriuretic peptide (BNP), Troponin, CKMB; C) BMP, LFTs

Traditional markers of cardiomyocyte lysis reveal elevated Troponin and CKMB. Biomarkers of increased ventricular wall stress and myocardial damage such as BNP and NT-proBNP are commonly elevated. Since natriuretic peptides are generally related to HF trending these biomarkers are more useful. Nonspecific serum makers of inflammation that may be elevated include ESR, CRP, and leukocyte count. Monitoring a BMP to assess electrolytes and kidney function and LFTs to assess liver involvement is indicated in myocarditis.

2. A) Biopsy; B) Electrocardiography; D) MRI; E) CT

Biopsy, electrocardiography, MRI, and CT tests are all indicated for this patient.

3. A) Initiation of bedrest

Acute myocarditis in children can rapidly progress to hemodynamic compromise, and in most cases of suspected myocarditis, an ICU with initiation of bedrest may be necessary to monitor cardiovascular status with close observation of the patient's rhythm. If hemodynamic compromise is suspected in the patient trajectory, transferring to a center that provides pediatric mechanical circulatory support (MCS) with extracorporeal membrane oxygenation (ECMO) and transplantation should be considered. Supportive care with milrinone for inotropy (squeeze of the heart) may be initiated as first-line therapy, however, if the patient has lower BP, milrinone should not be administered at that time. Dopamine and Epinephrine are inotropes with vasopressor properties that are reserved for patients with hypotension and compartment syndrome (CS) since they have more chronotropic (increase heart rate [HR]) and arrhythmogenic potential.

4. Which of the following interventions is most appropriate in this clinical situation?
   A. Administration of intravenous (IV) epinephrine
   B. Synchronized cardioversion
   C. 30 mL/kg normal saline solution (NSS) bolus
   D. Defibrillation

Following the cardioversion, the patient continues in a wide-complex ventricle tachycardia. She is no longer responsive and her carotid and femoral pulses are absent.

5. Which interventions should be performed at this time?
   A. Synchronized cardioversion
   B. Transthoracic pacing
   C. Defibrillation
   D. Administration of amiodarone

(See answers next page.)

4. B) Synchronized cardioversion

For acute events of unstable perfusing VT, immediate synchronized cardioversion with the electrical dose of 0.5 to 1 joules/kilogram (J/kg) is indicated.

5. C) Defibrillation

For life-threatening events such as pulseless VT, CPR should be initiated and defibrillation with the electrical energy of 2 to 4 J/kg should be given. If unable to obtain the return of spontaneous circulation (ROSC), intervention with mechanical circulatory support (MCS) such as extracorporeal membrane oxygenation (ECMO) should be initiated.

CASE STUDY 2

A 3-day-old presents to the ED with a 24-hour history of decreased feeding and tachypnea. The baby's mother reports that the newborn admission was unremarkable and the screening for critical congenital heart disease (CHD) was negative. The ED nurse performs an initial assessment and obtains the following vital signs and physical exam:

Vital Signs:
- Temp: 37.1°C, rectal 98.8°F
- Heart rate (HR): 158
- Respiratory rate (RR): 78
- SpO_2: 94%
- Blood pressure (BP): 65/35 (47) on left leg

Physical Exam
- General: Irritable
- Neurologic: Alert
- Cardiac: HR regular with systolic murmur heard best at left lower sternal border. Bilateral brachial pulses bounding. Femoral and pedal pulses are difficult to palpate with capillary refill time of 3 to 4 seconds.
- RR: Breath sounds clear bilaterally. Tachypnea with mild subcostal retractions at rest.
- Gastrointestinal (GI): Hepatomegaly with liver edge 1 cm below costal margin. Active bowel sounds.

1. The nurse is concerned the baby may have congenital heart disease (CHD). Based on the initial assessment the nurse suspects the following heart defect:
   A. Atrial septal defect (ASD)
   B. Coarctation of the aorta (CoA)
   C. Ventricular septal defect (VSD)
   D. Patent ductus arteriosus (PDA)

The nurse notifies the physician of their initial assessment findings. They arrive at the bedside and perform a physical assessment. The physician updates the mother with potential causes for her baby's presentation including a concern for CHD. The mother becomes upset and keeps saying she does not understand how this could be the case because the screening test was negative and is frustrated that she is just finding out her baby may have a heart problem.

2. Which of the following statements by the nurse would be the most effective in validating the mother's concern?
   A. "There's no need to worry about the screening test now, you brought your baby to the right place to get the help they need."
   B. "The screening test is not 100% accurate. No test is. That does not mean the birth hospital did anything wrong when performing your baby's test."
   C. "I am hearing you say you do not understand how the screening test could be negative but now you are being told your baby may have a heart defect. It is understandable to be frustrated. As your nurse I will be with you and your baby to provide information and care that your baby needs."
   D. "Let's forget the screening test results and focus on what we can do right now, today, to take care of your baby."

(See answers next page.)

ANSWERS TO CASE STUDY QUESTIONS

1. B) Coarctation of the aorta (CoA)

Based on the patient's physical exam of tachypnea, murmur, difficulty to palpate femoral and pedal pulses, and delayed capillary refill time (CRT), CoA is the most likely diagnosis.

2. C) "I am hearing you say you do not understand how the screening test could be negative but now you are being told your baby may have a heart defect. It is understandable to be frustrated. As your nurse I will be with you and your baby to provide information and care that your baby needs."

This answer summarizes what the nurse is hearing the mother say, recognizing the mother's emotion and offering their support and time to the mother and baby, which are all facilitators of therapeutic communication. The other three options are not examples of therapeutic communication. Telling the mother not to worry dismisses or minimizes the mother's concern. Repeating that the test is not 100% accurate is acting defensive about the accuracy of the screening test results. Telling the mother to forget about the results changes the subject and does not address the mother's concern.

While the nurse was supporting the mother, the physician ordered a stat chest x-ray (CXR) and consulted cardiology STAT.

3. What additional physical assessment do you anticipate the physician request you perform as the nurse while waiting for x-ray and cardiology consult?
   A. Four extremity blood pressure (BP) assessment
   B. Left arm and left leg BP assessment
   C. Left arm and right leg BP assessment
   D. Right leg and left leg BP assessment

The nurse completes a four-extremity BP assessment with the following results: right upper extremity (RUE): 99/65 (82) LUE: 95/60 (78), right lower extremity (RLE): 69/35 (52), left lower extremity (LLE): 65/30 (48). The portable x-ray technician arrives at the bedside and a chest x-ray (CXR) was performed and revealed generalized cardiomegaly and mild pulmonary venous congestion. Following the x-ray, the cardiologist arrived at the bedside to perform a physical assessment and echocardiogram, where the diagnosis of coarctation of the aorta (CoA) is confirmed.

4. Based on the diagnosis of coarctation of the aorta (CoA), what medication should the nurse anticipate that the physician will order to stabilize this patient's circulation?
   A. Milrinone
   B. Dopamine
   C. Indomethacin
   D. Prostaglandin (PGE$_1$)

The physician orders a continuous Prostaglandin (PGE$_1$) infusion at a dose of 0.1 mcg/kg/min and places an order for the baby to be admitted to the pediatric cardiac ICU.

5. The nurse in the ED starts the infusion and anticipates monitoring the patient for which of the following until transferring the baby?
   A. Hypotension
   B. Apnea
   C. Flushing
   D. Fever

(See answers next page.)

3. A) Four extremity blood pressure (BP) assessment

This is the only option that provides an assessment of preductal and post ductal upper extremity BP compared to the lower extremity BP assessment.

4. D) Prostaglandin (PGE₁)

Prostaglandin is indicated to open the ductus arteriosus and improve blood flow to the lower extremities. Indomethacin is not indicated because there is not a PDA that needs to be closed. You want to reopen the PDA. Milrinone is not indicated because this baby's increased upper extremity BPs are from a physical obstruction to blood flow and medication cannot address physical obstruction. Dopamine is not indicated because this patient continues to have adequate lower extremity BPs, however, in the setting of hypotension in the lower extremities dopamine or epinephrine may be used.

5. B) Apnea

While hypotension, flushing and fever may also be side effects of PGE₁ administration, apnea is the most common side effect and presence/severity is dose dependent (0.01 mcg/kg/min is a low dose).

KNOWLEDGE CHECK: CHAPTER 2

1. An 8-year-old patient with pulmonary vein stenosis has returned from the cardiac catheterization laboratory post a balloon dilation of her right upper pulmonary vein. The patient was accessed in their right femoral artery and a neurovascular assessment revealed a pale, cool right lower extremity with an absent dorsalis pedis pulse, and >3-second capillary refill time (CRT). The most likely etiology of this finding is
   A. Hematoma
   B. Hemorrhage
   C. Edema
   D. Thrombosis

2. A Doppler ultrasound has confirmed a right femoral arterial thrombosis. The patient has completed their postcardiac catheterization flat time and is sitting up in bed playing with their toys. In this situation, the nurse expects the initial treatment to consist of
   A. Administering intravenous morphine for pain
   B. Immobilizing the affected extremity
   C. Raising the right extremity above the level of the heart
   D. Subcutaneously administering Enoxaparin

3. A 2-day-old with undiagnosed Tetralogy of Fallot (TOF) presents with cool extremities and delayed capillary refill time. Which of the following clinical signs is the patient most likely to exhibit in cardiogenic shock (CS)?
   A. Hypertension and bradycardia
   B. Hypotension and bradycardia
   C. Polyuria and tachycardia
   D. Oliguria and tachycardia

4. A 4-year-old presents with a fever and rash. The child's father states they have had a high fever and has been unresponsive to antipyretics for 5 days. On physical examination, the child has red, edematous hands and feet, erythema of the palms and soles, and dry cracked lips. Which clinical finding supports the diagnosis of Kawasaki Disease (KD)?
   A. Conjunctivitis bilaterally
   B. Dyspnea on exertion
   C. Hepatomegaly
   D. Vesicular rash

5. A newborn diagnosed with hypoplastic left heart syndrome (HLHS) is on a prostaglandin (PGE$_1$) infusion through their right hand peripheral intravenous catheter (PIV). On assessment, the PIV insertion site is red, edematous, and leaking at the site. To continue the PGE$_1$ infusion, which of the following interventions is most appropriate at this time?
   A. Acquire a new PIV to ensure pulmonary blood flow through the patent foramen ovale
   B. Alert the physician to insert an umbilical venous catheter to maintain blood flow through the ductus venosus
   C. Obtain a new PIV to maintain systemic blood flow through the ductus arteriosus
   D. Reposition the patient's hand and flush the PIV to check patency of the catheter

6. A 3-year-old patient is being admitted to the critical care unit for suspected Kawasaki Disease (KD). Initial vital signs show a temperature of 39.1°C (102.3°F), heart rate (HR) of 125 beats/min, respiratory rate (RR) of 28 breaths/min, blood pressure (BP) of 81/48 mmHg, 99% SpO$_2$ on room air. Their echocardiogram reveals left ventricular dysfunction with coronary artery dilation. Which of the following is the appropriate treatment?
   A. Cyclosporine intravenously and ketorolac intravenously
   B. Gentamicin intravenously and acetaminophen orally
   C. Immunoglobulin intravenously (IVIG) and acetylsalicylic acid (aspirin) orally
   D. Methylprednisolone intravenously and ibuprofen orally

(See answers next page.)

1. D) Thrombosis

Thrombosis in an artery postcardiac catheterization will present with a pale, cool extremity with a delayed CRT and diminished or absent pulses. Hematomas can indicate internal bleeding and hemorrhage indicates external bleeding. The patient with hematoma and hemorrhage should be assed for signs of intravascular volume depletion such as hypotension, tachycardia, and delayed CRT. They may present with decreased peripheral perfusion, however, will remain with a pulse. Although some edema may occur locally after a cardiac catheterization, the patient should not present with distal changes such as absent pulse or greater capillary refill; the vessel should not occlude for this reason.

2. D) Subcutaneously administering Enoxaparin

Postcardiac catheterization thrombus will be treated with antithrombotic medication such as Enoxaparin. A thrombosis may take weeks to resolve. The treatment measures for hemorrhage postcatheterization include immobilization of the affected extremity or raising the extremity above the level of the heart. Patients with increased pain scores may require pain management but initial treatment should begin with a non-narcotic option.

3. D) Oliguria and tachycardia

In cardiogenic shock (CS), the compensatory response stimulates the sympathetic nervous system resulting in tachycardia to improve systemic perfusion and renal fluid retention evidenced by oliguria. The compensatory response can be counterproductive as tachycardia and oliguria cause a rise in the demand for myocardial oxygen, worsening hypoxemia, pulmonary venous congestion, and myocardial ischemia. Although the patient in CS will present with persistent hypotension that is not responsive to fluids and requires inotrope/vasopressor support to maintain BP the patients will not present with bradycardia, hypertension, or polyuria.

4. A) Conjunctivitis bilaterally

The patient has several features of KD including a high fever for 5 days duration, erythema of the hands and feet, and mucosal changes. An additional clinical finding to support a diagnosis of KD is bilateral conjunctivitis without exudate. A rash in KD is never vesicular and dyspnea on exertion and hepatomegaly are not common findings in KD.

5. C) Obtain a new PIV to maintain systemic blood flow through the ductus arteriosus

HLHS requires interatrial shunting (e.g., atrial septal defect) and a patent ductus arteriosus (PDA) to provide systemic blood flow. Preoperative care for ductal dependent congenital heart defects such as HLHS is to maintain a PDA with a prostaglandin (PGE$_1$) infusion until a surgical correction is performed. When an infant is born, lack of blood flow results in ductus venosus closure and this patient no longer requires the fetal duct to remain patent. Although the physician may choose to insert an umbilical venous catheter, this procedure will take time and the PGE$_1$ infusion needs to be urgently reinitiated. Infiltrated PIVs are evidenced by edematous, red, and leaking insertion sites, and flushing a catheter with PGE$_1$ will further cause skin irritation.

6. C) Immunoglobulin intravenously (IVIG) and acetylsalicylic acid (aspirin) orally

The mainstay of initial treatment for KD is a single high dose of IVIG with ASA to reduce inflammation, arterial damage, and thrombosis formation in those with coronary artery abnormalities. Administration of cyclosporine is considered in refractory KD patients when a second IVIG infusion, a course of steroids, or infliximab have failed. KD is unresponsive to antibiotics such as gentamicin and not recommended as a treatment option for KD. Administration of high-dose pulse steroids such as methylprednisolone may be considered as an alternative to the second IVIG infusion for patients with persistent fever; however, initial treatment with high-dose IVIG is the recommended primary treatment. Concomitant use of ibuprofen and aspirin should be avoided in children with coronary artery aneurysms due to its antiplatelet effects.

7. A 4-day-old infant weighing 3 kg has been returned to the critical care unit following open-heart surgery for transposition of the great arteries (TGA). Six hours later, the vital signs show a temperature of 37.8°C (100.4°F), a heart rate (HR) of 160 beats/min, a respiratory rate (RR) of 40 breaths/min, blood pressure (BP) of 55/35 mm Hg, and oxygen saturation of 95% on 100% oxygen supplied by mechanical ventilation. Based on this information, the critical care nurse anticipates which of the following interventions?
    A. Intravenous dopamine administration and a fluid bolus of 15 mL
    B. Intravenous milrinone administration and a fluid bolus of 30 mL
    C. Intravenous epinephrine administration and a fluid bolus of 45 mL
    D. Intravenous dobutamine administration and a fluid bolus of 60 mL

8. A 4-year-old with a large atrial septal defect (ASD) is admitted for surgical repair. Which of the following indicates how blood flow is shunted in patients with an ASD?
    A. Interatrial shunting from the right side of the heart to the left side of the heart
    B. Interatrial shunting from the left side of the heart to the right side of the heart
    C. Interventricular shunting from the right side of the heart to the left side of the heart
    D. Interventricular shunting from the left side of the heart to the right side of the heart

9. A 17-year-old patient is admitted to the critical care unit for increased work of breathing. They have a history of Duchenne's muscular dystrophy and have been wheelchair bound for 4 years. They typically use continuous positive airway pressure (CPAP) at night but during the day does not require respiratory support. Initial vital signs show a temperature of 38.2°C (100.7°F), heart rate (HR) of 108 beats/min, respiratory rate (RR) of 32 breaths/min, blood pressure (BP) of 122/46 mmHg, 92% SpO$_2$ on room air. Their echocardiogram revealed worsening left ventricular dilation with thinning of the left ventricular wall and mild, which is a significant change from his echo last year. Which of the following medications will be added to their daily regimen for their a now symptomatic heart failure (HF)?
    A. Furosemide
    B. Enalapril
    C. Atenolol
    D. Coumadin

10. The critical care nurse is caring for a 5-month-old patient 1 day post Tetralogy of Fallot (TOF) repair. The patient has been scheduled for Furosemide every 6 hours with a dose due now. Looking at the intake and output, the nurse sees that the patient has a negative 150 mL balance. The cardiac respiratory monitor keeps alarming frequently for premature ventricular contractions (PVCs). Which initial intervention should the critical care nurse expect to perform for this patient?
    A. Assess for hypovolemia
    B. Notify the frontline about the fluid balance
    C. Administer the scheduled Furosemide
    D. Check the potassium level

11. A 15-year-old patient presents to the ED with complaint of headache and blood pressure (BP) of 180/102. Which of the following is the most likely priority intervention?
    A. Oral chlorothiazide
    B. Continuous intravenous (IV) nicardipine
    C. Oral enalapril
    D. Intravenous morphine sulfate

12. A newborn infant is diagnosed with a congenital heart defect shortly after birth. As a part of the infant's diagnostic work up the patients PaO$_2$ was 60 on room air and 80 after 10 minutes of 100% FiO$_2$ delivery. Based on this information, what is the most likely cardiac defect?
    A. Hypoplastic left heart syndrome (HLHS)
    B. Patent ductus arteriosus (PDA)
    C. Atrial septal defect (ASD)
    D. Ventricular septal defect (VSD)

(See answers next page.)

7. A) Intravenous dopamine and a fluid bolus of 15mL

Following cardiac surgery requiring cardiopulmonary bypass (CPB), the patient is at risk for cardiogenic shock (CS) resulting from a low-cardiac output (CO) state with a peak impact of 6 to 18 hours after bypass. In CS, it is advisable to give small fluid boluses, such as 5 to 10 mL/kg, rather than aggressive fluid resuscitation as in other forms of shock. A smaller fluid bolus of 5 mL/kg (5 mL/kg × 3 kg = 15 mL) will avoid fluid overload and pulmonary edema, therefore eliminating the answers with a 15 mL/kg and 20 mL/kg fluid bolus. To treat myocardial dysfunction in CS, treatment focuses on improving CO and cardiac function. Medications that reduce systemic vascular resistance (SVR) and improve myocardial contractility include dopamine, milrinone, epinephrine, and dobutamine. Milrinone is eliminated in this response due to hypotension as a major side effect.

8. B) Interatrial shunting from the left side of the heart to the right side of the heart

An ASD is characterized as an acyanotic congenital heart defect (CHD) with increased pulmonary blood flow. In this defect blood at the atrial level will shunt (interatrial) from the high-pressure left side of the heart to the low-pressure right side of the heart.

9. B) Enalapril

First line therapy is to help the failing heart with forward flow. Angiotensin-converting enzyme (ACE) inhibitors will create less resistance for the heart to pump against. Dilated cardiomyopathy (DCM) is revealed in the echocardiogram, worsening left ventricular dilation with thinning of the left ventricular wall and mild, mitral valve (MV) regurgitation. This is a change from a year ago and this patient is now symptomatic. Furosemide, while helpful short term in patients with distress, will not be added daily at this point. Atenolol will help slow the heart rate (HR) but may decrease his diastolic blood pressure (BP) too much, not allowing his coronaries to fill effectively. Anticoagulation will be necessary as the disease progresses, but at this stage it is too soon.

10. D) Check the potassium level

The frequency of PVCs is concerning as this indicates that the heart is irritable. Potassium (K+) is excreted from the kidneys in the urine and this patient has a large negative fluid balance, which most likely indicates the K+ is low. Until the K+ level comes back, K+ cannot be replaced, which will treat the PVCs. Assessing for hypovolemia is a good answer, but not the initial intervention the nurse should perform. Notifying the front line about the fluid balance is a good choice but having the data of the potassium level to minimize phone calls is a better option. The PVCs are indicative of a low potassium level, which will need to be treated before administering further diuretics.

11. B) Continuous intravenous (IV) nicardipine

This patient is presenting in hypertensive crisis (BP greater than 140/90 in an adolescent over the age of 13) and requires IV medication management to address it. Nicardipine is the best option as the only IV antihypertensive medication listed. Chlorothiazide and enalapril are first line oral medications for the ongoing management of hypertension but would not be the priority intervention for the patient presenting in hypertensive crisis. Morphine is a pain medication and may be necessary to treat pain but would not be the priority intervention to address this patient's hypertensive crisis.

12. A) Hypoplastic left heart syndrome (HLHS)

HLHS is the only cyanotic, critical heart disease listed. PDA, ASD, and VSD are all acyanotic heart diseases that do not present with hypoxia.

13. A neonate with critical congenital heart disease (CHD) is receiving a prostaglandin (PGE$_1$) infusion to maintain the patency of the ductus arteriosus. What is the most worrisome side effect of this medication?
    A. Fever
    B. Flushing
    C. Rash
    D. Apnea

14. A 5-day-old infant returned from the operating room 4 hours ago following an arterial switch operation for transposition of the great arteries (TGA). Which of the following statements about the patient's chest tube output reflects significant postoperative bleeding?
    A. Dark red in color
    B. Light red, almost pink, color
    C. Has been 2 mL/kg/hr for the last 4 hours
    D. Has been 8 mL/kg/hr for the last 2 hours

15. The critical care nurse is administrating ordered medications to the patient in heart failure (HF). With maintaining a milrinone infusion, giving the scheduled furosemide and spironolactone, what is the goal of treatment?
    A. Decreasing preload by increasing urine output
    B. Symptom relief and remodeling of the heart
    C. Making it easier for the heart to pump blood to the body
    D. Maintaining hemodynamic stability

16. The critical care nurse is admitting a previously healthy, 13-year-old patient after collapsing while playing kickball at school. The patient achieved return of spontaneous circulation (ROSC) after receiving CPR and being defibrillated twice by teachers. What rationale for arrest during kickball seems likely in this patient?
    A. Ventricular fibrillation (V-fib) from the ball hitting the patient hard in the chest
    B. Undiagnosed hypertrophic cardiomyopathy (HCM)
    C. Dilated cardiomyopathy (DCM)
    D. Wolff-Parkinson-White Syndrome (WFW)

17. A 4-day-old infant presents to the ED with a 24 hour history of lethargy, decreased feeding, and pallor. On examination, the right upper extremity blood pressure (BP) is 90/50 and the right lower extremity BP is 55/35. Upper extremity peripheral pulses are bounding with brisk capillary refill and lower extremity peripheral pulses are +1 with delayed capillary refill. Which of the following is the most appropriate treatment?
    A. Initiate prostaglandin (PGE$_1$) infusion
    B. Administer 20 mL/kg bolus of normal saline solution (NSS)
    C. Initiate epinephrine infusion
    D. Administer 20 mL/kg bolus of Dextrose 10%

18. A critical care nurse is caring for a 3-year-old patient with restrictive cardiomyopathy (RCM) the day after a diagnostic cardiac catheterization. Which of the following medications is the nurse expecting the patient to have ordered for RCM management?
    A. Angiotensin-converting enzyme (ACE) inhibitor
    B. Aspirin
    C. Beta-blocker
    D. Digoxin

(See answers next page.)

13. D) Apnea
While all of these are potential side effects of prostaglandin (PGE$_1$), apnea is the most concerning side effect if not addressed when present.

14. D) The patient's chest tube output has been 8 mL/kg/hr for the last 2 hours
8 ml/kg/hr for 2 consecutive hours in the first 12 hours is concerning for significant postoperative bleeding. Dark red chest tube output is an expected finding immediately postoperative and does not necessarily indicate significant bleeding. A light red, almost pink, color output would indicate decreasing bleeding. 2 ml/kg/hr is an acceptable amount of bleeding following cardiac surgery.

15. B) Symptom relief and remodeling of the heart
The goal of treatment is to try and "remodel" the heart muscle with medications, preventing fulminant heart failure (HF). Through decreasing oxygen demand and the work for the heart with the use of medications, symptom relief can improve the quality of life for this patient. Decreasing preload by increasing urine output is correct, but symptom relief and heart remodeling is what decreasing preload will do. Making it easier for the heart to pump blood to the body is the afterload reduction that milrinone administration causes, but that does not address the furosemide and spironolactone. Maintaining hemodynamic stability is a goal of treatment but administrating diuretics and an afterload reducer may compromise this goal with hypotension.

16. B) Undiagnosed hypertrophic cardiomyopathy (HCM)
Blood was not able to leave the heart leading to myocardial ischemia and syncope. HCM prevents blood from filling the left ventricle (LV) and possibly ejecting well, compromising oxygenated blood flow to the coronaries leading to ischemia. This is the most common cause of sudden death in young adults and athletes. A kickball is less likely than a baseball or softball to cause Vfib as it is a soft rubber material. With DCM, there would be signs of congestive heart failure (HF), or pulmonary over-circulation well before sudden death from overexertion would occur. WPW is unlikely to cause sudden death without previous signs of arrhythmias. During puberty, WPW may become active after being dormant for many years since being a small child experiencing fast growth.

17. A) Initiate prostaglandin (PGE$_1$) infusion
This infant presents with an exam consistent with coarctation of the aorta (CoA). The most appropriate treatment to stabilize this patient is a PGE$_1$ infusion to open the ductus arteriosus and provide improved cardiac output (CO) to the lower extremities and areas distal to the area of coarctation. In obstructive shock, fluid boluses and epinephrine infusion do not address the primary cause of obstruction, which makes them less appropriate than PGE$_1$. Dextrose bolus is not indicated based on the information provided in this question and this is not the appropriate dosing.

18. B) Aspirin
The risk of thrombus formation is high due to the difficulty of the ventricles to pump the blood out due to diastolic dysfunction and decreased left ventricle (LV) compliance. ACE inhibitors are not typically indicated as decreasing afterload may cause hypotension due to the inability to compensate from restrictive filling. Beta-blockers may help manage arrhythmias, but the decreased heart rate (HR) response may lessen the ability of the heart to compensate when increased cardiac output (CO) may be needed. Digoxin is not correct as the ventricles are already restricted and the ability to contract more is not warranted.

19. A critical care nurse is caring for a 8-month-old patient 2 days following a Glenn procedure. The patient is on 5 mcg/kg/minute of dopamine, 0.02 mcg/kg/minute epinephrine, 1 mcg/kg/minute milrinone, and is on continuous positive airway pressure (CPAP) of 8. After the nurse changes the epinephrine syringe the patient experiences acute hypertension. What could explain why the patient becomes hypertensive?

  A. The patient has a headache and is noise sensitive
  B. The epinephrine was bolused inadvertently
  C. The patient has an air embolism
  D. The epinephrine was paused for too long

20. A 6-month-old infant had a double lumen central venous catheter (CVC) placed in the subclavian vein 2 days ago. Today the patient developed dyspnea, cough, facial swelling, and full jugular veins. Which of the following is responsible for this patient's symptoms?

  A. Pulmonary embolism
  B. Deep vein thrombosis (DVT)
  C. Superior vena cava syndrome (SVCS)
  D. Cor pulmonale

(See answers next page.)

19. B) The epinephrine was bolused inadvertently

Epinephrine has a fast half-life and is a powerful vasoconstrictor. This means that even small doses cause an extreme reaction. To avoid hypertension, the nurse needs to follow hospital guidelines when changing syringes. Postoperative Glenn procedure patients often have headaches due to the congestion of blood in the brain as it becomes used to the passive flow, but this should not cause acute hypertension. The patient should not have an air embolism as the nurse would make sure the tubing was filled with epinephrine solution and no air was present in the tubing. Epinephrine being paused too long would cause hypotension.

20. C) Superior vena cava syndrome (SVCS)

SVCS is less common in infants and children compared to adults but is most often seen in malignancy or in the setting of a CVC. Symptoms of SVCS include dyspnea, facial swelling, full jugular veins, and edema of the head, neck, and arms.

REFERENCES

Albisetti, A. & Chan, A. (2022). Venous thrombosis and thromboembolism (VTE) in children: Risk factors, clinical manifestations and diagnosis. In S. O'Brien & C. Armsby (Eds.), *UptoDate*. https://www.uptodate.com/contents /venous-thrombosis-and-thromboembolism-vte-in-children-risk-factors-clinical-manifestations-and-diagnosis? search=VTE%20in%20children&topicRef=5916&source=see_link

Alphonso, N., Angelini, A., Barron, D. J., Bellsham-Revell, H., Blom, N. A., Brown, K., Davis, D., Duncan, D., Fedrigo, M., Galletti, L., Hehir, D., Herberg, U., Jacobs, J., Januszewska, K., Karl, T., Malec, E., Maruszewski, B., Montgomerie, J., Pizzaro, C., . . . Simpson, J. M. (2020, September 1). Guidelines for the management of neonates and infants with hypoplastic left heart syndrome: The European Association for Cardio-Thoracic Surgery (EACTS) and the Association for European Paediatric and Congenital Cardiology (AEPC) Hypoplastic Left Heart Syndrome Guidelines Task Force. *European Journal of Cardio-Thoracic Surgery, 58*(3), 416–499. https://doi .org/10.1093/ejcts/ezaa188

Atles, K., Farber, J. S., Shields, K., & Lebet, R. (2022). Multisystem inflammatory syndrome in children in the critical care setting. *Journal of the American Association of Critical-Care Nurses, 42*(1), 13–22. https://doi.org/10.4037/ccn2021964

Callow, L. & Scheffer, A. (2019). Cardiovascular system. In M. C. Slota (Ed.), *AACN core curriculum for pediatric high acuity, progressive, and critical care nursing* (3rd ed., pp. 147–348). Springer Publishing Company.

Centers for Disease Control and Prevention. (2022a). *Data and statistics on congenital heart defects*. https://www.cdc .gov/ncbddd/heartdefects/data.html

Centers for Disease Control and Prevention. (2022b, September 27). *Myocarditis and pericarditis after mRNA COVID-19 vaccination*. https://www.cdc.gov/coronavirus/2019-ncov/vaccines/safety/myocarditis.html

Chandler, H. K., & Kirsch, R. (2016). Management of the low cardiac output syndrome following surgery for congenital heart disease. *Current Cardiology Reviews, 12*(2), 107–111. https://doi.org/10.2174 /1573403X12666151119164647

Chaudhry, M. A., Satti, S. D., & Friedlander, I. R. (2017). Lyme carditis with complete heart block: Management with an external pacemaker. *Clinical Case Reports, 5*(6), 915–918. https://doi.org/10.1002/ccr3.934

Das, D., Dutta, N., & Roy Chowdhuri, K. (2021). Total circulatory arrest as a support modality in congenital heart surgery: Review and current evidence. *Indian Journal of Thoracic and Cardiovascular Surgery, 37*(1), 165–173. https: //doi.org/10.1007/s12055-020-00930-3

De Carolis, S., Garufi, C., Garufi, E., De Carolis, M. P., Botta, A., Tabacco, S., & Salvi, S. (2020). Autoimmune congenital heart block: A review of biomarkers and management of pregnancy. *Frontiers of Pediatrics, 8*, 607515. https: //doi.org/10.3389/fped.2020.607515

Fida, N., Loebe, M., Estep, J. D., & Guha, A. (2015). Predictors and management of right heart failure after left ventricular assist device implantation. *Methodist Debakey Cardiovascular Journal, 11*(1), 18–23. https://doi.org /10.14797/mdcj-11-1-18

Kar, S. (2015). Pediatric cardiogenic shock: Current perspectives. *Archives of Medicine and Health Sciences, 3*(2), 252–265. https://doi.org/10.4103/2321-4848.171917

Law, Y. M., Lal, A. K., Chen, S., Čiháková, D., Cooper, L. T., Deshpande, S., Godown, J., Grosse-Wortmann, L., Robinson, J., & Towbin, J. A. (2021). Diagnosis and management of myocarditis in children. *Circulation, 144*(6), 123–135. https: //www.ahajournals.org/doi/full/10.1161/CIR.0000000000001001

Upsal, N. G. & Halbach, S. M. (2020). Approach to hypertensive emergencies and urgencies in children. In G. A. Woodward, F. B. Stapleton, J. F. Wiley, & L. Wilkie (Eds.), *UptoDate*. https://www.uptodate.com/contents/ approach-to-hypertensive-emergencies-and-urgencies-in-children?search=hypertensive%20crisis%20in %20children&source=search_result&selectedTitle=1~150&usage_type=default&display_rank=1

Respiratory System Review

Jaclyn Campbell, Jennifer Highfield, and Lisette Kaplan

Many children are admitted to the pediatric ICU (PICU) as a result of respiratory complications. It is paramount for the nurse to recognize respiratory decompensation before it proceeds to full cardiopulmonary arrest. A detailed assessment is key in recognizing impending respiratory complications prior to the child's decompensation and needing to be intubated. We can bridge that gap with some noninvasive oxygen delivery modalities.

▶ OXYGEN DELIVERY DEVICES

Oxygen therapy can be delivered via a variety of modalities divided into two basic categories: low-flow or high-flow systems. The determination for the type of device utilized is based on the assessment of the patient and individualized needs determined. Some oxygen delivery devices that are considered noninvasive are:

Low-Flow Devices
- nasal cannula
- simple face mask
- oxygen hood

High-Flow Devices
- non-rebreather mask
- continuous positive airway pressure (CPAP)
- bilevel positive airway pressure (BIPAP)
- High-flow nasal cannula (HFNC) oxygen (e.g., Optiflow™ or Vapotherm®): These delivery devices can accommodate higher liter flows up to 20 L/min. Reasonable flow rate is thought to be 1 to 2 L/kg/min, followed by increasing every 0.5 L/kg/min as tolerated. Adult liter flow can be up to 50 to 60 Lpm (Kwon, 2020).

Patients who continue to demonstrate respiratory distress and enter into respiratory failure may progress to intubation with mechanical ventilation or the placement of a tracheostomy if long-term ventilation is needed.

▶ INVASIVE MECHANICAL VENTILATION

The purpose of mechanical ventilation of the critically ill pediatric patient is to improve oxygenation and ventilation and reduce work of breathing.

Several ventilator modes, which describe the method of inspiratory support, are used in pediatric critical care. A few common **modes** of positive pressure ventilation (PPV) include:
- assist/control (A/C; mode formerly known as continuous mandatory ventilation [CMV])
  - has set respiratory rate and tidal volume (TV, Tv, or Vt)
  - If the child initiates a low-volume breath, the ventilator will finish the triggered breath at the set volume. If the child doesn't initiate a breath (or trigger), they will still receive a breath at a predetermined volume.
- synchronized intermittent mandatory ventilation (SIMV)
  - has set respiratory rate and TV
  - Child can take additional breaths on their own (not assisted by the ventilator) and of their own volume.
  - is more comfortable for the awake child

- pressure support ventilation (PSV)
  - is inspiratory assist ventilation
  - used if patient is breathing spontaneously with ventilatory effort
  - decreases inspiratory effort to overcome the resistance
  - can be used alone or with another mode like SIMV
- airway pressure release ventilation (APRV)
  - has elevated CPAP level with timed pressure releases
  - allows for spontaneous breathing
  - Breaths can be unsupported, pressure supported, or supported by automatic tube compensation.
  - generally used for patients that require recruitment of alveoli to maintain oxygenation, such as in acute respiratory distress syndrome (ARDS)

Delivery of mechanical ventilation can be by **PRESSURE** or **VOLUME**:

- pressure ventilation
  - delivers pressure greater than intraalveolar pressure
  - has preset maximum pressure
  - results in increased airway and intrathoracic pressure (can lead to decreased venous return)
- volume ventilation
  - delivers a preset flow and TV
  - peak inspiratory pressures (PIP) are variable according to lung compliance

Ventilator parameters are:

- FiO_2
  - inspired oxygen concentration
  - titrate oxygen to FiO_2 needed to achieve goal PaO_2
- rate
  - breaths per minute
- TV
  - amount of air that moves in or out of the lungs with each respiratory cycle
  - important to monitor closely; increases may cause barotrauma
- peak inspiratory pressure (PIP)
  - is the highest pressure in the lungs during a ventilator breath (inspiration)
  - normal is 10 to 12 mmHg (infant), 12 to 15 (children), under 20 (adolescents)
  - determinants of PIP include:
    - ❑ lung compliance
    - ❑ inspiratory time
    - ❑ airway resistance
    - ❑ TV
- mean airway pressure (MAP)
  - average (mean) airway pressure over a respiratory cycle
  - affects the PaO_2
- inspiratory time
  - Inspiratory:expiratory (I:E) ratio is determined by inspiratory time and rate
  - A longer I time generally improves oxygenation. Alveoli stay open longer and allows more time for gas exchange. A longer expiratory time allows more time for CO_2 to be removed from the lungs.
- flow rate
  - continuous flow of gas in L/min
- positive end expiratory pressure (PEEP)
  - used with any of the ventilator modes
  - positive pressure applied during expiration
  - keeps alveoli open to continue gas exchange
  - prevents early closure during expiration
  - improves compliance and ventilation perfusion (VQ) mismatching
- minute ventilation (MV)
  - total volume of gas inspired over a period of 1 minute MV = (respiratory rate × TV)

ALTERNATIVE THERAPIES

HIGH FREQUENCY VENTILATION

High frequency ventilation modes are used for patients with hypoxemia unimproved by conventional ventilation, pulmonary air leaks syndromes, ARDS, congenital diaphragmatic hernia, and persistent pulmonary hypertension (PPHN). Typical criteria for use of high frequency ventilation include:

- FiO_2 greater than .60 for more than 24 hours
- PIP greater than 40 cm
- PEEP greater than 12 cm
- air leak syndromes

High Frequency Oscillatory Ventilation

- gas disperses throughout lungs at high frequencies
- uses a MAP and high respiratory rates typically 60 to 3,600 per minute
- has small TVs
- exhalation is active
- helps expand alveoli
- decreases pulmonary vascular resistance
- improves VQ matching
- reduces the risk of barotrauma

High Frequency Jet Ventilation

- delivers small pulses of gas
- rates typically 60 to 600 pulses per minute
- exhalation is passive, monitor for air trapping

Extracorporeal Membrane Oxygenation

Extracorporeal membrane oxygenation (ECMO) is a temporary therapy for patients in respiratory or cardiovascular failure who have failed other therapies. The two types of ECMO are:

- **venoarterial (VA)**: provides respiratory and hemodynamic support
- **venovenous (VV)**: provides respiratory support only

In ECMO therapy, blood is oxygenated and carbon dioxide is removed through use of a cardiopulmonary bypass machine. Common indications for ECMO include:

- respiratory
  - persistent hypoxemia
  - pneumonia
  - ARDS
- cardiovascular
  - cardiogenic shock
  - septic shock
  - myocardial stunning
  - unable to remove from bypass

Not all patients are candidates for ECMO therapy and contraindications include:

- irreversible disease
- prematurity and low birth weight
- intraventricular or pulmonary hemorrhage
- unable to receive heparin

Clinical Pearl

Nurses caring for patients receiving mechanical ventilation must recognize and respond to rapid deterioration quickly. Common causes of deterioration may be attributed to one of the following, remembered by the mnemonic "DOPE": Displacement of endotracheal tube (ETT), Obstruction of the ETT, Pneumothorax, Equipment or ventilator failure.

VENTILATOR MANAGEMENT

Changes to ventilator settings are made in response to several factors. Arterial blood gases (ABG; see Chapter 12, "Multisystem Review," for the discussion of acid–base imbalance and ABG interpretation) are one tool helpful in monitoring improvements to oxygenation and ventilation.

STRATEGIES TO IMPROVE VENTILATION

- pressure ventilation
  - ↑ rate
  - ↑ PIP
  - ↓ I time for hyperinflation
- volume ventilation
  - ↑ rate
  - ↑ TV
  - ↓ I time for hyperinflation

STRATEGIES TO IMPROVE OXYGENATION

- pressure ventilation
  - ↑ FiO_2
  - ↑ PEEP
  - ↑ PIP
  - ↑ I:E ratio
- volume ventilation
  - ↑ FiO_2
  - ↑ PEEP
  - ↑ I:E ratio

TROUBLESHOOTING VENTILATORS

- high pressure alarm
  - endotracheal tube (ETT) kinked or circuit kinked
  - excess water in the tubing
  - patient biting the ETT
  - patient coughing, needs suctioning
  - patient agitated, needs sedation

LOW PRESSURE ALARM

- disconnected ventilator circuit (trace tubing from patient to the ventilator)
  - leaking around the ETT
  - leak in the ventilator circuit

DESATURATION/SIGNIFICANT CHANGE IN PATIENT CONDITION—DOPE PNEUMONIC

- **D**isplacement: Check ETT placement (auscultation, chest x-ray [CXR])
- **O**bstruction: Checking for mucous plug, kink in tubing
- **P**neumothorax: Auscultation, CXR
- **E**quipment failure: Disconnect patient and bag manually (call for help)

AIRWAY PATENCY

Maintaining a patent and clear airway is crucial. Assisting with airway clearance through suctioning is a vital nursing intervention in the pediatric patient.

Types of suctioning devices for a noninvasive airway include:

- nasal aspirator (i.e., Little Sucker® or Neosucker®)
- Yankauer
- suction catheter

These can be used to clear the nasal, oral, or nasopharngeal passages.

Types of suctioning devices for an invasive (ETT or tracheostomy) airway include:

- **Suction catheter (sterile one-time use or a closed suction system)** A sterile one-time-use catheter is what we would consider standard suctioning.

- A closed suctioning system: A closed suction system allows a suction catheter to be inserted into the ETT through a one-way valve, with no need to disconnect the patient from the ventilator. This is especially helpful if the patient is dependent on the ventilator for a pre-set respiratory rate. Advantages of using this system are:
  - improved oxygenation
  - decreased clinical signs of hypoxemia
  - maintenance of PEEP
  - smaller loss of lung volume
  - decreased incidence of contamination

Clinical Pearl

Capnography is a quick assessment of ventilation that measures carbon dioxide (CO_2; normal is 35–45 mmHg). Not affected by motion or artifact.

▶ ACUTE PULMONARY EDEMA

Acute pulmonary edema involves abnormal collection of extravascular fluid within the lungs. There are two primary types of pulmonary edema:

- **Noncardiogenic pulmonary edema**: The primary cause is related to lung injury. This causes an increase in pulmonary vascular permeability, subsequently leading to the shift of fluids into the interstitial and alveolar regions.
- **Cardiogenic type**: The pulmonary edema occurs due to a rapid elevation in the pressure of the pulmonary capillaries. The origination is related to disorders such as left ventricular systolic/ diastolic dysfunction, valvular issues, and rhythm disturbances.

SIGN AND SYMPTOMS

- tachypnea
- diminished breath sounds
- shortness of breath
- cough
- crackles
- murmur
- cyanosis
- diaphoresis
- anxiety
- agitation
- confusion
- jugular venous distention
- pink frothy secretions

PATHOPHYSIOLOGY

The increased extravascular fluid within the lungs is caused by a variety of physiologic processes that disrupt the delicate balance of filtration fluid and solutes across the pulmonary capillary membrane. This imbalance can be attributed to a variety of causes such as an increase in intravascular hydrostatic pressure; increase in interstitial hydrostatic pressure; lymphatic insufficiency; increased oncotic pressure (related to malnutrition, protein losing states, hepatic or renal issues); endothelial or epithelial injury or increased negative interstitial pressure.

NURSING IMPLICATIONS AND TREATMENT

ASSESSMENT

Upon examination, the clinician will need to perform a comprehensive cardiopulmonary assessment as physiological impacts will primarily affect these systems. Concern for pulmonary edema should be heightened when tachypnea, dyspnea, rales, or crackles coupled with hypoxia are present. In cardiogenic edema, cough with pink frothy secretions can be associated with hypoxemia (stemming from alveolar flooding).

LABS AND DIAGNOSTICS

Laboratory testing can include:

- **Brain natriuretic peptide (BNP)** can be utilized to identify increased ventricular blood volume or increased intracardiac pressures in instances where the level is elevated. Natriuretic peptide is released by the ventricles of the heart in response to increased wall tension. It is not as easy to determine a cardiac cause versus a pulmonary cause in children, like it is in adults.
- **Electrolytes** including renal function, albumin, and serum osmolarity will enable the clinician to manage patient needs.
- **X-rays** (lateral and postero-anterior views) can assist in identifying effusions, central edema, peribronchial cuffing, enlarged heart size, and septal lines common in cardiogenic etiologies. In the noncardiogenic type, radiographic findings might include patchy edema patterns, consolidations and ground-glass appearing opacities.
- **Echocardiograms** are utilized to identify ventricular systolic dysfunction or valvular dysfunction.

TREATMENT AND MANAGEMENT

Treatment is aimed at identifying the cause of the pulmonary edema and treating the underlying condition. Typical management strategies encompass ventilator support (noninvasive and invasive) focusing on increasing oxygenation, reducing the work of breathing, managing hypercarbia (thereby reversing acidosis) and assisting with guiding fluids into the capillaries. In patients with ventricular failure, diuretics are common as well as vasodilators, positive inotropes, and digoxin as indicated by patient condition.

COMPLICATIONS

The most common complications are related to those directly correlating to the pathophysiology noted. In addition, progressive respiratory distress leading to respiratory failure requiring ventilator support can be cited as a complication.

▶ ACUTE PULMONARY EMBOLUS

A pulmonary embolus occurs when a thrombus (which originated somewhere in the body) migrates to the pulmonary artery or its branches and occludes blood flow. Common causes of pulmonary embolus include:

- deep vein thrombosis (DVT)
- bacterial endocarditis
- septic thrombophlebitis
- osteomyelitis

Acute pulmonary embolus occurs when there is a sudden blockage of a major artery in the lungs. A patient may be at higher risk for a pulmonary embolism secondary to surgery or after a trauma.

SIGNS AND SYMPTOMS

- hypoxemia
- tachypnea
- dyspnea
- acute chest pain
- fever in the absence of other signs of infection

PATHOPHYSIOLOGY

This clinical condition occurs when clots break off and migrate into the pulmonary circulation. There are typically multiple emboli involved with more frequent involvement of lower lobes vs. upper and bilateral lung impact most commonly. Due to obstruction of the pulmonary vasculature impaired gas exchange is common secondary to a mismatch of the ventilation to perfusion ratios (alveolar ventilation remains normal but pulmonary capillary blood flow is decreased, leading to hypoxemia and dead space ventilation).

NURSING IMPLICATIONS AND TREATMENT

ASSESSMENT

The clinician should complete a thorough assessment and obtain a thorough history that examines potential risk factors for a pulmonary embolus. Risk factors include fractures of the lower extremities, trauma, central venous lines, chemotherapy, infection, heart disease, oral contraceptive use, cancer, and immobility. Assessment findings may include hypoxemia, tachypnea, **dyspnea**, or **acute chest pain**. Many of these findings are nonspecific, therefore, the history is essential.

LABS AND DIAGNOSTICS

Common diagnostic tests for patients suspected of having an acute pulmonary embolus include:

- **CXR** (may show nonspecific abnormalities)
- **CT**
- **pulmonary angiogram**: the "gold standard" but impractical for many pediatric patients
- **VQ scan** or **helical (spiral) CT scan**: most common diagnostic tool; quick and noninvasive
- **laboratory analysis**: labs are limited in their usefulness for this diagnosis. ABGs are most helpful in evaluating hypoxemia and effectiveness of treatment.

> ### Clinical Pearl
>
> *Ventilation Perfusion (VQ) matching is the ratio between the amount of air getting into the alveoli and the amount being sent to the lungs. Each alveolus should have comparable ventilation and perfusion. Ventilation = air ventilating the alveoli, perfusion = blood perfusing the alveoli. If there is a VQ mismatch, either there is not enough blood or not enough ventilation. As a result, CO_2 may be increased.*

TREATMENT AND MANAGEMENT

Initial treatment for pulmonary embolus involves supportive therapy, such as the provision of supplemental oxygen for hypoxemia, with escalation to mechanical ventilation as the clinical picture warrants. Anticoagulation and potentially thrombolytic therapy are mainstays in treatment with titration of medication to achieve therapeutic goals. In some cases, fibrinolytic agents or catheter directed therapy may be indicated. Inferior vena cava filters may be indicated in adolescents. Thrombectomy may be warranted to restore pulmonary vessel patency. Nursing management is focused on managing oxygen delivery therapies as well anticoagulation medication titration and effects.

COMPLICATIONS

Complications of pulmonary embolus include:

- recurrence of pulmonary embolus (PE)
- hemorrhage from the anticoagulation
- right heart failure
- cardiogenic shock
- potential death if early treatment is not initiated

▶ ACUTE RESPIRATORY DISTRESS SYNDROME

ARDS consists of acute onset of edema, parenchymal opacification, and significant oxygen impairment. ARDS has multiple potential causes and can result from **direct** or **indirect lung injury**. Top causes are:

- pneumonia
- pulmonary aspiration
- sepsis
- shock
- cardiopulmonary bypass

NURSING IMPLICATIONS AND TREATMENT

ASSESSMENT

The patient develops increased accessory muscle use, hypoxia, hypocarbia initially, and tachypnea in an attempt to increase MV. As respiratory mechanics worsen and atelectasis increases, hypercarbia develops. Once the patient develops hypercarbia, PPV is needed to open the atelectatic alveoli. There may be decreased lung sounds, rales, or wheezing on exam.

- CXR reveals diffuse alveolar infiltrate and air bronchograms, +/− pleural effusion, diffuse atelectasis.
- SvO_2 (mixed venous oxygen saturation) measures the oxygen content of the blood returning to the right side of the heart and is impacted by oxygen delivery and oxygen consumption. If oxygen supply is inadequate, as is the case in ARDS, the SvO_2 will be decreased.
- percentage of oxygen saturation in pulmonary arterial blood
- normal is 65% to 75%
- measures the end result of oxygen consumption and delivery
- evaluates adequacy of tissue oxygenation
- detects changes and evaluations effectiveness of O_2 delivery and consumption

TREATMENT AND MANAGEMENT

- Management is mostly supportive care with an emphasis on PPV. Low TV (5 to 8 mL/kg), mechanical ventilation, and prone positioning are the only components of supportive care that have significantly decreased mortality.
- PEEP is utilized for lung recruitment when managing ARDS and a cuffed ETT should be utilized to help maintain PEEP. A PEEP as high as 15 may be required when treating ARDS and should be increased and decreased slowly while monitoring oxygen delivery, compliance, and hemodynamics.
- In patients with moderate to severe respiratory failure due to ARDS, high-frequency oscillatory ventilation (HFOV) may be considered. Patients on HFOV require neuromuscular blockade medications as spontaneous respirations interrupt ventilation. The benefit of HFOV is low TV ventilation with an open lung strategy where the alveoli remain open without collapsing or becoming overdistended.
- Prone positioning is utilized for severe ARDS with persistent hypoxemia refractory to changes in ventilation modalities. Prone positioning facilitates the recruitment, or opening of the dependent, collapsed alveoli; therefore, improving VQ mismatch and improving oxygenation and ventilation. Once the collapsed alveoli have opened, secretions may mobilize, allowing for clearance strategies to become more effective.
- Patients may require suctioning of the ETT but this must be done with caution to prevent derecruitment. Routine use of saline with ETT suctioning is not recommended and should be avoided.
- Patients should have targeted sedation and valid, reliable sedation scales should be used to titrate sedation. In certain cases where sedation is not enough to achieve adequate ventilation, neuromuscular blockade may be used. Doses should be adjusted to goal effect based on effective ventilation, clinical movement, and train-of-four response.
- Steroids, fluid resuscitation, surfactant, prone positioning, and inhaled nitric oxide (INO) may benefit some patients.
- Lower saturations may be acceptable depending on the degree of lung disease. If PEEP has been optimized, saturations of 88% to 92% may be acceptable.
- A blood transfusion should be considered for a patient with a hemoglobin less than 7 g/dL.
- Patients should receive total fluids to maintain adequate intravascular volume, end-organ perfusion, and optimal oxygen delivery, but a positive fluid balance should be avoided.

Clinical Pearl

Inhaled nitric oxide (iNO) acts on vascular smooth muscle cells causing pulmonary vasodilation and improved oxygenation. It may be prescribed to patients with ARDS. Onset is 1 to 3 minutes and iNO has a half-life of 3 to 6 seconds. When caring for a patient receiving iNO, it is important to avoid interruptions due to the short half-life.

▶ ACUTE RESPIRATORY FAILURE

Acute respiratory failure can be defined as the inability to maintain sufficient oxygenation. This process may or may not involve retention of carbon dioxide. It can have a gradual or acute onset and is the most common cause of cardiopulmonary arrest in children. Though respiratory failure can lead to respiratory arrest, it should be noted that respiratory arrest differs from respiratory failure in that respiratory arrest is the complete cessation of breathing.

SIGNS AND SYMPTOMS

Common early signs and symptoms include:
- restlessness
- tachypnea
- tachycardia
- diaphoresis

Other early signs and symptoms include:
- change in mental status
- headache
- hypertension/increased cardiac output
- dyspnea
- nasal flaring
- retractions
- grunting
- wheezing

Late and ominous signs and symptoms include:
- hypotension
- somnolence/coma
- decreased respiratory rate or shallow respirations
- bradycardia
- cyanosis

PATHOPHYSIOLOGY

Respiratory failure is characterized by the inability of the pulmonary system to provide adequate oxygenation to the tissues, with or without retention of carbon dioxide. The mechanism by which this occurs can have many causes that may be a result of either direct or indirect lung injury. **Direct lung injury** includes but is not limited to:
- pneumonia
- aspiration
- pulmonary contusion
- pulmonary embolism
- inhalation injury

Indirect pulmonary injury includes:
- sepsis
- shock
- cardiopulmonary bypass
- blood transfusions

Acute respiratory failure is typically seen as a result of an abrupt onset of a severe respiratory disorder that increases the work of the respiratory system, leading to eventual ventilator muscle fatigue. This can cause hypoxia, hypercapnia, and acidosis. Patients who experience acute respiratory failure will likely need support from mechanical ventilation.

NURSING IMPLICATIONS AND TREATMENT

ASSESSMENT

Symptoms of acute respiratory failure may vary from patient to patient and can be nonspecific, making it potentially difficult to identify without training. However as soon as respiratory distress is recognized, the primary focus should be on ensuring the patient is maintaining adequate oxygenation and ventilation.

This may require administering supplemental oxygen, positioning the patient, and suctioning any secretions from the airway. Early intubation may be warranted if the patient cannot adequately maintain a patent airway or is at risk for further respiratory compromise. A thorough respiratory assessment includes:

- respiratory rate
- respiratory effort (presence of retractions, nasal flaring)
- respiratory sounds (grunting, wheezing, stridor, lung sounds)
- skin color (pallor, cyanosis)
- mentation
- pulse oximetry

When caring for a patient who is experiencing acute respiratory failure, the primary goal is to maintain adequate ventilation and oxygenation and minimize end organ damage, while identifying and correcting the underlying cause.

LABS AND DIAGNOSTICS

There are some lab and diagnostic tests that may be beneficial in diagnosing or guiding management of patients experiencing acute respiratory failure.

- **Blood gas**: ABG is preferred; shows oxygen content in the blood, as well as carbon dioxide retention.
- **Lactate test**: Lactic acid is produced as a result of anerobic metabolism. It is a good indicator of poor end-organ perfusion and oxygenation.
- **CXR**: may be useful in determining the cause of acute respiratory failure; can depict atelectasis, consolidation, pulmonary edema, and pulmonary fibrosis. Though there are many limitations to the accuracy of a CXR, it continues to be one of the most commonly used diagnostic imaging tests for acute respiratory failure.
- **Chest CT**: considered the *gold standard imaging test*. A chest CT scan can give a more accurate picture of physiology and disease process. However, in most cases, this requires transportation of a critically ill patient as well as exposure to a higher amount of radiation, along with higher cost.
- **Lung ultrasound**: noninvasive, can be performed at the bedside, and can be a useful diagnostic tool.

TREATMENT AND MANAGEMENT

Management of patients with acute respiratory failure focuses on maintaining adequate ventilation and oxygenation, which may require intubation. Once a patent airway is established and adequate oxygenation is ensured via signs of adequate end organ perfusion and improving blood gas values, it is imperative to identify and treat the underlying cause of the respiratory failure.

COMPLICATIONS

Acute respiratory failure can progress to respiratory arrest. Respiratory arrest is the cessation of spontaneous respiration that leads to cardiopulmonary collapse. In this case, CPR should be immediately initiated.

Acute respiratory failure with a persistent or irreversible cause can lead to chronic respiratory failure. Children with chronic respiratory failure require chronic ventilator support, most often via a tracheostomy.

▶ ACUTE RESPIRATORY INFECTIONS

Acute epiglottitis is a rapidly progressing infection of the epiglottis and surrounding area and is a severe life-threatening medical emergency. The most common organism that causes epiglottitis is *Haemophilus influenza type b (Hib)* and the incidence has decreased significantly since the Hib vaccine. When it does occur, it is most common in children 2 to 5 years old.

Acute laryngotracheobronchitis (LTB) is often referred to as **croup** and is caused by swelling of the submucosa in the subglottic area resulting in stridor, cough, and hoarseness. LTB typically affects children under 5 years old and can be bacterial or viral in etiology but viral etiology is much more common.

Bacterial tracheitis is an infection of the mucosa of the upper trachea occurring most commonly in children younger than 3 years old. Although rare, it is the most common potentially life-threatening upper airway infection as the marked subglottic edema, erythema, pseudomembranous formations of the tracheal surface and tenacious secretions may lead to airway obstruction. Tracheitis may be a complication of LTB; common organisms are *S. aureus, Moraxella catarrhalis, S. Pneumoniae*, and *H. influenza.*

Bronchitis is a nonspecific inflammation of the bronchioles and may be acute, which is most commonly viral—parainfluenza, respiratory syncytial virus (RSV), rhinovirus—or may be chronic from other conditions. Secondary bacterial infections may develop.

Bronchiolitis most commonly occurs between winter and early spring. 60% to 85% of cases are caused by RSV. Bronchiolitis is an acute inflammatory disease of the lower respiratory tract leading to obstruction of the small airways. Increased secretions and edema of the submucosal layer cause obstruction of the small airways leading to atelectasis and VQ mismatch. Children with comorbidities are at highest risk of severe disease.

Pneumonia is a lower respiratory tract infection causing inflammation of the lung parenchyma associated with fever and respiratory symptoms. The most common organism varies by age and whether it is community or hospital acquired. Immunocompromised patients, or children with comorbidities are at highest risk of developing pneumonia.

Pertussis or "whooping cough" is caused by *Bordetella pertussis* or *Bordetella parapertussis* and is highly contagious and dangerous for infants. Pertussis can lead to encephalopathy, seizures, and pneumonia. It is most common in the spring and summer. Pertussis is spread by aerosol droplets and causes inflammation, congestion, and infiltration of the respiratory mucosa with lymphocytes and granulocytes leading to the accumulation of tenacious secretions in the bronchi, bronchial obstruction, and atelectasis.

Tuberculosis (TB) is caused by *Mycobacterium TB*, an acid-fast bacillus, and children are susceptible to the human and bovine organisms. Cases are higher in urban, low-income areas, and high-density living arrangements. TB is spread person-to-person via inhalation of infected airborne particles after a cough, sneeze, or even by talking or laughing. The droplets can remain suspended in the air for hours, making TB highly contagious. The majority of children who inhale these infected droplets develop latent TB as opposed to active infection. Younger children are at increased risk of developing severe disease after the typical 3 to 8 week asymptomatic incubation period.

SIGNS AND SYMPTOMS

Acute epiglottitis: The symptoms present acutely and include high fever, sore throat, dyspnea, and rapidly progressive airway obstruction. The swollen epiglottis leads to a narrowing of the airway and turbulent gas flow; this airway obstruction can lead to postobstructive pulmonary edema. The patient will sit upright in the *tripod position* and may have dysphagia, drooling, dysphonia, irritability, and anxiety; stridor is a late sign. Characteristic red and inflamed throat with a cherry-red edematous epiglottis on exam.

Acute laryngotracheobronchitis has a gradual onset of symptoms including rhinorrhea, coryza, and low-grade fever. The hallmarks of LTB are stridor and a barky, hoarse cough.

Bacterial tracheitis presents with a typical upper respiratory infection (URI) prodrome: rhinorrhea, low grade fever, cough, sore throat, and hoarse voice. Symptoms progress to respiratory distress exhibited by increased work of breathing, airway compromise, higher fever, and toxic appearance.

Bronchitis has an initial phase of upper respiratory symptoms, may have a dry, brassy cough that may or may not be productive and coarse breath sounds or rhonchi on exam.

Bronchiolitis typically presents after 3 to 7 days of URI symptoms that progresses into cough, sneezing, rhinorrhea, and respiratory distress exhibited by tachypnea, retractions, wheezing, prolonged expiration, rales, and irritability. The patient may have poor feeding, low grade fever, apnea, and cyanosis. Viral bronchiolitis typically peaks between 2 to 3 days and can last 7 to 10 days. *Tachypnea is the most consistent clinical manifestation.*

Pneumonia occurs from the inspiration of microorganisms, aspiration of oropharyngeal secretions or systemic circulation; the location of the pneumonia on an x-ray may help to determine the cause. The patient may present with URI, fever, cough and chest pain. Infants may have poor oral intake (PO), fever, irritability, and respiratory distress. Fine crackles, dullness, or diminished breath sounds may indicate pneumonia. Wheezing is more common in viral pneumonia. The patient may have abdominal distention from swallowed air secondary to respiratory distress.

Pertussis typically begins with URI symptoms and continues for 1 to 2 weeks when the dry hacking cough develops. The cough is the most prevalent symptom and occurs most at night and is characterized by rapid, short coughs followed by sudden inspiration "whoop." The coughing paroxysm can last until a thick mucus plug becomes dislodged; the child may be flushed or cyanotic. Infants may not have the characteristic whoop but may have hypoxemia secondary to the secretions.

Tuberculosis can be asymptomatic or have a wide range of symptoms. Symptoms are progressive and include tachypnea, poor lung expansion, diminished breath sounds and crackles, persistent fever, pallor, anemia, weakness, weight loss, and generalized symptoms.

NURSING IMPLICATIONS AND TREATMENT (ASSESSMENT, LABS AND DIAGNOSTICS, TREATMENT AND MANAGEMENT, COMPLICATIONS)

Acute epiglottitis *assessment:* The airway should not be assessed unless there are providers skilled in difficult intubation. Noxious stimuli should be avoided to prevent worsening of symptoms. *Labs and diagnostics:* Lateral neck x-ray is indicated, and blood cultures should be obtained after the airway is secure. *Treatment and management:* The patient should be taken to the operating room for direct laryngoscopy and intubation. Ceftriaxone or cefotaxime should be given until cultures result.

Acute laryngotracheobronchitis *assessment:* The degree of respiratory distress and accessory muscle use depends on the degree of obstruction. *Labs and diagnostics:* A CXR reveals the **"steeple sign,"** a narrowing of the upper trachea. *Treatment and management:* Supplemental oxygen, cool mist, single dose of oral dexamethasone, Heliox, racemic epinephrine to reduce mucosal edema. Intubation is rare but may be needed for significant distress. Heliox is a helium-oxygen gas mixture; the lower density helium allows the oxygen to flow through a narrowed airway.

Bacterial tracheitis should be diagnosed by bronchoscopy and bronchial alveolar lavage (BAL). Blood cultures should be obtained to identify the specific organism and a lateral x-ray will reveal subglottic swelling. The majority of patients will require intubation for 3 to 7 days with frequent suctioning and intravenous (IV) antibiotics for 10 to 14 days. Mortality rate is 18% to 40% and there is significant morbidity associated depending on presentation: respiratory arrest, cardiac arrest, shock, ARDS, and multiple organ dysfunction syndrome (MODS).

Bronchitis management is mostly supportive and includes hydration, analgesia, antivirals or antibiotics as indicated, cough suppressants, and bronchodilators.

Bronchiolitis: Radiographic or laboratory studies are not routinely indicated. Rapid viral tests may be ordered to determine which virus is leading to the symptoms. While most cases can be managed in the outpatient setting with supportive care, severe cases may require mechanical ventilation for apnea, hypoxemia, or respiratory failure. The management of bronchiolitis includes nasal suctioning, nasogastric (NG) feeding or IV fluids, and heated and humidified high flow nasal cannula to deliver PEEP and prevent atelectasis. Hypertonic, 3% saline may be used in the inpatient setting, bronchodilators are not routinely recommended and are rarely helpful. Guidelines do not recommend the routine use of systemic corticosteroids, chest physiotherapy, or antibiotics.

Pneumonia does not require x-ray images for diagnosis but may be indicated in certain cases such as severe disease, failure to improve, and to rule out other causes such as heart disease or foreign body aspiration. CXR may reveal a pleural effusion or empyema and will show an infiltration, although the CXR may lag behind the clinical picture. Rapid viral panel, blood, and sputum cultures may be used for diagnostic purposes. Bronchial alveolar lavage (BAL) or lung biopsy may be indicated in special populations. Complications of pneumonia include lung abscess, necrotizing pneumonia, pneumatocele, empyema, pleural effusions, bronchopleural fistula and pneumothorax. Prevention includes immunization against Hib and *S. pneumoniae*. Bactrim prophylaxis is needed for immunocompromised patients. Adequate hydration and respiratory support with mechanical ventilation for respiratory failure and antibiotics are used for the management of pneumonia.

Pertussis can be managed at home in most cases. Preventative care includes immunization, boosters, and prophylactic antibiotics after known exposure. Supportive care includes hospitalization, humidified oxygen, adequate fluid intake and mechanical ventilation as needed. Complications can include pneumonia, apnea, atelectasis, otitis media, seizures, hemorrhage, weight loss, dehydration, hernias, prolapsed rectum, syncope, sleep disturbance, rib fractures, and incontinence. Pertussis symptoms usually last for 6 to 10 weeks but can persist for longer.

Tuberculosis is diagnosed by physical exam and history, TB skin test, blood testing, CXR, and cultures. The TB skin test is usually positive 2 to 10 weeks after the initial infection but does not confirm the presence of active disease. Latent TB infection indicates a positive skin test but no active symptoms, while active TB describes a child with clinical symptoms or radiographic findings caused by the TB organism. For children with latent TB, adequate nutrition and hydration and avoidance of other infections are encouraged. For the child with active TB, anti-TB medications are indicated including ethambutol (Myambutol), isoniazid (Niazid), pyrazinamide, and rifampin (Rifadin). These drugs are given for 6 months, with there often being concerns for nonadherence to the prescribed treatment regimens. Most children are managed in the outpatient setting, but if they have respiratory symptoms and are admitted to the hospital, they require a negative pressure room and for personnel to wear an N95 mask (airborne precautions). Active TB is very serious in the first 2 years of life, during adolescence, and in children who are HIV positive. Because of the new antibiotic regimens, death rarely occurs except in cases of TB meningitis.

▶ AIR LEAK SYNDROMES

An air leak is defined as movement of air from a cavity that contains air to a cavity that does not normally contain air. Air leak syndromes are a group of disorders that are a result of overdistention of the terminal air spaces. This can occur with PPV, atelectasis of the alveoli such as in respiratory distress syndrome, and barotrauma or volutrauma. Ventilatory support is a significant risk factor for developing an air leak syndrome.

SIGNS AND SYMPTOMS

Air leak syndrome can have varying causes, and specific clinical presentation differs based on the underlying cause. In general, patients with an air leak syndrome present in respiratory distress with a significantly deteriorating clinical course.

- **Pneumomediastinum**: may be asymptomatic or have mild respiratory distress, unless accompanied by pneumothorax. Increased anteroposterior diameter of the chest may be seen on CXR.
- **Pneumothorax**: Presentation can vary from mild tachypnea and increased oxygen requirement to more severe respiratory distress, including grunting, retractions, nasal flaring, and more pronounced tachypnea. Other signs include decreased breath sounds on the affected side and uneven chest wall movement. Patients who are already on ventilator support may have a more rapid clinical deterioration that is characterized by hypoxemia, cyanosis, hypotension, bradycardia, and respiratory acidosis.
- **Pulmonary interstitial emphysema**: typically presents as a gradual deterioration including hypoxemia, hypercarbia, and acidosis that leads to an increase in ventilator support.
- **Pneumopericardium**: Signs and symptoms vary depending on the degree of pneumopericardium, from asymptomatic to those of cardiac tamponade, which can lead to cardiopulmonary arrest. Hallmark signs include narrow pulse pressure and/or hypotension, tachycardia, and distant heart sounds.
- **Pneumoperitoneum and pneumoretroperitoneum**: typically a result of pneumothorax, pneumomediastinum, or pulmonary interstitial edema, and present as respiratory distress. There may be abdominal findings present as well.
- **Subcutaneous emphysema**: presents as bubbling or bulging in the skin, typically on the chest or neck area, and is detected by palpation of subcutaneous air (crepitus) under the affected area.

PATHOPHYSIOLOGY

Air leak typically begins with an overdistended alveolus that eventually ruptures. The air then shifts into a different space, such as the pleural space, pericardial space, or subcutaneous tissue. Depending on where the air travels to, varying types of air leak syndrome may occur.

- **Pneumomediastinum**: Air travels to the mediastinal space; often preceded by pulmonary interstitial edema.
- **Pneumothorax**: air between the visceral and parietal pleura
- **Pulmonary interstitial edema**: air trapped in the interstitial tissues of the lungs themselves, often the precursor to other types of air leak syndromes
- **Pneumopericardium**: Preceded by some other type of air leak such as pneumothorax, this is a collection of air in the pericardial space.
- **Pneumoperitoneum or pneumoretroperitoneum**: air in the peritoneal or retroperitoneal space; often follows an abdominal procedure
- **Subcutaneous emphysema**: air in the subcutaneous tissues, often a sign of a more serious underlying air leak

NURSING IMPLICATIONS AND TREATMENT

ASSESSMENT

Assessment of a patient with an air leak syndrome will vary depending on the type, but typically includes auscultating for diminished lung sounds and assessing for signs of respiratory distress such as tachypnea, hypoxemia, and accessory muscle use. Oftentimes air leak syndromes are asymptomatic.

LABS AND DIAGNOSTICS

X-ray is the most useful diagnostic test for air leak syndromes, as air is easily seen on radiograph. X-ray is used to make a definitive diagnosis of different types of air leak syndromes.

TREATMENT AND MANAGEMENT

Treatment and management vary based on the type of air leak syndrome:
- **Pneumomediastinum**: typically just managed with close observation, as attempting to drain is typically not beneficial; oxygen may be administered for clinically significant cases.
- **Pneumothorax**: Management varies based on degree of severity; in a mildly symptomatic child who presents with a spontaneous pneumothorax, usually 100% oxygen therapy is initiated, and the pneumothorax will resolve on its own. For pneumothoraces that are clinically significant or causing more severe symptoms, evacuation of the pneumothorax is necessary by needle decompression and/or chest tube placement.
- **Pulmonary interstitial edema**: Attempting to decrease ventilator support is preferred, though may be difficult. Sometimes HFOV is used effectively to treat this type of air leak.
- **Pneumopericardium**: Draining the air via pericardiocentesis is considered effective treatment for this type of air leak.
- **Pneumoperitoneum or pneumoretroperitoneum**: typically closely observed before air removal is attempted
- **Subcutaneous emphysema**: typically resolves without any intervention once underlying cause (such as other type of air leak syndrome) is treated

COMPLICATIONS

Complications depend on a multitude of factors, including the age of the patient, underlying conditions, and whether the air leak is detected and treated early. Certain air leaks, such as pulmonary interstitial edema and pneumothorax, can progress into other air leaks or cause other disorders.

▶ APNEA OF PREMATURITY

Apnea of prematurity is a common phenomenon that occurs in at least 25% of all infants born prematurely. It is considered a developmental disorder of not only the respiratory system but also the neurologic system that did not fully mature in utero. Apnea is commonly defined as a period of at least 20 seconds in which no breaths are taken.

SIGNS AND SYMPTOMS

Apnea of prematurity is displayed by periods of **absence of breathing for at least 20 seconds** in the preterm neonate. Apneic periods may be associated with color change, desaturation on pulse oximetry, and decline in heart rate.

PATHOPHYSIOLOGY

Apnea is typically characterized as one of three types: central, obstructive, or mixed.
- **Central apnea**, the most common type of apnea of prematurity, is caused by immature respiratory control centers in the brain.
- **Obstructive apnea** is caused by physical obstruction of airflow. This can be a result of neck position, nasal occlusion, or laryngospasm.
- **Mixed apnea** is a combination of both central and obstructive apnea.

In most cases, apnea of prematurity resolves as the infant grows and is most often completely resolved by 44 weeks postmenstrual age. In cases of extreme prematurity, apneic episodes may persist. It was previously thought that gastroesophageal reflux disease was a cause of apnea in premature infants, however this is no longer believed to be true and should not be considered an explanation for apneic episodes.

It is important to mention that though apnea of prematurity is common in premature neonates, there may be other more serious cause of apnea that should be investigated in the premature neonate experiencing apneic episodes, including metabolic diseases, infectious causes, cardiac abnormalities, neurologic conditions, and thermoregulation disorders.

NURSING IMPLICATIONS AND TREATMENT

ASSESSMENT AND DIAGNOSIS

The preterm neonate should be assessed for breathing patterns, respiratory rate, and effort. Typically, premature neonates will be monitored in the neonatal ICU (NICU) and will be placed on a cardiopulmonary monitor. These monitors can be set to detect periods of apnea lasting longer than 20 seconds. However, these monitors can sometimes be inaccurate due not picking up true apnea accurately. Heart rate and pulse oximetry monitoring should also be employed. Diagnosis of apnea of prematurity can be made when the neonate has repeated monitored episodes of apnea with no other identifiable cause.

TREATMENT AND MANAGEMENT

Stimulation is the first line of treatment for apneic spells. Stimulation treatment is usually enough to stop the apneic episode.

Medication is often used to treat apnea of prematurity with **caffeine citrate** being the most commonly prescribed. Caffeine is a respiratory stimulant and is considered safe with few side effects. It can be administered orally or via IV, and therapeutic levels can be monitored. Once caffeine is prescribed to treat apnea, it is usually continued until the neonate is without apneic episodes for at least 5 to 7 days.

If stimulation and medication are employed and the apneic episodes persist, or the neonate has severe events, PPV should be considered. Typically, continuous PPV is the ventilation strategy of choice to treat apneic episodes.

When a neonate who was diagnosed with apnea of prematurity is discharged to the home, parents should be educated on signs and symptoms of apnea as well as how to intervene (i.e., providing stimulation, repositioning, performing CPR in the event the infant stops breathing, or becomes unresponsive). Home monitoring with pulse oximetry or a home cardiorespiratory monitor is not routinely recommended. The infant will be required to pass a car seat test prior to discharge.

▶ ASPIRATION

When describing aspiration one can say that this complication can fall under two general categories—**foreign body aspiration** or **aspiration pneumonia**.

Foreign body aspiration occurs when an object (semisolid or solid) is aspirated and becomes lodged in the trachea or the larynx. This diagnosis can be a life-threatening emergency dependent upon a variety of factors such as level of obstruction, location, and the object that has become obstructed.

SIGNS AND SYMPTOMS

- choking
- coughing
- wheezing (late sign)
- pneumonia (late sign)
- fever (late sign)

PATHOPHYSIOLOGY

Physiological symptoms manifest dependent upon the anatomical location of the obstruction, size of the foreign body, material type, and the timeframe of obstruction.

NURSING IMPLICATIONS AND TREATMENT

ASSESSMENT

Upon examination the clinician may assess diminished air entry, rhonchi, wheezing, or stridor. If the obstruction is at the level of the larynx, then the patient may present with dyspnea, cough, stridor, voice changes, or cyanosis.

LABS AND DIAGNOSTICS

Neck and CXRs should be obtained to assist in ruling out a foreign body obstruction. The obstruction itself may not be readily identifiable. Instead, findings secondary to the obstruction may be evident. Some of these findings can include abnormal air patterns, pneumonia, or pneumothorax.

TREATMENT AND MANAGEMENT

Patients with an identified foreign body obstruction should be maintained in a quiet environment until the object removal can take place. The patient should be continuously monitored for increased respiratory distress, desaturation, respiratory rate, heart rate, and overall coloring.

COMPLICATIONS

Complications from a foreign body aspiration are typically related to a life-threatening airway obstruction. In this scenario, basic life support management should be employed, followed by an emergent bronchoscopy procedure to remove the foreign body if a resolution is not achieved.

▶ ASPIRATION PNEUMONIA

Aspiration pneumonia is an infectious process affecting the lungs, which occurs when the lungs are infiltrated by secretions, food, liquids, or other substances. Anatomical variances of the esophagus or trachea can increase the likelihood that this will occur for some patients.

SIGNS AND SYMPTOMS

- cough
- fever
- wheezing
- increased respiratory rate
- increased work of breathing
- retractions

PATHOPHYSIOLOGY

Initially injury is sustained by the parenchyma due to damage inflicted to the epithelium by the infiltration of the foreign matter. Additional injury occurs related to the inflammatory response and activation of the complement system.

NURSING IMPLICATIONS AND TREATMENT

ASSESSMENT

The clinician should perform a full respiratory assessment inclusive of obtaining a complete history to ascertain the type of aspirated contents.

LABS AND DIAGNOSTICS

Laboratory studies can include ABGs to gain understanding of severity and facilitate interventions. If a tracheal aspirate specimen can be elicited, cultures can be pursued, which can ensure appropriate antibiotic selection. CXR should be utilized to identify infiltrates, opacifications, and other abnormalities. These should be followed through the course of treatment. Frequency is determined by the patient's overall status.

TREATMENT AND MANAGEMENT

Treatment strategies are dependent upon the quantity and type of material aspirated coupled with clinical assessment of symptomatology. Materials aspirated with a normal pH lead to a milder course with primary issues being hypoxia and/or pulmonary edema. For acidotic materials the clinical sequelae can include bronchospasm, airway irritation, hemorrhage, or necrosis. These types of responses occur as a result of the material causing burns, which lead to increased alveolar capillary membrane permeability with extravasation to surrounding structures.

Management is supportive in nature with titration of oxygen, oxygen delivery devices, and/or ventilator support as indicated. Antibiotics should be ordered directly corresponding with the cause of the aspiration. If reflux aspiration is the causative agent, common management includes keeping the head of the bed elevated, gastrointestinal (GI) medications (motility agents and antacids), and feeds limited in size and thickened.

COMPLICATIONS

Complications from aspiration pneumonia can include empyema, lung abscess, effusion, ARDS, or respiratory failure.

▶ CHRONIC PULMONARY CONDITIONS

PATHOPHYSIOLOGY

Cystic fibrosis (CF) is an autosomal recessive disorder of the cystic fibrosis transmembrane regulation gene (CFTR). The mutation of the CFTR leads to an imbalance of electrolytes and fluids at the cell surface, which results in abnormal secretions and inflammatory processes. These dry, viscous secretions are found in the upper and lower airways, vas deferens, gut, liver, and pancreas.

Obstructive sleep-disordered breathing is a combination of structural and neuromuscular variables that lead to a prolonged period of complete or partial upper airway obstruction during sleep that disrupts normal respirations and normal sleep. Childhood sleep apnea is often associated with adenotonsillar hypertrophy.

Bronchopulmonary dysplasia (BPD; chronic lung disease of prematurity) is the response of the lung to acute injury at critical times of lung growth. BPD may be mild, moderate, or severe and is characterized by disruption of normal lung development, oxygen requirement, and chest radiograph abnormalities. Prematurity, volutrauma or barotrauma, oxygen toxicity, pulmonary vascular damage and edema, and deficiency or dysfunction of surfactant are all contributing factors for BPD.

SIGNS AND SYMPTOMS

Cystic fibrosis: Newborns with CF may present with meconium ileus. Infants may have failure to thrive, recurrent of chronic pulmonary infections, large, bulky and foul-smelling stools, and salty-tasting skin. The physical exam may reveal wheezing or crackles, nasal polyps, digital clubbing, rectal prolapse.

Obstructive sleep-disordered breathing commonly includes night snoring, paradoxical chest and abdominal movement, interrupted or disturbed sleep, enuresis, and daytime neurobehavioral problems. Obese children may exhibit daytime sleepiness.

Bronchopulmonary dysplasia may cause tachypnea, retractions, failure to thrive, inability to wean ventilator support, hypoxia, hypercapnia, crackling, wheezing, bronchospasm, and respiratory acidosis. Exacerbations of BPD are usually triggered by viral infections.

NURSING IMPLICATIONS (LABS, DIAGNOSTICS, TREATMENT, MANAGEMENT, COMPLICATIONS)

Cystic fibrosis is included in newborn screening for all 50 states. Genetic analysis of CFTR is available. *Pilocarpine iontophoresis sweat test is the gold standard for diagnosis of CF.* Treatment usually includes nutritional support, pancreatic enzymes, airway clearance techniques, and inhaled antibiotics. Respiratory disease is the main cause of morbidity and mortality and some patients may undergo lung transplant.

Obstructive sleep-disordered breathing is diagnosed by polysomnography and is commonly treated by adenotonsillectomy if indicated. CPAP and BIPAP may be a helpful long-term solution in older children and require frequent reassessments and adjustment of settings. If untreated it can lead to growth failure, corpulmonale, pulmonary hypertension, poor learning, behavioral problems, attention deficit hyperactivity disorder (ADHD) and death.

Bronchopulmonary dysplasia: CXR can show bilateral changes with atelectasis or edema, large airway collapse may be seen. CT scan can show multifocal hyperaeration as well as opacities. Serial pulmonary function testing may be performed. Tracheomalacia or bronchomalacia may be seen during bronchoscopy. Treatment includes supplemental oxygen to maintain saturations 90% to 95%. Home ventilation and tracheostomy may be required. Patients on a home ventilator and/or with a tracheostomy should be monitored at home with continuous pulse oximetry and all caregivers must be trained to manage routine care as well as emergencies. All trach/vent dependent patients must always have emergency equipment available including but not limited to spare trach (same size and one size smaller), spare trach ties, lubricant, normal saline, suction equipment, manual resuscitator bag, and oxygen. Adequate nutrition is preferred via enteral route and with increased calorie and protein to meet increased metabolic demands. Fluid management is critical as BPD infants tend to accumulate extra fluid in their lungs leading to hypoxemia, hypercapnia, and prolonged ventilator use. Bronchodilators are used during acute exacerbations of airway obstruction, and corticosteroids are reserved for infants with severe BPD or acute exacerbation. Diuretics are used to mobilize fluid and improve lung compliance. RSV prophylaxis with vaccine palivizumab. Complications include more frequent respiratory issues in childhood and, as a result of decreased oxygenation, they may be neurodevelopmentally delayed.

▶ CONGENITAL AIRWAY ABNORMALITIES

Congenital airway abnormalities comprise a group of disorders that are present at birth. Incidence varies and the cause is typically unknown. Prognosis and treatment varies depending on the type and degree of severity of the abnormality.

SIGNS AND SYMPTOMS

- **Congenital diaphragmatic hernia**: Typically diagnosed in utero, signs and symptoms can vary greatly. The newborn typically presents with a scaphoid abdomen and a funnel shaped chest, and there may be tracheal deviation to the opposite of the affected side. The baby may have retractions and apneic episodes or may experience profound respiratory distress. Sometimes upon auscultation, bowel sounds may be heard in the chest.
- **Tracheoesophageal fistula (TEF)**: an abnormal opening between the trachea and esophagus. As a result, swallowed liquids or formula can be aspirated (inhaled) into the child's lungs. There are 5 types of TEF depending on the location of the fistula. It is often accompanied by maternal polyhydramnios.
- **Choanal atresia**: Signs and symptoms may vary depending if one or both nostrils are affected. Unilateral choanal atresia may present minimal symptoms if the unaffected nostril is patent and unobstructed. Bilateral choanal atresia is more problematic.
- **Tracheomalacia**: Presenting signs and symptoms vary, and diagnosis requires direct visualization of the airway via bronchoscopy. Stridor is a common symptom.
- **Tracheal stenosis**: presentation varies; may present within first few hours of life or around 1 year of age, depending on severity. Less severe forms may be diagnosed incidentally and presents with wheezing with activity; more severe forms present with stridor, cough, and cyanosis.

PATHOPHYSIOLOGY

- **Congenital diaphragmatic hernia**: During fetal development; the diaphragm fails to completely form, resulting in abdominal organs herniating into the thoracic cavity and compressing the lungs. This herniation affects growth and development of the fetal lungs not only on the affected side but causes a mediastinal shift, thereby compressing the lungs on the opposite side as well.
- **Tracheoesophageal fistula**: an abnormal connection between the trachea and the esophagus that occurs during fetal development. There are five different variations of tracheoesophageal abnormalities with the most common being esophageal atresia with a distal TEF. In this type, the upper portion of the esophagus is atretic and the lower portion is connected to the trachea via a small hole, or fistula.
- **Choanal atresia**: abnormal formation of one or both nares, causing unilateral or bilateral obstruction
- **Tracheomalacia**: occurs when the cartilage in the windpipe or trachea has not developed properly or was damaged. This weakened part of the trachea may collapse, causing airway obstruction. It can be due to an intrinsic abnormality of the trachea or as a result of external compression and is very often associated with other congenital anomalies. Tracheomalacia often resolves within the first 1 to 2 years of life without intervention if significant airway collapse doesn't occur. Otherwise the infant/child may need a temporary tracheostomy.
- **Tracheal stenosis**: narrowing of the trachea, typically either generalized or segmented to a specific portion. Tracheal stenosis may often be associated with other congenital anomalies.

NURSING IMPLICATIONS AND TREATMENT

ASSESSMENT AND MANAGEMENT

- **Congenital diaphragmatic hernia**: Immediately after birth, the neonate's respiratory effort should be assessed. Management should focus on preventing hypoxemia and acidosis. Medical management focuses on stabilizing the patient and optimizing respiratory function, requiring intubation and ventilation. Noninvasive ventilation should be avoided as it may case gastric distention. Care should be bundled when possible. Surgical correction is typically delayed until the baby is more stable and has gained weight.
- **Tracheoesophageal fistula**: On assessment, the nurse may find copious saliva from the mouth. Attempts at passing a NG or orogastric (OG) tube will result with the tube coiling in the blind esophageal pouch, making NG or OG tube placement unsuccessful. The patient should be medically stabilized until surgical repair is performed. Postoperative care focuses on ensuring surgical anastomosis maintains integrity, which may be achieved by adequately sedating and using a

neuromuscular blocking agent in the intubated patient. Suctioning the mouth or nose should only happen under orders from the surgeon, monitoring any chest tube output for change in amount, color, or consistency, and maintaining gastric decompression via surgically placed NG or OG tube to suction pre- and postsurgical repair.

- **Choanal atresia**: In the patient who requires intubation or oral airway placement, care must be taken to maintain a patient endotracheal or oral airway. Surgical repair will relieve the obstruction and tubes to maintain patent airways are sutured in place during surgery. These tubes remain in place for approximately 1 month.
- **Tracheomalacia**: Assessment should include patient's work of breathing and any abnormal breath sounds. The patient will likely present with stridor. It should be noted if the stridor is brought on by a particular triggering event, such as coughing, crying, agitation, and so on. Care should be taken not to agitate the child when possible. If the patient is sent home without surgical intervention, parents should be taught infant CPR. More severe cases may require medical or surgical intervention. For example, tracheomalacia caused by a vascular ring can be relieved by vascular ring repair. Alternatively severe tracheomalacia without an extrinsic cause may require tracheostomy. Intervention depends on the severity and the cause of the tracheomalacia.
- **Tracheal stenosis**: On assessment, the nurse may expect to find stridor and cyanotic spells in the neonate or wheezing and increased work of breathing in the infant. Though some patients outgrow tracheal stenosis, surgical repair may be indicated. Slide tracheoplasty is the preferred surgical repair technique.

LABS AND DIAGNOSTICS

- **Congenital diaphragmatic hernia**: often diagnosed in utero during prenatal appointments via maternal ultrasound. It can be definitively diagnosed on CXR after birth.
- **Tracheoesophageal fistula**: may be diagnosed in utero; after birth OG or NG tube coiled in blind esophageal pouch may be seen on x-ray.
- **Choanal atresia**: Though CT scan can diagnose choanal atresia, MRI will determine if intracranial connections are present.
- **Tracheomalacia**: Echocardiogram may be useful to determine if an associated cardiac anomaly such as vascular ring is contributing to the tracheomalacia.

COMPLICATIONS

- **Congenital diaphragmatic hernia**: Prognosis overall is poor, though outcome may be slightly more favorable in some cases, such as in isolated left-sided hernias, intra-abdominal stomach, and diagnosis after 24 weeks' gestation. Typically, these neonates have prolonged hospitalizations, which put them at greater risk of an iatrogenic complication as well. In neonates who survive surgical repair, the underdeveloped lung may or may not become normal.
- **Tracheoesophageal fistula**: may have stricture or recurrent fistula, as well as persistence of respiratory symptoms likely due to gastroesophageal reflux
- **Choanal atresia**: most common complication is restenosis of the chonae requiring repeated dilations

▶ FAILURE TO WEAN FROM MECHANICAL VENTILATION

Weaning from mechanical ventilation requires the child to be able to support their own work of breathing without the assistance of the ventilator as well as have neurological control of their airway reflexes. Though tools have been developed to aid in the prediction of extubation readiness, these tools are not 100% accurate and it is not uncommon that the child fails ventilator weaning.

SIGNS AND SYMPTOMS

The child who is failing or who has failed an attempt at weaning from mechanical ventilation may display any of the following signs and symptoms:

- hypoxia
- hypercapnea
- lethargy
- tachypnea
- retractions/increased work of breathing
- hemodynamic instability
- unmanageable agitation
- cardiopulmonary collapse

PATHOPHYSIOLOGY

Failure to wean from mechanical ventilation can be caused by a multitude of different factors. Some common causes include decreased cardiac output, infection or sepsis, seizure disorder, neurologic impairment, respiratory muscle dysfunction, and oversedation.

NURSING IMPLICATIONS AND TREATMENT

ASSESSMENT

When weaning a child from mechanical ventilation, the following may be seen when the child is not tolerating the wean:

- increased respiratory rate from baseline
- decreased respiratory rate from baseline (late finding)
- use of accessory muscles for breathing
- color change including pallor or cyanosis
- fatigue or lethargy
- hypoxia and or hypercapnia seen on blood gas analysis

In general, criteria that indicates a patient is ready for weaning from mechanical ventilation include the following:

- decreased FiO_2 less than 50% and decreased PEEP of less than or equal to 5 cm H_2O
- PIP less than 20 cm or greater than 25 cm H_2O
- spontaneous TV greater than 5 mL/kg
- normal pH
- normal or baseline $PaCO_2$
- hemodynamic stability
- normal work of breathing
- adequate strength and tone
- intact gag reflex and cough
- not requiring the use of excessive sedation
- normal respiratory drive
- good aeration throughout lung fields
- air leak present
- resolution of the etiology of respiratory failure requiring intubation

LABS AND DIAGNOSTICS

In addition to clinical assessment, blood gas monitoring, pulse oximetry, end-tidal CO_2 measurements, and CXR may be used as monitoring tools during and after weaning from mechanical ventilation to determine if the child has failed weaning.

TREATMENT, MANAGEMENT, AND COMPLICATIONS

There are different strategies that can be used to avoid failure to wean from mechanical ventilation. A frequently used method is spontaneous breathing trials with minimal pressure support. Different ventilator modes may be employed to achieve this goal.

Sometimes children may be successfully extubated but still require noninvasive positive pressure ventilation (NIPPV). NIPPV has benefits over invasive mechanical ventilation, including allowing the child to maintain speech, cough and gag reflexes, lower sedation requirements, ability to pause the therapy if needed, less incidence of tracheal or laryngeal damage, and lower pneumonia rates.

Children with a chronic respiratory condition who are unable to be weaned from mechanical ventilation may require tracheostomy placement and use of a long-term ventilator. This decision comes with risks including increased morbidity and mortality rates.

▶ PULMONARY HYPERTENSION

PATHOPHYSIOLOGY

- Pulmonary hypertension (PH) is rare in the pediatric population but is associated with high morbidity and mortality. It is defined as a resting pulmonary arterial pressure (PAP) greater than 25 mmHg.

- Pulmonary vascular reactivity is maintained by a complex interaction of vasoactive hormones; nitric oxide (vasodilator), prostacyclin (vasodilator) and endothelin (vasoconstrictor).
- Over time, impaired production of these mediators adversely affects vascular tone and promotes vascular remodeling.
- PH is caused by vasoconstriction of the pulmonary vascular bed as well as proliferation of endothelial and smooth muscle cells.
- Risk factors include congenital heart disease, PPHN of the newborn, bronchopulmonary dysplasia, chronic lung disease, diaphragmatic hernia, meconium aspiration, sleep disordered breathing, and chronic kidney disease.

SIGNS AND SYMPTOMS (ASSESSMENT, CLINICAL MANIFESTATIONS)

- **Infants**: present with signs of low cardiac output-tachypnea, tachycardia, poor PO, failure to thrive, diaphoresis, irritability, or lethargy
- **Infants and older children**: cyanosis with exertion
- **Children**: syncope if no patent foramen ovale or mechanism for shunting
- **Older children**: exertional dyspnea and chest pain. Patients with PH may have a prominent S_2 on auscultation, jugular vein distention, hepatomegaly, ascites and peripheral edema, clubbing and/or cyanosis, and exertional dyspnea.
- **Acute pulmonary hypertensive crisis**: hypoxia, hypercarbia, tachycardia, hypotension, increased central venous pressure
- Hypercarbia, acidosis, acute infection, airway secretions, noxious stimuli, and agitation can precipitate a pulmonary hypertensive crisis.

TREATMENT (LABS, DIAGNOSTICS, AND COMPLICATIONS)

- Echocardiogram is the noninvasive test of choice to diagnose and evaluate PH.
- Cardiac catheterization is used to confirm the diagnosis of PH and evaluate the severity as well as to assess the response to vasodilators prior to starting therapy.
- MRI is the gold standard for assessing the right ventricle (RV).
- Exercise tests and proBNP may be performed to monitor cardiac function.
- Sleep study may be performed to evaluate for obstructive sleep apnea as a cause of PH.

MANAGEMENT

- Maintain vaccines up to date including flu and pneumococcal.
- Treat hyperthermia to prevent increased metabolic demands.
- Medications:
  - **sildenafil (Viagra;** monitor for priapism and adjust dosing as needed)
  - **bosentan (Tracleer; Safebo;** monitor liver function)
  - **epoprostenol (Flolan, Veletri;** monitor for systemic hypotension)
- Aggressive and immediate therapy is needed for pulmonary hypertensive crisis as the patient may progress to cardiac arrest.
- **Acute PH in the ICU**: minimal stimulation, oxygen, inhaled nitrous oxide (iNO), acute hyperventilation to decrease CO_2, sodium bicarbonate to treat acidosis, sedation, neuromuscular blockade. Fluid administration may help to support the RV by offering more preload during PH crisis.

▶ STATUS ASTHMATICUS

Asthma is characterized by limitations in airflow that are caused by a variety of physiologic conditions such as **edema** of the airway, **bronchoconstriction**, exaggerated responsiveness of the airway, and potentially permanent structural changes to the airway. **Inflammation** is another hallmark finding in identifying asthma as a diagnosis. The inflammation and the airflow limitations combine to manifest into episodes of wheezing, coughing, and shortness of breath, which clinicians identify as asthma.

Status asthmaticus is the exacerbation of asthma symptoms unresponsive to conventional outpatient or emergency department management.

SIGNS AND SYMPTOMS

The most common signs and symptoms include:
- cough
- wheezing
- prolonged/forced expiratory phase
- increased work of breathing
- hypoxemia

It's critical the pediatric critical care nurse recognized and responds to signs of impeding respiratory failure:
- absent or distant breath sounds
- inability to speak in more than monosyllables
- diaphoresis
- inability to lie flat
- change in mental status (Flasch et al., 2019)

Clinical Pearl

Pulses paradoxus is a decrease in systolic blood pressure during inspiration of more than 10 mmHg. Pulses paradoxus can be observed in the waveform of an arterial line and can occur in severe asthma.

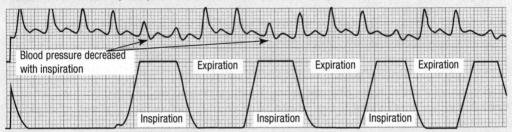

Source: Healio Learn the Heart (n.d.). "Pulsus Paradoxus Topic Review." https://www.healio.com/cardiology/learn-the-heart/cardiology-review/topic-reviews/pulsus-paradoxus.

NURSING IMPLICATIONS AND TREATMENT

ASSESSMENT AND CLINICAL MANIESTATIONS

Nursing assessment of a patient with asthma includes a complete respiratory assessment inclusive of auscultation and visual inspection of work of breathing. In addition, a complete physical inspection should be done in part focused on identification of overall color, chest, and facial features common in patients with long term asthma exacerbation.

LABS AND DIAGNOSITICS

- Chest x-ray may show hyperinflation, flattened diaphragm, and possible infiltrates.
- Arterial blood gas will show respiratory acidosis.

TREATMENT AND MANAGEMENT

The goals of management of status asthmaticus are to relieve airway obstruction and to restore oxygenation and ventilation. Nurses caring for children with status asthmaticus should expect to administer oxygen, give fluids, monitor inputs and outputs (I&Os), and administer prescribed medications (Flasch et al., 2019).

Medications commonly administered include the following:
- **Beta-2 agonists** produce smooth muscle relaxation. Common beta-2 agonists include albuterol (inhalation) and terbutaline (SQ or IV). Monitor for tachycardia, arrythmias, hypertension, and prolonged QT interval.
- **Anticholinergics** (ipratropium bromide) promote bronchodilation.
- **Corticosteroids** (methylprednisolone) decrease airway inflammation, inhibit vascular leak, decrease mucous production, and modify lymphocyte activation.
- **Magnesium sulfate** is administered intravenously and causes smooth muscle relaxation by inhibiting calcium uptake.

- **Methylxanthines** (theophylline/aminophylline) help augment diaphragmatic contractility. Monitor closely for toxicity.
- **Ketamine** has bronchodilatory effects and may be considered as induction for intubation.
- **Heliox**

Patients may be managed on noninvasive ventilation (BiPaP) to improve oxygenation and ventilation and ease work of breathing. Severe cases of status asthmaticus may be require intubation, but generally, intubation is avoided for as long as possible due to complications such as:

- hypotension from intrathoracic pressure changes and reduced systemic venous return
- difficulty ensuring oxygenation and ventilation
- development of pneumothorax or subcutaneous emphysema

Inhaled anesthetics such as isoflurane (a potent bronchodilator) may be administered to intubated patients to support ventilator synchrony.

▶ THORACIC AND AIRWAY TRAUMA

There is increased morbidity and mortality for patients with thoracic trauma that is also associated with head, abdominal, and spinal trauma.

- **Rib fractures** are unusual in pediatric patients due to the elasticity of the bone and cartilaginous framework. Multiple rib fractures may be indicative of nonaccidental trauma and should be evaluated carefully. Chest wall trauma can lead to pulmonary and cardiac contusions, pneumothoraces, or hemothorax. Flail chest is a serious complication that results from 2 to 3 aligned rib fractures that lead to impaired respiratory mechanics.
- **Traumatic pneumothorax** can be traumatic, simple, tension, or open, but are rare in children. A tension pneumothorax occurs when there is an imbalance in the amount of air entering versus exiting the pleural space, which results in mediastinal shift, significant lung compression, major vessel compression, and shock. This may be caused by chest or lung wall trauma or esophageal rupture.
- **Hemothorax** involves blood in the pleural space, which can occur from high pressure from the chest wall or low pressure from the pulmonary vessels.
- **Tracheobronchial trauma** is rupture of the trachea or bronchus from severe compression or blunt trauma to the neck.
- **Posttraumatic atelectasis** is defined by pulmonary contusions leading to increased tracheobronchial secretions, but elimination of secretions is impaired by airway obstruction, pain, and cough suppression.
- **Injuries to the esophagus** can be developed by the neonate at delivery from excessive positive pressure or suction with a stiff catheter. Older infants and children can have rupture from ingestion of lye, or foreign body aspiration.
- **Traumatic blunt rupture of the diaphragm** may occur in severe trauma, more commonly on the left than the right with significant cardiopulmonary compromise. If not diagnosed early, late-stage intestinal obstruction may be what leads to diagnosis.

SIGNS AND SYMPTOMS (ASSESSMENT, CLINICAL MANIFESTATIONS)

- **Overall**: There may not be outward evidence of abdominal/thoracic trauma so careful evaluation must be performed with rapid assessment of the patient's airway and breathing.
- **Rib fractures**: Point tenderness to affected rib that intensifies with movement; area may be ecchymotic and edematous.
- **Traumatic pneumothorax**: Severe respiratory distress, distended neck veins, poor systemic perfusion, tachypnea, dyspnea, cyanosis, absence or transmission of lung sounds, dislocation of the trachea and point of maximal impulse.
- **Hemothorax**: Blood will eventually clot in the pleural space. Patient will develop respiratory distress, may have hemoptysis, tachycardia, and hypotension secondary to decreased venous return to the heart.
- **Tracheobronchial trauma**: Rapidly progressive interstitial emphysema, pneumomediastinum, tension pneumothorax, and hemoptysis. Stricture at the site of rupture leads to sepsis and atelectasis with progressive loss of lung function.
- **Posttraumatic atelectasis**: Dyspnea, cyanosis, unrelenting unproductive cough accompanied by wheezing, rhonchi, and rales.

- **Injuries to the esophagus**: Hyperthermia, hypotension, chest and neck pain, pneumomediastinum, tension pneumothorax, subcutaneous emphysema, and hematemesis.
- **Traumatic blunt rupture of the diaphragm**: Abdominal tenderness, rigidity, rebound tenderness.
- **Aortic and great vessel injuries**: Mid-scapular back pain, unexplained hypotension, upper extremity hypertension, bilateral weak/absent femoral pulse, large chest tube output upon placement, sternal fracture, widened mediastinum on CXR.

TREATMENT (LABS, DIAGNOSTICS, TREATMENT, AND COMPLICATIONS)

Chest Tube Placement

- Management of traumatic pneumothorax or hemothorax often requires chest tube placement. After placement, the tube is connected to either a wet or dry drainage system, based on facility equipment.
- wet system
  - suction to −25 cm H_2O
  - water in suction control chamber and air leak meter (water seal chamber)
- There is a suction chamber where the level of fluid inserted is ordered from −10 cm H_2O to 25 cm H_2O. The suction control chamber is filled to the desired height with sterile fluid and the short suction tubing is connected to a suction source, which is adjusted to produce gentle bubbling in the suction control chamber. This chamber must be closely monitored as fluid can evaporate over time, and the suction level must be regulated to ensure proper amount of suction as ordered.
- dry system
  - suction to 40 mmHg
  - water only in air leak meter (water seal chamber)
- Dry suction systems are regulated by a dial and suction regulator. A dry system is connected to the wall suction regulator. The wall suction is turned up until the orange indicator pops into the suction control window.
- **caring for a patient with a chest tube**
  - The drainage collection tubing should be free of dependent loops and should remain below the level of the patient to facilitate drainage.
  - The drainage tubing should not hang over a bedrail or crib-rail as this will impede drainage.
  - If the drainage system is knocked over and the fluid collected overflows to another chamber, the drainage system must be changed.
  - Within the drainage system there is an air leak detection chamber, for a pneumothorax you would expect to see bubbling of the fluid in the air leak detection chamber as the purpose of the tube is to evacuate the entrained air in the pleural space. There should not be an air leak in the presence of a hemothorax or pleural effusion as the tube is intended to drain fluid, whether blood or serous fluid.
  - Equipment to keep at the bedside of a patient with a chest tube includes:
    - ❏ bottle of sterile water
    - ❏ occlusive dressing
    - ❏ chest tube clamps
    - ❏ 4-inch tape or dressing material

Clinical Pearl

Monitoring for an air leak includes:
- evaluating for dislodgement or displacement of the chest tube at the level of the patient
- disconnections in the system, or a breakdown of the integrity of the system that is allowing air to enter the drainage collection system
- The presence of subcutaneous air may indicate migration of the chest tube or occlusion of the drainage system.
- A CXR may be indicated to evaluate the tube placement and lung fields and surrounding tissues.

Thoracentesis

Alternatively to chest tube placement, a thoracentesis may be performed to evacuate the fluid without leaving a chest tube in place. In this procedure, a needle is inserted into the pleural space and the fluid is drained. It may be therapeutic to evacuate the fluid. The fluid may also be used for diagnostic purposes.

Fluid may be sent for culture if there is concern for infection or for cytology if there is a concern of malignancy. Following a thoracentesis, the site should be monitored for leaking of fluid or bleeding. The patient's work of breathing and oxygenation should be closely followed.

- **Rib fractures**: CXR-rib and thoracic spine fractures, pain management to prevent hypoventilation, thoracentesis, and chest tube placement for pneumothorax or hemothorax
- **Traumatic pneumothorax**: CXR-unilateral hyperlucency with collapsed underlying lung and deviated trachea and mediastinum shifted to opposite side of affected lung, chest tube insertion is indicated for tension or simple pneumothorax, which should provide immediate relief. For large open chest wounds causing a pneumothorax, management includes prompt occlusion with bulky sterile dressings while chest tube is placed followed by surgical washout and debridement of the open wound.
- **Hemothorax**: CXR-complete opacification of the hemothorax, fluid is dependent, but diagnosis is confirmed by thoracentesis and chest tube placement to evacuate the blood.
- **Tracheobronchial trauma**: Bronchoscopic examination of the rupture is required. Initial management is securing the patient's airway and decompression of any pneumothorax or pneumomediastinum.
- **Posttraumatic atelectasis**: frequent position changes, oxygen, humidification, antibiotics, diuretics, coughing, and deep breathing. Minimize medications that may suppress cough.
- **Traumatic blunt rupture of the diaphragm**: Secure the patient's airway and circulation, gastric decompression.
- **Injuries to the esophagus**: Tension pneumothorax must be quickly evacuated, esophageal defect must be closed, and mediastinum drained as indicated with dosing of antibiotics.
- **Aortic and great vessel injuries**: Angiography is the diagnostic test of choice, CXR-widened mediastinum, blurring of aortic knob, tracheal deviation, widened peritracheal stripes, increased heart size with tamponade.

THORACIC SURGERY

▶ PECTUS EXCAVATUM

- a deformity of the chest wall characterized by a sternal depression, often referred to as "funnel chest"
- 3 to 5 times more prevalent in males than females and may be associated with Marfan syndrome, Ehlers-Danlos syndrome, Noonan Syndrome, Turner syndrome, Neurofibromatosis type 1, osteogenesis imperfecta, and neuromuscular disease
- believed to be a result of abnormal cartilage development

SIGNS AND SYMPTOMS (ASSESSMENT, CLINICAL MANIFESTATIONS)

- Sternal depression, exercise intolerance, chest pain, resting tachypnea in 98% of cases. Poor endurance, shortness of breath. Pectus excavatum (PE) rarely improves after 6 years of age and usually progresses during adolescence.

TREATMENT (LABS, DIAGNOSTICS, TREATMENT, AND COMPLICATIONS)

- Although uncommon, patients with severe PE or respiratory/cardiac involvement should be evaluated with CT scan.
- Cosmetic concerns are usually the most common reason for surgical consultation. Patients with severe pectus excavatum should under pulmonary function testing and cardiac evaluation.
- Surgical correction is optimal during late childhood or early adolescence.

▶ VIDEO-ASSISTED THORACOSCOPIC SURGERY

Video-assisted thoracoscopic surgery (VATS) is a type of minimally invasive surgery that uses small incisions to insert a camera called a thoracoscope. This procedure is used in pediatrics for management of recurrent pneumothoraxes, chylothorax, pericardial window for pericardial effusion, patent ductus arteriosus closure, and others.

NURSING IMPLICATIONS AND TREATMENT

COMPLICATIONS

Complications of VATS include bleeding, infection, pain, atelectasis, and recurrent pneumothorax.

▶ CARING FOR THE INTUBATED PATIENT

OVERVIEW

When caring for the intubated patient supported on mechanical ventilation, the primary goal is to maintain proper position and patency of the ETT. As a safety measure, an ambu bag with an appropriate size face mask along with suctioning equipment must be kept at the bedside at all times.

NURSING IMPLICATIONS AND TREATMENT

ASSESSMENT

An overall assessment of the intubated child should include monitoring their color, perfusion, level of consciousness, and work of breathing. Auscultation should be performed to note the presence and quality of lung sounds. The nurse should take note of the insertion depth of the ETT as well as ventilator settings and presence of an air leak. Presence and quality of airway secretions should be noted. Finally, palpation of the chest should be performed to note any crepitus or other abnormalities.

Monitoring

Monitoring parameters for the intubated patient should include the following:
- Blood gases: Arterial are preferred but venous or capillary (least invasive) can also be used.
- pulse oximetry
- end-tidal CO_2
- transcutaneous CO_2
- alarms, including EKG alarms and ventilator alarms
- CXRs
- level of sedation and neuromuscular blockade if applicable
- ventilator parameters:
  - TV
  - PIP
  - PEEP/auto-PEEP
  - pressure support
  - set rate
  - patient effort (rate)

TREATMENT AND MANAGEMENT

The nurse caring for an intubated patient is responsible for the following:
- understanding equipment function and emergency management
- monitoring fluid and electrolyte levels
- maintaining optimal nutrition of the patient
- performing routine repositioning and taking care to protect bony prominences or other at-risk areas of skin
- suctioning the ETT to maintain a patient airway
  - Patients should always be preoxygenated prior to suctioning.
  - Care should be taken to avoid suctioning below the tip of the ETT.
  - Sterile technique should be maintained throughout suctioning.
  - Routine use of saline with ETT suctioning is not recommended and should be avoided.
- managing pain and sedation
- evaluating psychosocial needs of the patient and family

▶ HIGH-FREQUENCY OSCILLATORY VENTILATION

- HFOV is often considered a rescue ventilation strategy as it is most often used when conventional ventilation has failed. It delivers small TVs with a constant MAP and high respiratory rate to achieve both oxygenation and ventilation.
- Special considerations should be taken when an intubated patient requires the use of an HFOV.
- Assessment of the patient on HFOV may be somewhat limited as breath sounds are difficult to distinguish. One of the most important physical assessment parameters is the presence of a chest wiggle.
- These patients are prone to developing pneumothorax. Care should be taken when repositioning and suctioning.
- Patients on HFOV need adequate sedation and will likely require neuromuscular blockade.
- HFOV may not be as effective in treating respiratory disorders with increased airway resistance such as asthma.

NURSING IMPLICATIONS AND TREATMENT

COMPLICATIONS

Complications of mechanical ventilation can include the following:

- oxygen toxicity
- alveolar overdistension
- barotrauma
- pneumonia
- atelectasis
- dislodgement
- obstruction
- pneumothorax
- equipment failure

CASE STUDY

A 5-year-old presents to the ED with a 4-day history of fever, cough, and malaise. For the last day, they have not wanted to eat or drink anything. They have no past medical history. They recently visited their cousins who were sick with the flu. The patient's vital signs upon arrival include a heart rate (HR) of 140, respiratory rate (RR) of 40, blood pressure (BP) of 95/55, temperature of 39.5°C (103.1°F), and oxygen saturation of 90% on room air. They respond to commands but appear lethargic.

CASE STUDY QUESTIONS

1. What is the nurse's first priority after a brief primary assessment?
   A. Obtain a chest x-ray (CXR)
   B. Draw blood cultures
   C. Place the patient on supplemental oxygen via simple face mask and monitor closely
   D. Prepare for intubation

2. After placing the patient on a simple face mask with 6 L/minute of flow, the nurse performs a more thorough assessment of the patient. Which of the following assessment findings would be the most concerning?
   A. Nasal flaring
   B. Decline in mental status
   C. Tachypnea
   D. Left lower lobe crackles

3. Given the assessment findings of a decline in mental status and decrease in respiratory rate (RR) to 15 bpm in the patient, which of the following is the next most appropriate action?
   A. Prepare to emergently intubate the patient using rapid sequence intubation
   B. Obtain a chest x-ray (CXR)
   C. Administer a nebulized respiratory treatment
   D. Administer antibiotics

(See answers next page.)

ANSWERS TO CASE STUDY QUESTIONS

1. C) Place the patient on supplemental oxygen via face mask and monitor closely

Obtaining a CXR and blood cultures will be an important part of the assessment after the patient's oxygenation status is stabilized and it is ensured their airway will remain patent. Though they may ultimately require intubation, they are still responsive and maintaining their own airway, so they should be placed on supplemental oxygen and monitored. However, if their respiratory effort or vital signs become compromised, the nurse should be prepared to intubate the patient.

2. B) Decline in mental status

Nasal flaring and tachypnea are expected findings in this patient given their presentation. A decline in mental status can indicate a worsening in condition; specifically, in acute respiratory failure, a decline in mental status is due to a decrease in oxygenation and retention of carbon dioxide. Additionally, a significant decrease in respiratory drive or effort in a patient in respiratory distress or respiratory failure is an ominous sign and can indicate imminent respiratory arrest. The presence of crackles is abnormal but not the most concerning finding.

3. A) Prepare to intubate the patient using rapid sequence intubation

Rapid sequence intubation is appropriate when the patient's last mealtime is unknown or there is any concern for aspiration. Preoxygenation is achieved using a nonrebreather mask and the goal is to secure the airway with an endotracheal tube (ETT) expediently. This method is only to be employed when there is no evidence of a difficult airway. Obtaining a CXR will be a useful diagnostic tool, however, the patient's airway is compromised and must first be stabilized. Administering antibiotics will be important given the patient's fever and should not be delayed, but the first priority is establishing a secure airway. Administering a nebulized respiratory treatment is not warranted at this time.

KNOWLEDGE CHECK: CHAPTER 3

1. Baby Smith is a 1-week-old neonate who was born at 34 weeks' gestation. They are currently working on tolerating taking feedings by mouth. The nurse performs a shift assessment and notices that they are having periods of breath holding that last 20 to 25 seconds. What is the likely cause of these apneic spells?
   A. Tracheomalacia
   B. Choanal atresia
   C. Apnea of prematurity
   D. Bronchopulmonary dysplasia

2. A 1-week-old neonate is diagnosed with apnea of prematurity. What is the first line treatment for this diagnosis?
   A. Noninvasive ventilation via nasal continuous positive airway pressure (CPAP)
   B. Oral caffeine
   C. Stimulation and monitoring
   D. Intravenous (IV) caffeine

3. The nurse is caring for a 13-year-old patient who was struck by a car while walking home from school. Their vital signs are:
   Heart rate (HR): 110
   Respiratory rate (RR: 35
   Blood pressure (BP): 87/55
   Temp: 36.5°C (97.7°F [oral])
   Oxygen saturation: 85% on 6 L/minute oxygen via simple face mask.
   Upon examination the nurse notices small bubbling of the skin on the patient's right chest that makes a crackling noise on palpation. What do these bubbles indicate?
   A. Pulmonary interstitial edema
   B. Pneuperitoneum
   C. Pneumothorax
   D. Subcutaneous emphysema

4. In a patient who is in acute respiratory failure, the primary focus of management is:
   A. Obtaining a chest CT
   B. Obtaining a chest x-ray (CXR)
   C. Intubating the patient who cannot maintain a patent airway
   D. Treating the underlying cause

5. Which of the following is a risk factor for failure to wean from mechanical ventilation?
   A. Use of medication for analgesia or sedation
   B. Age younger than 1 year
   C. Intact cognitive function
   D. Invasive hemodynamic monitoring

6. A 6-year-old is admitted to the pediatric ICU (PICU) after a 1-day history of difficulty breathing. The parents say that the child was out of town visiting extended family and began coughing a few hours after arriving home. Additionally, the mother says that the coughing is persistent and at times accompanied by a whistling sound. Upon assessment the nurse finds the following vital signs:
   Heart rate (HR): 145
   Respiratory rate (RR): 45
   Saturation (Sat): 88% on room air
   On auscultation, the nurse finds wheezing bilaterally with subcostal and suprasternal retractions. What additional information related to the chief complaint should be obtained from the family?
   A. Environmental allergies
   B. Previous history of breathing difficulties
   C. Family history of wheezing
   D. Food allergies

(See answers next page.)

1. C) Apnea of prematurity
Premature infants are prone to apnea of prematurity, which can be due to central, obstructive, or mixed causes. While premature neonates are at risk for apnea of prematurity, it is important to rule out other possible causes of apnea as well. Other common causes of apnea in the neonate include, but are not limited to, metabolic diseases, infectious causes, cardiac abnormalities, neurologic conditions, and thermoregulation disorders. Choanal atresia, tracheomalacia and bronchopulmonary dysplasia do not typically cause breath holding spells.

2. C) Stimulation and monitoring
Oftentimes, stimulation alone is enough to resolve an apneic episode. If stimulation alone does not resolve the apneic episodes, the patient may be prescribed enteral or IV caffeine. Noninvasive ventilation is used for severe apneic episodes not responsive to stimulation or medication.

3. D) Subcutaneous emphysema
Crackling on palpation and bubbling of the skin are signs of subcutaneous emphysema. The signs and symptoms of pulmonary interstitial edema, pneumoperitoneum, and pneumothorax include respiratory distress, hypoxia, and hypercarbia.

4. C) Intubating the patient who cannot maintain a patent airway
Maintaining adequate oxygenation and ventilation is the main focus of managing a patient in acute respiratory failure. Therefore, intubating the patient who cannot maintain their own airway is the primary goal. While treating the underlying cause is necessary, failure to establish adequate oxygenation and ventilation right away can lead to respiratory arrest. Chest CT and CXR are useful diagnostic tools and may be used but are not the primary management strategies for the patient.

5. A) Use of medication for analgesia or sedation
The use of analgesic or sedating medications, while necessary, can make weaning from mechanical ventilation difficult as they can impair the patient's intrinsic respiratory drive and effort. Intact cognitive function would indicate that a patient may tolerate weaning from mechanical ventilation. Age is not a factor in determining readiness to extubate. Though stable hemodynamics make a child's outcome more favorable when attempting to wean from mechanical ventilation, the presence of invasive hemodynamic monitoring is not considered a risk factor and may provide more real time monitoring of hemodynamics during the weaning process.

6. A) Environmental allergies
Obtaining a complete but focused history is essential in diagnosing and treating the patient appropriately. Environmental allergies are typically a trigger for patients with asthma. It is essential to understand the underlying history related to any other pulmonary exacerbations to understand patterns and treatment strategies employed previously. Family history of asthma and food allergies can be deferred while focusing on treating the primary presenting cause.

7. A 6-year-old presents with bilateral wheezing and subcostal and suprasternal retractions, and has vital signs of:
   Heart rate (HR): 145
   Respiratory rate (RR): 45
   Saturation (Sat): 88% on room air
   Upon further inquiry, the child's mother mentions they were around an aunt who is a heavy smoker and that the child has previously displayed sensitivity to cigarette smoke. The physician writes orders for treatment. Which of these should be the first order to be performed?
   A. Chest x-ray (CXR)
   B. Albuterol 5mg (ProAir HFA, Ventolin HFA) via nebulization up to 3 times
   C. Laboratory studies: complete blood count (CBC), basic metabolic panel (BMP), magnesium (Mg)
   D. Acetaminophen

8. A postoperative patient in the cardiovascular ICU begins to acutely desaturate 6 hours after returning from the operating room. Upon further assessment, the nurse finds the patient to be cyanotic, tachypneic, and short of breath. The first step in treating the patient is to:
   A. Provide albuterol (ProAir HFA, Ventolin HFA)
   B. Call for a STAT chest x-ray (CXR)
   C. Provide oxygen
   D. Obtain an arterial blood gas (ABG)

9. A postoperative patient in the cardiovascular ICU begins to acutely desaturate 6 hours after returning from the operating room following a mitral valve replacement. Upon further assessment, the nurse finds the patient to be cyanotic, tachypneic, and short of breath. The healthcare team provides oxygen which helps minimally but the patient continues to deteriorate. The physician decides to intubate the patient. Upon intubating, the patient the team notes pink, frothy secretions coming up through the endotracheal tube (ETT). The most likely diagnosis for this patient is:
   A. Pulmonary edema
   B. Pneumothorax
   C. Pulmonary interstitial emphysema
   D. Acute pulmonary embolus

10. A 2-year-old presents with a history of choking and coughing over the last 2 hours. The mother recounts that right before the child starting exhibiting symptoms, the older sibling was playing with small plastic toy bricks. Considering the most likely cause of the patient's respiratory distress, what would be contraindicated in the care of this patient?
    A. Oxygen administration
    B. Monitor heart rate, respiratory rate, and oxygen saturation
    C. Remove the child from the mother's arms and secure them on the stretcher
    D. Neck and chest x-rays (CXRs)

11. A 10-year-old trauma patient has sustained a variety of facial and oral injuries and has had a nasogastric (NG) tube placed to optimize his nutrition. When minimizing his risk of aspiration, what measure should be avoided by the team?
    A. Evaluate the patient for a history of gastroesophageal reflux disease (GERD)
    B. Maintain the head of the bed elevated during feedings
    C. Start prophylactic antibiotics
    D. Verify feeding tube position

12. Pulmonary embolism risk factors include all of the following except:
    A. Trauma
    B. Myocarditis
    C. Central venous catheter
    D. Immobility

(See answers next page.)

7. B) Albuterol 5mg (ProAir HFA, Ventolin HFA) via nebulization up to 3 times

The priority should be administration of Albuterol due to the child's respiratory status (tachypnea and desaturation noted on assessment). A chest x-ray (CXR) and laboratory studies are relevant to the workup for the child with this presentation but are secondary to the initial treatment necessary to pursue improvement in the patient's respiratory status. There is no history provided, nor assessment finding that indicates that acetaminophen should be administered as a first line treatment.

8. C) Provide oxygen

The first assessment finding that should be addressed is the patient's hypoxemia; with provision of oxygen, the shortness of breath, tachypnea, and cyanosis could resolve. Albuterol is not indicated based on the assessment findings. Obtaining a CXR important but is not the priority when addressing the imminent clinical needs of the patient. An ABG may be performed as a secondary step in determining additional treatment strategies.

9. A) Pulmonary edema

Pink, frothy secretions are a hallmark sign of pulmonary edema. Additionally, this patient presented with hypoxemia, shortness of breath, tachypnea, and a history of a mitral valve surgery which are common signs and symptoms as well as being potential causes for cardiogenic pulmonary edema. The patient's signs and symptoms are not consistent with pneumothorax, pulmonary interstitial emphysema, or pulmonary embolus.

10. C) Remove the child from the mother's arms and secure them on the stretcher

Prior to removal of the foreign body, the patient should be maintained in a calm, quiet state. Removing the child from the parent's arms would likely induce anxiety and crying, all of which could potentially cause the foreign object to dislodge. Oxygen administration, monitoring of vital signs, and radiographic studies are all considered part of initial treatment and assessment for a suspected foreign body aspiration.

11. C) Start prophylactic antibiotics

Prophylactic antibiotics are not indicated unless the patient develops aspiration pneumonia. Prophylactic antibiotics should be avoided to limit the patient from developing antibiotic resistance. Evaluating the patient for a history of GERD allows for the team to consider ordering antacids or gastrointestinal (GI) motility enhancing agents or potentially transpyloric feeds. Maintaining the head of the bed elevated helps to promote gastric motility and minimize risk of reflux. Feeding tube positioning should be verified to ensure that placement is appropriate in the stomach and that migration nor misplacement has occurred.

12. B) Myocarditis

Bacterial endocarditis, not myocarditis, is a risk factor for developing a pulmonary embolus. Central venous catheters are understood to be a risk due to the increased risk of thrombus formation related to the body's inflammatory response to foreign material (as well as the catheter itself becoming a site for clot formation to occur). Trauma patients are predisposed related to their injuries and the clotting factors that get activated as a result of the healing process. Immobility generates a risk of clot formation thereby leaving this broad group of patients at risk.

13. Which of the following is reserved as a last resort treatment for patients presenting in status asthmaticus?
    A. Administration of beta agonists
    B. Oxygen administration
    C. Endotracheal intubation
    D. Corticosteroid administration

14. Which of the following statements is true regarding congenital diaphragmatic hernia?
    A. The patient should be medically optimized immediately after birth, which may include the use of high frequency oscillatory ventilation (HFOV).
    B. The patient should undergo emergency corrective surgery immediately after birth.
    C. Patients with congenital diaphragmatic hernia often have a good prognosis with uncomplicated hospital course.
    D. Patients with congenital diaphragmatic hernia present with a scaphoid shaped abdomen and tracheal deviation toward the affected side.

15. A 3-year-old presents with a 4-day history of productive cough, fever, and decreased activity. They had been recovering from a viral illness diagnosed the week prior. Their vital signs are:
    Temp: 41.1°C (105.9°F)
    Heart rate (HR): 135 bpm
    Respiratory rate (RR): 45
    Saturation (Sat): 84% on room air
    The patient is listless, and their extremities are cool to the touch. Breath sounds are diminished over the right lung and diffuse crackles are heard over the left lung. What should be the first intervention?
    A. Start antibiotics
    B. Provide oxygen
    C. Obtain a chest x-ray (CXR)
    D. Review immunization history

16. A 16-year-old involved in a motor vehicle accident complains of acute chest pain and shortness of breath several days following admission. The nurse notifies the attending physician and can anticipate the most definitive diagnostic study will include:
    A. D-dimer test
    B. Arterial blood gas (ABG)
    C. Chest x-ray (CXR)
    D. Pulmonary angiogram

17. What nursing interventions can minimize common complications of anticoagulation therapy?
    A. Padding the bed rails
    B. Closely monitoring laboratory studies
    C. Counseling the patient on risky activities
    D. Providing mouth care

18. A 7-year-old is intubated in the ICU for acute respiratory failure secondary to sepsis. The nurse notes that the patient is beginning to desaturate and the ventilator is alarming high pressure. On assessment, the nurse notes thick secretions in the endotracheal tube (ETT). Which of the following should the nurse do next?
    A. Sedate the patient and increase the FiO_2
    B. Preoxygenate the patient, don sterile gloves, and suction the ETT
    C. Instill normal saline in the ETT, don sterile gloves, and suction the ETT
    D. Notify the physician that the patient is desaturated and anticipate ventilator changes

(See answers next page.)

13. C) Endotracheal intubation

Endotracheal intubation is typically reserved as a last resort treatment for patients presenting in status asthmaticus. Intubation can worsen bronchospasm and trigger laryngomalacia. Intubation carries an increased risk of mortality in this patient population. Beta agonists such as Albuterol and corticosteroids are first line treatments for patients with asthma. Oxygen administration is a typical mainstay of treatment for patients presenting with hypoxemia related to asthma exacerbation.

14. A) The patient should be medically optimized immediately after birth, which may include the use of high frequency oscillatory ventilation (HFOV).

Patients with congenital diaphragmatic hernia should be medically optimized immediately after birth. Efforts to stabilize the baby will likely include the use of inotropic support and mechanical ventilation and may escalate to the use of the HFOV or extracorporeal membrane oxygenation (ECMO). Immediate corrective surgery is no longer indicated and surgical intervention is typically postponed until the patient is stabilized, sometimes for days or weeks. Patients with congenital diaphragmatic hernia have a poor prognosis and typically have a long, complicated hospital stay. In patients with congenital diaphragmatic hernia, the presentation consists of scaphoid abdomen, funnel-shaped chest, and tracheal deviation to the opposite side of the affected area.

15. B) Provide oxygen

Providing oxygen to the hypoxic patient is the first priority to prevent further decompensation. Antibiotics may be indicated if the differential includes pneumonia or other causes but should be secondary to first line interventions and assessments. A CXR is a definitive part of the workup for a patient presenting with the clinical picture depicted. Immunization status is an influential component of the history obtained as it could provide essential information about protection against certain organisms.

16. D) Pulmonary angiogram

Based on the presenting history, this patient likely has an acute pulmonary embolus and the most definitive diagnostic test is a pulmonary angiogram. A D-dimer is not clinically useful in pediatrics. An ABG can provide data to help provide treatment and support but will not specifically confirm the diagnosis. Although a CXR is commonly ordered due to ease and accessibility, in cases of pulmonary embolism the film will likely be inconclusive and lead to additional work-up.

17. B) Closely monitoring laboratory studies

Close monitoring of laboratory studies and titration will ensure that therapeutic ranges are actively pursued and out of range lab values are addressed thereby minimizing the risk of the patient developing bleeding due to mismanagement of the anticoagulation. Padding the bed rails would assist in minimizing risk in a select segment of the patient population such as those with a seizure disorder, agitation, etc. Explaining the risk of bleeding to the patient is important to ensure their understanding and compliance but it is not the most significant action out of the list provided. Mouth care is essential for all patients but not a particular focus to minimize risk of bleeding.

18. B) Preoxygenate the patient, don sterile gloves, and suction the ETT

When secretions are visibly present in the ETT the patient requires suctioning. The patient should be preoxygenated to avoid any further desaturation while the ventilator circuit is disconnected for suctioning. When suctioning is performed by opening the circuit (not via in-line suctioning), sterile gloves should be donned. Care should be taken not to suction beyond the tip of the ETT. The patient may require sedation or an increase in FiO_2; however, the need for either of these interventions should be assessed further. If the patient is interfering with the ventilator or appears uncomfortable or agitated, sedation would be warranted. Increasing the FiO_2 may be indicated if clearing the secretions from the ETT does not mitigate the desaturation. If the patient continues to have worsening symptoms, the physician should be notified, but when secretions are visibly seen in the ETT, the patient should be suctioned before additional settings are adjusted. Normal saline is not routinely instilled during suctioning.

19. A 12-year-old is admitted to the pediatric ICU (PICU) after a motor vehicle accident. The patient arrives at the PICU intubated, sedated, and with a right sided pleural chest tube for a traumatic hemothorax. Shortly after arrival, the patient's father accidentally kicks over the drainage system and the collected blood spills over into the next fluid column. The appropriate intervention to correct this mistake is to:

A. Tilt the collection system to navigate the fluid back into one chamber
B. Replace the collection system
C. Manually drain the fluid from the collection system
D. Increase the suction on the drainage system

20. A 3-year-old patient intubated earlier in the day for worsening respiratory distress begins to desaturate acutely. Upon assessment of the patient, the nurse discovers that the patient is thrashing around, the end-tidal CO_2 tracing is flat, and they can hear crying around the endotracheal tube (ETT). The first action by the nurse should be to:

A. Attempt to suction the patient
B. Manually ventilate the patient via the ETT
C. Remove the ETT and manually ventilate the patient
D. Educate the family regarding sedation options

(*See answers next page.*)

19. B) Replace the collection system

Once the collected fluid spills over into another fluid column, there is no way to accurately quantify the output and the collection system must be changed. Tilting the system would not mobilize the fluid back to the correct column and it is not an appropriate intervention. The fluid cannot be manually drained from the system. Increasing the suction to the drainage system requires an order and would not move the fluid back to the correct column.

20. C) Remove the endotracheal tube (ETT) and manually ventilate the patient

Due to the assessment of desaturation, lack of end-tidal CO_2, and audible crying, it is evident that the patient has self-extubated and therefore the ETT must be removed and the patient manually ventilated to stabilize the saturations. Attempting to suction the patient is not a first-line intervention with the assessment depicted. Ventilation via the ETT is contraindicated due to the tube displacement. Family education is not a priority at this time in light of the acute desaturation.

REFERENCES

Flasch, E., Brueck, N., Lynn, J., & Henninfeld, J. (2019). Pulmonary system. In M. C. Slota (Ed). *AACN core curriculum for pediatric high acuity, progressive, and critical care nursing* (3rd ed.; pp. 35–145). Springer Publishing Company.

Kwon, J.-W. (2020). High-flow nasal cannula oxygen therapy in children: A clinical review. *Clinical and Experimental Pediatrics, 63*(1), 3–7. https://doi.org/10.3345/kjp.2019.00626

ADDITIONAL RESOURCES

Bevis, R. (2019, October). *Mechanical ventilation: weaning pediatric patients (Respiratory Therapy).* https://www.elsevier.com/__data/assets/pdf_file/0009/1000233/Mechanical-Ventilation-Weaning-Pediatric-Patients-Skill-Respiratory-Therapy-COVID-19-toolkit_070420.pdf

Chiumello, D., Papa, G. F. S., Artigas, A., Bouhemad, B., Grgic, A., Heunks, L., Markstaller, K., Pellegrino, G. M., Pisani, L., Rigau, D., Schultz, M. J., Sotgiu, G., Spieth, P., Zompatori, M., & Navalesi, P. (2019). ERS statement on chest imaging in acute respiratory failure. *European Respiratory Journal, 54*(3), 1900435. https://doi.org/10.1183/13993003.00435-2019

Eichenwald, E. C., Committee on Fetus and Newborn, Watterberg, K. L., Aucott, S., Benitz, W. E., Cummings, J. J., Goldsmith, J., Poindexter, B. B., Puopolo, K., Stewart, D. L., & Wang, K. S. American Academy of Pediatrics. (2016). Apnea of prematurity. *Pediatrics, 137*(1), e20153757. https://doi.org/10.1542/peds.2015-3757

Louisdon, P., Pringle, E. J., & Care, C. (2018). *Pediatric fundamental critical care support.* Society Of Critical Care Medicine.

Malek, R., & Soufi, S. (2021). Pulmonary edema. In *StatPearls* [Internet]. StatPearls Publishing. https://www.ncbi.nlm.nih.gov/books/NBK557611/

Nichols, D. G., & Shaffner, D. H. (2016). *Rogers' textbook of pediatric intensive care.* Wolters Kluwer.

Sanivarapu, R., & Gibson, J. (2021). Aspiration pneumonia. In *StatPearls* [Internet]. StatPearls Publishing. https://www.ncbi.nlm.nih.gov/books/NBK470459/

Slota, M. C. (2019). *AACN core curriculum for pediatric high acuity, progressive, and critical care nursing.* Springer Publishing Company.

Vyas, G. (2022). Acute pulmonary embolism. In *StatPearls* [Internet]. StatPearls Publishing. https://www.ncbi.nlm.nih.gov/books/NBK560551/

Wallbridge, P., Steinfort, D., Ren Tay, T., Irving, L., & Hew, M. (2018). Diagnostic chest ultrasound for acute respiratory failure. *Respiratory Medicine, 141*, 26–36. https://doi.org/10.1016/j.rmed.2018.06.018

Endocrine System Review

Maryann Godshall and Jennifer Cannon

The endocrine system is responsible for maintaining homeostasis by regulating:
- growth
- reproduction
- metabolism
- fluid and electrolyte balance
- coordination of the body's stress response

The components of the endocrine system include:
- **cells**: send chemical message through a hormone
- **target cells and organs**
  - receive those message
  - include blood, lymphatic system, extracellular fluids (ECF)

Hormones that influence the reabsorption/excretion of sodium to control fluid balance are:
- **antidiuretic hormone (ADH; Vasopressin)**
  - formed in hypothalamus, stored in posterior pituitary
  - increases reabsorption of water in the collecting ducts of the kidneys
  - affects water returning to the intravascular space
  - can increase blood return
  - decreases water loss in the urine
- **aldosterone**
  - secreted by the adrenal cortex and acts on the renal tubules
  - conserves sodium and water
  - decreases urine production
  - increases renal secretion of potassium and hydrogen ions
- **atrial natriuretic**
  - produced by cells of the atria of the heart
  - has vasoactive effects on blood vessels including the glomerular filtration
  - can increase urine production and salt excretion

▶ ADRENAL INSUFFICIENCY

The adrenal gland is located on top of the kidney and consists of two parts: the cortex and the medulla, with the cortex being 80% of the gland. The adrenal medulla has sympathetic and parasympathetic innervation, the cortex does not. Adrenal insufficiency is a deficiency of glucocorticoid (cortisol) and mineralocorticoids (aldosterone).

The **CORTEX** is comprised of three separate zones:

1. **zona glomerulosa:** outer most layer (15%)
   - Secretes **mineralocorticoids** and **aldosterone** in response to:
     - ❑ sodium depletion
     - ❑ decreased renal perfusion
     - ❑ dehydration
     - ❑ increased angiotensin II
     - ❑ hyperkalemia

2. **zona fasciculate**: middle layer (75%)
   - Secretes **glucocorticoids** mostly **cortisol** and small amount of androgen
     - ❑ **cortisol**
       - ○ produced and secreted by the adrenal cortex
       - ○ regulated by the anterior pituitary
       - ○ released in response to perceived stress
       - ○ decrease causes the secretion of adrenal corticotropic hormone (ACTH)
     - ❑ Inadequate response of cortisol can lead to:
       - ○ hypotension
       - ○ electrolyte imbalances
       - ○ myocardial depression
3. **zona reticularis**: innermost layer (10%)
   - Secretes androgen, estrogen, and small amount of glucocorticoids

The **MEDULLA** contains cells called chromaffin cells, which store catecholamines. Two types of catecholamines are:

- epinephrine
- norepinephrine

Both are dependent on cortisol level. They are responsible for:

- maintaining blood pressure (BP) by increasing heart rate (HR)
- vascular tone
- myocardial contractility

Clinical Pearl

Autonomic nervous system:
- *sympathetic: fight or flight*
- *parasympathetic: rest and digest*

In times of stress, the medulla is stimulated by the hypothalamus and stimulates the sympathetic centers to increase catecholamine levels in the blood. This produces a "fight or flight" reaction in the body: increased HR, BP, and glucose concentration.

Adrenal insufficiency can occur any time there is an *inadequate response to stress* perceived by the body such as, infection, trauma, illness, or surgeries. A deficiency in the cortisol and aldosterone can lead to adrenal crisis.

Aldosterone deficiency can cause:

- decrease in sodium and water reabsorption
- increased potassium reabsorption, leading to
  - profound hypotension
  - electrolyte imbalances
  - cardiac depression
  - loss of vascular tone

The two types of adrenal insufficiency are primary and secondary.

- **Primary** cause is due to the adrenal's inability to produce cortisol and aldosterone.
- **Secondary** is associated with congenital adrenal hypoplasia, adrenal hemorrhage, and tuberculous adrenalitis.

Clinical signs and symptoms include:

- hyperkalemia
- hyponatremia
- nausea, vomiting, diarrhea
- shock (from profound hypotension)
- hypoglycemia

Treatment of adrenal insufficiency:

- improve fluid status, prevent shock
- vasoactive agents
- reversal of hyperkalemia (calcium gluconate, sodium bicarb, glucose, insulin, kayexalate)
- replace glucocorticoids (stress dose hydrocortisone intravenous [IV])
- replace mineral corticoids (flurocortison [Florinef] by mouth [PO] when able)

> ### Clinical Pearl
>
> ■ *Use of etomidate in patients with adrenal insufficiency can reduce the intrinsic production of cortisol and trigger an adrenal crisis.*
> ■ *Patients with profound hypotension and shock who are not responsive to fluid and vasoactive agents should always consider adrenal insufficiency (Elshimy et al., 2022).*

▶ DIABETES INSIPIDUS

Diabetes insipidus (DI) is a condition where the body is unable to concentrate urine, leading to high volumes of dilute urine with high serum osmolality and hypernatremia. This is a result of either an insufficient secretion of ADH (central) or failure of the kidneys to respond to ADH (nephrogenic), which are the two types of DI.

■ central
  ● most common
  ● deficiency of ADH
  ● can be genetic, congenital, or acquired
■ nephrogenic
  ● normal secretion of ADH, lack of response to it
  ● distal tubule and collecting duct in the kidney are resistant to its effects
  ● most difficult form to treat
  ● can be congenital or acquired
  ● associated with renal disease
  ● caused by medications, such as:
    ❏ lithium (Lithobid, Eskalith)
    ❏ amphotericin B (Fungizone, Amphocin)
    ❏ phenytoin (Phenytek)
    ❏ diuretics
    ❏ rifampin (Rifadin)

> ### Clinical Pearl
>
> *Osmolality is a factor that regulates fluid balance between the intracellular fluid (ICF) and extracellular fluid (ECF). Normal plasma osmolality ranges from 275 to 290 mOsm/L. Sodium is the major cation (+ charged ion).*

SIGNS AND SYMPTOMS

■ high urine output of dilute or clear urine is the first sign (>4 mL/kg/hr)
■ hypernatremia
■ serum hyperosmolality occurs with osmolality >300 mOsm/kg
■ polyuria with specific gravity <1.005
■ polydipsia (if able to report)
■ signs of dehydration:
  ● low central venous pressure (CVP)
  ● tachycardia
  ● hypotension
  ● poor skin turgor
  ● dry mucous membranes
  ● weight loss
■ altered mental status with lethargy, confusion, and coma (related to sodium changes)

NURSING IMPLICATIONS AND MANAGEMENT

TREATMENT AND MANAGEMENT

■ correct dehydration and fluid deficits (isotonic fluids if in shock)
■ correct hyponatremia slowly (1–2 mEq/hr over 24 hr)

- control free water loss by kidneys
- prevent neurologic sequalae
- desmopressin (DDAVP)
- vasopressin: powerful vasoconstrictor

▶ SYNDROME OF INAPPROPRIATE SECRETION OF ANTIDIURETIC HORMONE

Syndrome of inappropriate secretion of antidiuretic hormone (SIADH) is a common disorder in pediatric critical care. Causes of SIADH include:

- central nervous system (CNS) injury
- infection
- pituitary/hypothalamus injury
- holoprosencephaly
- spinal cord disease
- liver disease

In SIADH, the body makes *too much* ADH. This will cause the body (kidneys) to hold on to water. It results in a high serum sodium level and impaired water excretion.

SIGNS AND SYMPTOMS

- low urine output related to excessive reabsorption of water (<1 mL/kg/hr)
- hyponatremia (Na <135; extra fluid on board dilutes Na)
- anorexia and fatigue
- possible nausea and vomiting
- headache, confusion, or altered level of consciousness
- weight gain without peripheral edema
- elevated CVP (6–10 cm H_2O)
- hypervolemia
- hypertension, tachycardia, and coma are late signs
- can lead to life threatening fluid and electrolyte imbalances

NURSING IMPLICATIONS AND TREATMENT

LABS AND DIAGNOSTICS

- blood chemistries
  - Na <135
  - serum osmolality <275
  - calculate by 2 × Na + (glucose/18 + blood urea nitrogen (BUN)/2.8)
- urine for electrolytes
  - urine Na >20
  - urine Osmolality >900

MANAGEMENT AND TREATMENT

- eliminate excess water
- increase serum osmolality
- fluid restrictions (30%–75% of maintenance)
- hypertonic saline (3%) for severe cases
  - initial goal of 125 to 130 mEq/L
  - Na should rise by 0.5 mEq/L/hour

Clinical Pearl

DI is HIGH: high urine output and high serum sodium
SIADH is LOW: low to no urine output and low sodium

▶ CEREBRAL SALT WASTING

Cerebral salt wasting (CSW) occurs in children with CNS diseases. A frequent cause of CSW is subarachnoid hemorrhage. Loss of renal salts causes increased urine output and decreased serum sodium.

SIGNS AND SYMPTOMS

- increased urine output
- hyponatremia (Na <135)
- dry mucous membranes
- tachycardia and poor perfusion
- weight loss and poor skin turgor

NURSING IMPLICATIONS AND TREATMENT

LABS AND DIAGNOSTICS

- blood chemistries
  - Na <135
  - serum osmolarity <280 mOsm/kg
- urine for electrolytes
  - urine sodium >40
  - urine osmolarity >100 mOsm/kg (concentrated)

TREATMENT AND MANAGEMENT

- 3% hypertonic saline intravenously (IV) to increase serum sodium
- fluid replacement with IV fluids
  Please see Table 4.1 for a comparison of DI, SIADH, and CSW.

Table 4.1: Comparing Diabetes Insipidus (DI) and Syndrome of Inappropriate Antidiuretic Hormone Secretion (SIADH) and Cerebral Salt Wasting (CSW)

	DI	SIADH	CSW
Serum sodium	↑ >145 mEq/L	↓ <135 mEq/L	↓ <135 mEq/L
Urine output	↑ >4 mL/kg/hr	↓ low	2–3 mL/kg
Serum osmolality	↑ >300 mOsm/kg	↓ <280 mOsm/kg	↓ <280 mOsm/kg
Urine osmolality	Dilute <300 mOsm/kg	Concentrated >300 mOsm/kg	Concentrated >300 mOsm/kg
Urine specific gravity	<1.005	>1.025	>1.025
BUN/creatinine	Increased	Decreased	

BUN, blood urea nitrogen; CSW, cerebral salt wasting; DI, diabetes insipidus; SIADH, syndrome of inappropriate antidiuretic hormone secretion.

▶ ACUTE HYPOGLYCEMIA

Hypoglycemia is defined as a serum blood level less than 50 mg/dL in all ages. There is an imbalance between the production and use of glucose. Glucose is the fuel for the body, especially the brain. Causes can include:

- **endogenous**: inborn errors of metabolism
- **exogenous**: alcohol or diabetic agents
- **functional**: body uses up sugar such as during a seizure

Hypoglycemia causes the stimulation of counter regulatory hormones like:

- **EGGG**:
  - Epinephrine
  - Glucagon
  - Glucocorticoids
  - Growth hormone (GH)

These hormones inhibit the storage of glucose, the formation of glycogen, glycolysis, and lipogenesis. Causes can include:

- infants of diabetic mothers (large for gestational age with macrosomia)
- small for gestational age (SGA) infants with intrauterine growth retardation
- stress or acute illness
- infants/children with no IV access and nothing by mouth (NPO) status
- increase metabolism or catabolic state
- poor nutrition of feeding habits
- medications:
  - beta blockers (block the response or release of epinephrine)
  - angiotensin-converting enzyme (ACE) inhibitors
  - sulfonylureas
  - salicylates
  - alcohol ingestion
- liver disease
- congenital hyperinsulinism (Slota, 2019)

SIGNS AND SYMPTOMS

- shakiness
- trembling
- tachycardia
- anxiety
- sweating and diaphoresis
- weakness
- hunger
- nausea and vomiting
- mental confusion
- headache
- changes in vision
- possible seizures leading to coma

NURSING IMPLICATIONS AND TREATMENT

LABS AND DIAGNOSTICS

- Blood sugar <50 mg/d in children. If glucose is measured by a glucometer, correlate with a laboratory glucose level.

TREATMENT AND MANAGEMENT

- 15 g of carbohydrate if awake and alert
- D10 (2.5 mL/kg) infant
- D25 or D50 (older child) if unconscious (watch for rebound hypoglycemia)
- Glucagon 0.5 mg intramuscular (IM) for those under 12 years old; 1 mg for those older than 12 years old
- Recheck blood glucose (BG) in 30 minutes and repeat treatment if needed.
- Identify and treat underlying cause.
- Maintain normothermia.
- Continue to monitor BG levels.
- Emergency foods for hypoglycemia include:
  - 4 oz juice or soda
  - 2 packets of sugar
  - 6 Lifesavers
  - 3 glucose tablets
  - 2 to 3 graham crackers

▶ DIABETES MELLITUS TYPES 1 AND 2

Diabetes mellitus (DM) is characterized by an absolute or relative insulin deficiency. Lack of insulin or insulin responsiveness can lead to clinical issues as a result of alterations in carbohydrate, fat, and protein metabolism. There are two main types of diabetes: type 1 and type 2.

TYPE 1 DIABETES AKA INSULIN DEPENDENT DIABETES

TYPE 1A: AUTOMIMMUNE-MEDIATED DISEASE

- 90% of cases of childhood diabetes
- T cell mediated destruction of beta cells triggered by environmental (likely viral) or genetic factors
- Clinical symptoms appear when beta cells secretion is ≤20%.
- Insulin replacement therapy is needed.

TYPE 1B: IOPATHIC DISEASE

- less common
- usually found in people of Asian or African descent
- can be a result of other diseases like pancreatitis
- Insulin replacement therapy is needed.

TYPE 2 DIABETES

TYPE 2: TYPICAL OR ATYPICAL TYPE 2 DIABETES MELLITUS

- 10% of children with diabetes
- previously referred to as adult-onset diabetes
- associated with obesity, strong family history of diabetes, and older age
- numbers rising in pediatric population related to rising obesity rates
- occurs as a result of insulin resistance
- insidious (slow) onset
- can be treated with oral agents, diet modification, and exercise

MATURITY-ONSET DIABETES OF YOUTH

- accounts for only 1% to 2% of cases
- consider in children with strong family history (two generations)
- consider in children who do not have the phenotype of classic type 2 diabetes mellitus such as obesity or acanthosis nigricans
- Six specific types of autosomal dominant mutations can occur (Slota, 2019).

▶ HYPERGLYCEMIA

The American Diabetes Association guidelines recommend the use of insulin-based treatment in hospitalized patients to achieve BG level of 140 to 180 mg/dL. Hyperglycemia in hospitalized patients correlates with poor outcomes and increased hospital length of stay.

SIGNS AND SYMPTOMS

- polyuria
- polydipsia
- blurred vision
- headache
- fatigue
- weakness
- anorexia

- abdominal pain
- flushed skin
- evidence of dehydration

Progressive deterioration may occur and lead to a decrease level of consciousness. If ketoacidosis is present, the patient may have deep and rapid breathing (Kussmaul respirations) and the breath may have a fruity odor (acetone). A fasting blood sugar (FBS) or glucose level should be monitored. Norms are:

- FBS between 70 and 100 mg/dL = normal
- FBS between 100 and 125 mg/dL = prediabetes
- FBS over 126 mg/dL = diabetes

NURSING IMPLICATIONS AND TREATMENT

LABS AND DIAGNOSTICS

- serum glucose
- fasting blood glucose level
- hemoglobin A1C: long term BG test
- test to measure pancreatic function (Urden et al., 2022)

TREATMENT AND MANAGEMENT

Treatment and management will depend on how high the patient's blood sugar measures.

- decrease blood sugar
- weight loss
- diet modifications
- medications oral hypoglycemics versus insulin
- monitoring for complications

▶ DIABETIC KETOACIDOSIS

Diabetic ketoacidosis (DKA) is a life-threatening condition where there is an absence of insulin. The body is unable to use glucose for fuel so it starts breaking down fats instead. As a result of lipolysis and overproduction of ketone bodies, such as beta-hydroxybutyrate and acetoacetates, bicarbonate buffering does not occur and there is a rusting metabolic acidosis. Counterregulatory hormones (glucagon, cortisol, catecholamines, and GH) are released in times of stress. These contribute to the hyperglycemia. Glycosuria happens with osmotic diuresis after the renal threshold for glucose is exceeded. Electrolyte loss (magnesium phosphorus, sodium) occurs secondary to diuresis. One of the biggest concerns is the loss of potassium. Hyperosmolality happens as a result of hyperglycemia and water loss with diuresis. Dehydration occurs secondary to osmotic diuresis and vomiting. The fluid shift in the body from the intracellular space to the extracellular space helps to compensate for the dehydration. Nausea and vomiting occur when related to ketoacidosis and make electrolyte imbalances worse. Increasing osmolarity puts patients at risk for developing cerebral edema and stroke (Slota, 2019).

SIGNS AND SYMPTOMS

- **serum glucose >250 to 300 mg/dL (hyperglycemia)**
- pH <7.30 **(ketoacidosis)**
- polyuria
- polydipsia
- polyphagia
- HCO_3 <15
- tachycardia
- nausea/vomiting
- **ketonuria**
- metabolic acidosis
- glycosuria
- acetone breath
- **dehydration/shock**
- Kussmaul breathing
- dry mucous membranes
- abdominal pain
- hypotension

- Na and K imbalance
- mental status changes

NURSING IMPLICATIONS AND MANAGEMENT

LAB AND DIAGNOSTICS

- serum glucose levels
- glycosuria
- pH <7.30
- ketonuria
- serum osmolality >300 mOsm/L

TREATMENT AND MANAGEMENT

Treatment Goals

- Correct fluid and electrolyte imbalances.
- Correct metabolic acidosis.
- Prevent neurological complications.
- glucose control (<180 mg/dL)

Initial Treatment

- hourly glucose monitoring
- volume replacement (start intravenous fluids before insulin therapy)
  - Normal saline solution (NSS) or Lactated Ringer's (LR; if chloride is elevated)
  - If Na >145% to 0.45% NSS
  - If Na <140 NSS
- Add glucose to IVF when glucose <300.
- Insulin drip: Start at 0.1 units/kg/hr until acidosis is resolved.
- Monitor electrolytes.
- Monitor acidosis (arterial blood gasses or venous blood gasses).
- Monitor accurate input and output.
- Glucose: **Decrease glucose levels slowly, no more than 50 to 100 mg/dL every hour.**
  - Add dextrose (use a two-bag system) if dropping to fast to prevent cerebral edema.

Preventing Cerebral Edema

This can be accomplished by dropping glucose and osmolality slowly. Avoid using $NaHCO_3$. This can increase CO_2 production and make the acidosis worse. Rehydrate slowly.

Clinical Pearl

A patient in DKA is frequently given large amounts of NSS. Careful observation by the pediatric ICU nurse should look for the development of hyperchloremic acidosis from a patient receiving too much sodium chloride intravenously. The clinical significance of hyperchloremia in DKA is still unknown and should be monitored closely (Ferreira et al., 2020).

Clinical Pearl

An anion gap is a way to check acid-base balance in the blood. It should be zero. It is designated as a + or − number on the blood gas. DKA is resolved when:
(1) plasma glucose is <200 to 250 mg/dL;
(2) serum bicarbonate concentration is ≥15 mEq/L;
(3) venous blood pH is >7.3; and
(4) anion gap is ≤12. In general, resolution of hyperglycemia, normalization of bicarbonate level, and closure of anion gap is sufficient to stop insulin infusion.

▶ INBORN ERRORS OF METABOLISM

Inborn errors of metabolism (IEMs) are rare inherited (genetic) disorders where the body cannot properly turn food consumed into energy for use. These disorders are usually characterized by a defect in a specific protein (enzyme) that help break down (metabolize) foods. They can also be characterized by defects in cellular energy production or the accumulation of toxic metabolites. IEM occurs in 1 in every 800 to 2,500 births, and most (not all) are diagnosed by state newborn screening programs (Gold et al., 2021).

The standard diagnostic approach to IEMs is to first recognize the symptoms and routine laboratory abnormalities followed by biochemical and/or genetic testing. IEMs have a wide range of presentations from acute to chronic. Clinical manifestations can arise at any time from neonatal through adulthood. Patients who present with nonspecific neurological findings, including intellectual disability, global developmental delays, or autistic spectrum disorder should follow recommendations by governing bodies like the American Academy of Neurology and Pediatrics (Liu et al., 2021). Diagnosis can be lengthy as numerous blood test must be done to both include and rule out disorders.

CLASSIFICATION OF INBORN ERRORS OF METABOLISM

IEMs are divided into three groups based on their clinical and physiologic characteristics.
- **Directly affect the synthesis or degradation of specific molecules or compounds.** This leads to excessive accumulation of a substance or compounds with intoxicating **effects** (that is, vomiting or becoming obtunded). This is exemplified by those with organic acid disorders or urea cycle defects.
- **Directly affect energy metabolism.** This disruption to the metabolic process that affects one type of fuel leads to an increased need for another type of fuel. This compensatory shift can lead to a pattern of abnormal metabolites which can be seen in these patients and is key to making the diagnosis. It also causes symptoms in organs that are more medically active like the brain (coma, brain malformations) as can be seen in respiratory chain disorders or pyruvate dehydrogenase complex deficiency.
- **Defects in the catabolism of complex molecules in the cell organelles.** These can be seen in lysosomal storage disorders or peroxisomal disorders (Kwon, 2018).

Some examples of IEM include:
- fructose intolerance
- galactosemia
- maple syrup urine disease
- phenylketonuria (most common IEM)
- fatty acid oxidation defects
- lysosomal storage disorders
- mitochondrial disorders

SIGNS AND SYMPTOMS

Signs and symptoms vary but can include:
- hypoketotic hypoglycemia
- lactic acidosis
- metabolic acidosis
- ketosis
- hyperammonemia
- metabolic acidosis in combination with hyperammonemia

Evaluating these blood and urine test results in combination with the child's clinical presentation can narrow the focus toward a particular subset of metabolic disorders (Guerrero et al., 2018).

NURSING IMPLICATIONS AND TREATMENT

LABS AND DIAGNOSTICS

Diagnosing IEM can be very difficult. Appropriate testing should be driven by a combination of the patient's symptoms and the results of "first tier" laboratory testing. This can help guide additional specific testing.
- complete blood cell count with differential
- comprehensive chemistry panel
- glucose
- liver function tests/transaminases
- renal function tests
- calcium
- uric acid

- ammonia
- lactate
- pyruvate
- urinalysis
- urine for organic acids
- urine and blood ketones
- blood gasses
- plasma amino acids
- plasma acylcarnitine profile

A critically ill neonate with a history of deterioration following an uncomplicated pregnancy, episodes of being sick, or fluctuating symptoms of lethargy may indicate the presen of an IEM. Neurological symptoms precipitated by intercurrent illness or stress, multisystem involvement, failure to thrive, developmental delay, progressive neurological signs, or bizarre neurological symptoms with or without psychological problems in patients in whom the usual etiologies have been excluded should also raise suspicion of an IEM (Guerrero et al., 2018).

TREATMENT AND MANAGEMENT

Treatment varies widely based on the results of laboratory testing. If a deficiency can be corrected, that would be the course of treatment. Some disorders may present with life-threatening conditions such as metabolic acidosis. The child should be stabilized and maintained until laboratory results are confirmed. Other children may present with mild symptoms like skin blistering after sunlight exposure and/or neurological manifestations. Treatment will depend on presenting symptomology. Remember that not all IEMs are picked up on the newborn screening, so the pediatric ICU (PICU) nurse should be alert to these conditions or latter acute presentation.

CASE STUDY

A 6-year-old was admitted to the pediatric ICU (PICU) 2 days ago after suffering a traumatic brain injury (TBI) sustained from being an unrestrained passenger in a motor vehicle collision. An external ventricular drain was placed on admission to monitor intracranial pressure (ICP). The night shift RN is receiving the report on this patient. The day shift RN reports extended periods of elevated ICPs, hypotension with mean arterial pressure (MAP) of 50, and decreased urine output. The patient was given hypertonic saline and their labs are now:

Serum sodium: 157 mEq/L with a serum osmolarity of 322 mOsm/kg
ICP: 24 mmHg
Urine output: 8 mL/kg/hr

CASE STUDY QUESTIONS

1. What is most likely the cause of the patient's symptoms?
   A. Cerebral salt wasting (CSW)
   B. Syndrome of inappropriate antidiuretic hormone (SIADH)
   C. Diabetes insipidus (DI)
   D. Diabetes mellitus (DM)

2. How would the nurse calculate this patient's cerebral perfusion pressure (CPP)?
   A. MAP – urine output = CPP
   B. MAP – ICP = CPP
   C. Serum sodium – ICP = CPP
   D. ICP – MAP = CPP

(See answers next page.)

ANSWERS TO CASE STUDY QUESTIONS

1. C) Diabetes insipidus (DI)

Patients with traumatic brain injuries (TBIs) will often experience DI as result of the injury and swelling in the brain. It can present as an elevation in serum sodium levels, serum osmolality, and a large output of dilute urine. Urine specific gravity is typically less than 1.005, urine osmolality is less than 200 mOsm/kg, and urine sodium is less than 30. Symptoms can present hours to days after injury and can be transient in nature or permanent due to unregulated antidiuretic hormone (ADH) from the pituitary.

2. B) MAP – ICP = CPP

CPP can indicate how well the brain is perfusing. Periods of increased ICP and hypotension can indicate inadequate blood flow to the brain tissue which can lead to herniation and death. The goal for CPP in children is age related. An infant should maintain a CPP greater than 40 mmHg, children greater than 50 mmHg, and adults greater than 60 mmHg.

● KNOWLEDGE CHECK: CHAPTER 4

1. The pediatric ICU (PICU) receives a report from the ED on an 8-year-old patient diagnosed with syndrome of inappropriate antidiuretic hormone secretion (SIADH). The nurse anticipates this patient presented with a chief complaint of:
   A. Tetany
   B. Hypoglycemia
   C. Excessive urine output
   D. Seizures

2. What is the importance of drawing a hemoglobin (Hgb)-A1c in the patient with diabetes mellitus (DM)?
   A. It measures the effectiveness of insulin therapy.
   B. It measures the level of insulin resistance in a patient.
   C. It provides a mean measurement of blood sugars over a 6 month period.
   D. An Hgb-A1c is not important in the management of DM.

3. Children with inborn errors of metabolism (IEMs) often have:
   A. Neurologic abnormalities
   B. Short stature
   C. Excessive weight gain
   D. Poor feeding

4. Desmopressin (DDAVP) has been ordered for a patient. What condition are is being treated?
   A. Adrenal insufficiency
   B. Hypercalcemia
   C. Diabetes insipidus (DI)
   D. Cushing syndrome

5. What is the first thing the nurse should do for patient who is admitted with diabetic ketoacidosis (DKA) who begins to complain of a severe headache and declining mental status?
   A. Elevate the head of the bed to 30 degrees.
   B. Call neurosurgery.
   C. Administer a 20 mL/kg bolus of 0.9% normal saline.
   D. Give the PRN acetaminophen that is ordered.

6. Adrenal insufficiency can be caused by:
   A. Uncontrolled hypertension
   B. Abrupt withdrawal of steroids after long term use
   C. Administering high dose insulin therapy
   D. Injury to the hypothalamus

7. An infant presents to the ED lethargic and vomiting. The mother reports the baby has not been able to keep any of their formula down for the last 12 hours. What would the RN be most concerned for in this infant?
   A. Diabetic ketoacidosis (DKA)
   B. Rotavirus
   C. Inborn errors of metabolism (IEM)
   D. Hypoglycemia

8. The adrenal cortex responds to stress by:
   A. Increasing the secretion of glucocorticoids
   B. Decreasing the secretion of aldosterone
   C. Stimulating the posterior pituitary gland
   D. Decrease catecholamine levels in the blood

(See answers next page.)

1. D. Seizures

Common symptoms of a child with SIADH include low urine output and low sodium. As a result of low sodium levels, it may precipitate seizures. Tetany and hypoglycemia are not hallmark signs of SIADH. Excessive urine output would be as a result of diabetes insipidus (DI; the opposite of SIADH).

2. C. It provides a mean measurement of blood sugars over a 6 month period.

An Hgb-A1c glycated hemoglobin is a form of hemoglobin that is chemically linked to sugar. The Hgb-A1c measures the amount of blood sugar that is attached to the hemoglobin molecule over the past 2 to 3 months. A normal Hgb-A1c is <5.7%. By monitoring this test, you can tell how well the patient is managing their blood sugar over time. It does not measure the effectiveness of insulin or the level of insulin resistance in a patient. It is very important in monitoring long term compliance in patients with DM.

3. A. Neurologic abnormalities

Children with IEM frequently have neurological abnormalities. These abnormalities of nonspecific neurological symptoms, intellectual disability, or global developmental delays frequently are a que to further work the patient up for IEM. Not all IEM are picked up on standard newborn screenings done at birth. Short stature, excessive weight gain, and poor feeding are not symptoms demonstrated by children with IEM.

4. C. Diabetes insipidus (DI)

DDAVP is used to treat DI. DDVAP is a synthetic hormone. It replaces the missing ADH and decreases urination. It can be given intravenously or intranasally. DDAVP is not used to treat adrenal insufficiency, hypercalcemia, or Cushing syndrome. Adrenal insufficiency is a lack of cortisol in the body.

5. A. Elevate the head of the bed to 30 degrees.

One of the simplest things a nurse can do to decrease intracranial pressure (ICP) in this case associated with cerebral edema from DKA is to raise the head of bed to 30 degrees. You would not want to give a bolus of intravenous (IV) fluid as that would increase ICP and cerebral edema. Neurosurgery would not be indicated initially. PRN acetaminophen would not help this increasing ICP from cerebral edema in this case and would not be the first thing done.

6. B. Abrupt withdrawal of steroids after long-term use

Adrenal sufficiency can be caused by abruptly stopping steroids. Cortisol is produced by the adrenal glands. When a person is taking steroids, it lulls the adrenals into not making as much cortisol. Steroids need to be tapered off slowly not abruptly stopped to let the adrenals wake up and make adequate amounts of cortisol. Adrenal insufficiency is not caused by uncontrolled hypertension, administering high dose insulin therapy, or injury to the hypothalamus.

7. D. Hypoglycemia

In an infant who is vomiting and unable to keep any formula down, the risk for dehydration and hypoglycemia is very high. It is not likely the infant has DKA. Rotavirus usually causes watery diarrhea. IEMs do not usually present in this manner.

8. A. Increasing the secretion of glucocorticoids

The adrenal cortex responds to stress by increasing the secretion of hormones, including adrenaline and cortisol, as well as glucocorticoids. It does not decrease the secretion of aldosterone. Aldosterone is regulated by the renin-angiotensin system and is released when there is a drop in blood pressure (BP). It does not stimulate the posterior pituitary. Catecholamines would be secreted and increased in a stress response, not decreased.

9. Impaired glucose tolerance and insulin resistance are characteristic of what endocrine disorder?
   A. Type 1 diabetes mellitus
   B. Addison disease
   C. Type 2 diabetes mellitus
   D. Pancreatitis

10. A mother says her 6-week-old has been extremely lethargic, will not eat, and has lost weight. The nurse notices a dysmorphic presentation of the head. The baby had a normal newborn screen. They are being worked up for a possible inborn error of metabolism (IEM). Which of the following tests would the nurse anticipate being ordered?
    A. Ammonia level
    B. Cardiac enzymes
    C. An upper gastrointestinal (GI) series
    D. Stool for viral panel

(See answers next page.)

9. C. Type 2 diabetes mellitus

Impaired glucose tolerance and resistance are indicative of type 2 diabetes mellitus (DM). In type 1, insulin is not produced. Pancreatitis decreases the amount of insulin released. Addison disease is a disorder as a result of adrenal insufficiency.

10. A. Ammonia level

An ammonia level is typical in an IEM that affects amino acid transport. Ammonia is formed in the body when proteins are broken down. This would explain why the infant is not gaining weight and possibly not tolerating formula. A high level of ammonia could lead to seizures. Cardiac enzymes would not be correct in this situation. An upper GI series would be done if a GI issue was suspected like reflux. A stool for viral panel would be done if a viral illness was suspected. In this question it indicates the child was being worked up for an IEM. A "normal" newborn screen does not rule out all IEMs.

REFERENCES

Elshimy, G., Chippa, V., & Jeong, J. (2022). *Adrenal crisis. In StatPearls* [Internet]. StatPearls Publishing. https://www.ncbi.nlm.nih.gov/books/NBK499968/#_NBK499968_pubdet_

Ferreira, J. P., Hamui, M., Torrents, M., Carrano, R., Ferraro, M., & Toledo, I. (2020). The influence of chloride for the interpretation of plasma bicarbonate during the treatment of diabetic ketoacidosis. *Pediatric Emergency Care, 36*(3), e143–e145. https://doi.org/10.1097/PEC.0000000000001245

Gold, N., Kritzer, A., Weiner, D., & Michelson, K. (2021). Emergency laboratory evaluations for patients with inborn errors of metabolism. *Pediatric Emergency Care, 37*(12), e1154–1159.

Gosmanov, A., Gosmanova, E., & Dillard-Cannon, E., (2014). Management of adult diabetic ketoacidosis. *Diabetes Metabolic Syndrome & Obesity, Dove Press, 7*, 255–264. https://doi.org/10.2147/DMSO.S50516

Guerrero, R., Salazar, D., & Tanpaiboon, P. (2018). Laboratory diagnostic approaches in metabolic disorder. *Annals of Translational Medicine, 6*(24), 470. https://doi.org/10.21037/atm.2018.11.05

Kwon, J. (2018). Testing for inborn errors of metabolism. *Child Neurology, 24*(1), 37–56.

Liu, N., Xiao, J., Gijavanekar, C., Pappan, K. L., Glinton, K. E., Shayota, B. J., Kennedy, A. D., Sun, Q., Sutton, V. R., & Elsea, S. H. (2021). Comparison of untargeted metabolomic profiling vs traditional metabolic screening to identify inborn errors of metabolism. *JAMA Network Open/Pediatrics, 4*(7), e2114155. https://doi.org/10.1001/jamanetworkopen.2021.14155

Ning, L., Xiao, J., Gijavanekar, C., Pappan, K., Glinton, K., Shayotia, B., Kennedy, A., Sun, Q., Sutton, V., & Elsea, S. (2021). Comparison of untargeted metabolomic profiling vs traditional metabolic screening to identify inborn errors of metabolism. *JAMA Network Open, 4*(7), e2114155. https://doi.org/10.1001/jamanetworkopen.2021.14155

Slota, M. C. (2019). *AACN core curriculum for pediatric high acuity, progressive, and critical care nursing* (3rd ed.). Springer Publishing Company.

Urden, L., Stacy, K., & Lough, M. (2022). *Critical care nursing: Diagnosis and management* (9th ed.). Elsevier.

Hematology and Immunology Review

Emily D. Johnson

Hematologic disorders affect the production of blood and its components including blood cells, blood proteins such as hemoglobin (Hgb), platelets, methods of coagulation, and bone marrow. **Immunologic disorders** affect the components of the immune system including lymphocytes, phagocytes, and compliment. **Hematopoiesis** is the process by which blood cells are formed.

Primary sites of hematopoiesis vary throughout one's lifespan. Hemopoietic stem cells undergo a complex process of differentiation creating mature and functional red blood cells (RBCs), white blood cells (WBCs), and platelets. Growth factors and cytokines such as erythropoietin, thrombopoietin, and granulocyte colony stimulating factor guide this process. Five committed **precursor cell** types exist: proerythroblasts, megakaryoblasts, myoblasts, monoblasts, and lymphoblasts. These precursor cells further differentiate into their more commonly known counterparts:

- proerythroblasts → erythrocytes (RBCs)
- megakaryoblasts → thrombocytes (platelets)
- myoblasts → granulocytes (neutrophils, eosinophils, and basophils, types of WBCs)
- monoblasts → monocytes (type of WBC)
- lymphoblasts → lymphocytes (type of WBC).

Congenital and acquired hematologic disorders can occur at any point of differentiation in any cell line.

Plasma factors describe more than 40 different substances in the blood, some with procoagulant properties and other anticoagulant properties, that contribute to the clotting cascade. Many of these proteins are produced in the liver and require vitamin K for adequate synthesis. Proper coagulation depends on a balance between these substances, with a natural predominance toward anticoagulation until vessel or tissue injury occurs. Names of coagulation factors are listed in Table 5.1.

WBCs serve as the interconnections between the hematologic and immunologic systems, as they are created in the bone marrow and provide crucial pieces of the body's immune response upon maturation.

Table 5.1 Procoagulant and Anticoagulant Factors

Procoagulants	Anticoagulants
Factor Proteins	Antithrombin III
I- Fibrinogen	Protein C*
II- Prothrombin*	Protein S*
III- Tissue factor	
IV- Calcium	
V- Proaccelerin	
VI- Accelerin	
VII- Proconvertin*	
VIII- Antihemophiliac	
IX- Christmas factor	
X- Stuart-Prower factor	
XI- Plasma thromboplastin antecedent*	
XII- Hageman factor	
XIII- Protransglutaminase	

*Needs vitamin K for synthesis

Source: Slota, M. (Ed.). (2019). *AACN core curriculum for pediatric high acuity, progressive, and critical care nursing* (3rd ed.). Springer Publishing Company.

Immune system functions are divided into innate and adaptive responses, with adaptive immunity being further divided into humoral and cell-mediated forms.

Innate immunity is characterized as rapid system of self versus non-self-recognition by granulocytes and serves as the first line of defense against infectious microorganisms and malignant degeneration. Innate immunity also maintains the balance between the proinflammatory mechanisms of host defense and the anti-inflammatory responses that return the host to a healthy baseline. **Adaptive immunity** is a more specific immune response mediated by lymphocytes. Within adaptive immunity, **humoral immunity** refers to antibody production and the coinciding processes that accompany it. Plasma cells, derived from B lymphocytes synthesize five different types of antibodies, IgG, IgA, IgM, IgD, IgE, also called immunoglobulins (Igs). Humoral immunity is important for protection from encapsulated pyogenic bacteria. **Cell-mediated immunity** is mediated by T lymphocytes. Cytotoxic T cells interact directly with and secrete substances into microorganisms leading to cellular destruction. Cell-mediated immunity is important in the elimination of cells infected with pathogens that replicate intracellularly (e.g., viruses, mycobacteria, and some bacteria) and cells exhibiting aberrant differentiation.

The **complement system** works through innate and adaptive immunity to locally destroy microorganisms. It consists of nine plasma proteins, C1 to C9, and can be activated by three independent pathways: classical, alternative, and lectin (Spruit, 2019). Conditions that lead to dysregulation within these complex systems will be discussed in this chapter.

▶ MYELOSUPRESSION

Myelosuppression is a general term for decreased bone marrow activity resulting in fewer RBCs, WBCs, and platelets. It can be a symptom of acquired disease such as malignancy or infection, a side effect of medication such as chemotherapy, as well as a result of an inherited bone marrow failure syndrome. Myelosuppression is classified by the cell lineage affected:

- erythopenia—decreased RBCs
- thrombocytopenia—decreased platelets
- leukopenia—decreased WBCs
- pancytopenia—decrease in all cell lines
  Common types of myelosuppression are described as follows.

▶ ANEMIA

Anemia is one of the most common blood disorders in pediatrics. It represents an imbalance between the production and removal of RBCs. RBCs typically survive for 120 days before they are removed from circulation by the phagocytic cells in the liver and spleen. About 1% of circulating RBCs are cleared from the blood stream each day, necessitating reticulocytes and immature RBCs to be continually produced and released from the bone marrow at the same rate. When a deficit in circulating RBCs occurs, the body's oxygen carrying capacity is compromised. In pediatrics, anemia is defined as a reduction in hematocrit (Hct) or Hgb by more than two standard deviations below the mean for relative age, sex, and ethnicity. For RBC indices, the lower limit of normal is critically dependent on the population used to establish the normal range of values (Brugnara et al., 2015).

Anemia can have significant and long-standing consequences, especially in critically ill children. These complications can be acute and life-threatening, such as hemorrhagic shock or sickle cell crisis, as well as lifelong such as chronic fatigue and neurodevelopmental disabilities. Iron deficiency remains the most common cause of anemia worldwide (Warner & Kamran, 2021).

Clinical Pearl

Anemia is a symptom of an underlying process rather than a disease itself.

Anemia is reflective of either impaired production or increased destruction of RBCs, or blood loss. Common etiologies are listed in Table 5.2.

Table 5.2 Etiology of Anemia Classified by Functional Defect

Functional Defect	Etiology of Anemia
Impaired production of RBCs	Bone marrow pathology—Diamond-Blackfan, aplastic anemia, malignancy Chronic kidney disease Hypothyroidism Infection Inflammation Lead poisoning Nutrient deficiencies—folate, iron, vitamin B_{12} Thalassemia
Increased destruction of RBCs	Hemolytic anemias Defects in RBC membrane integrity—spherocytosis, elliptocytosis Defects in RBC metabolism—G6PD deficiency, PK deficiency Disorders of Hgb—sickle cell disease Hypersplenism Immune mediated Infection Lead poisoning Microangiopathic
Blood loss	Acute—hemorrhage, surgery, trauma Chronic—heavy menstrual bleeding, gradual losses through gastrointestinal and genitourinary systems, phlebotomy

RBCs, red blood cells; G6PD, glucose-6-phosphate dehydrogenase; Hgb, hemoglobin; PK, pyruvate kinase.
Source: Brugnara, C., Oski, F. A., & Nathan, D. G. (2015). *Nathan and Oski's hematology and oncology of infancy and childhood* (8th ed.). Saunders, an imprint of Elsevier Inc.

During anemic states, healthy bone marrow increases immature RBC production through a process known as reticulocytosis. The absolute **reticulocyte count** is helpful in understanding the underlying pathogenic process for the anemia. Anemia with reticulocytosis shows that the bone marrow is undergoing hematopoiesis so blood loss or peripheral destruction of the RBCs is likely. Anemia without reticulocytosis indicates a poor bone marrow response, which is more indicative for nutritional deficiencies, infection, or other causes of bone marrow suppression. Anemia can present independently or be a component of other hematologic pathologies, such as pancytopenia seen in certain malignancies.

SIGNS AND SYMPTOMS

- Fever, weight loss, and night sweats are associated with anemia caused by malignancy.
- Jaundice, scleral icterus, hepatosplenomegaly, and dark urine are associated with hemolytic processes.
- Pica, neurodevelopmental, and cognitive disabilities are seen with iron deficiency anemia and can permanent even after iron stores are repleaded.
- In critical illness, anemia contributes to hypoxia and hypovolemia leading to impaired tissue perfusion.
  See Table 5.3 for additional signs and symptoms.

Table 5.3 Symptoms and Laboratory Findings Consistent With Anemia

Abnormal RBC Indices	Evidence of Hemolysis	Patient Symptoms

↓ HCT/Hgb
↓ or ↑ MCV
↓ or ↑ MCH
Variation in RBC size (RDW)
↓ or ↑ reticulocyte count
Atypical findings on peripheral
  smear—sickle cells, spherocytes,
  schistocytes, Heinz bodies, etc.
	↑ LDH
	↓ haptoglobin
	↑ unconjugated/indirect bilirubin
	Hgb in urinalysis
	Positive Coombs test/DAT
		Tachycardia ± hypotension
		Dyspnea
		Tachypnea
		Hypoxia
		Fatigue
		Decreased exercise tolerance
		Pallor
		Dizziness
		Irritability
		Headache
		Pica

DAT, direct antiglobulin test; HCT, hemocrit; Hgb, hemoglobin; LDH, lactate dehydrohenase; MCH, mean corpuscular hemoglobin; MCV, mean corpuscular volume; RBC, red blood cell; RDW, red cell distribution width.
Source: Slota, M. (Ed.). (2019). *AACN core curriculum for pediatric high acuity, progressive, and critical care nursing* (3rd ed.). Springer Publishing Company; Brugnara, C., Oski, F. A., & Nathan, D. G. (2015). *Nathan and Oski's hematology and oncology of infancy and childhood* (5th ed.). Saunders, an imprint of Elsevier Inc.

NURSING IMPLICATIONS AND TREATMENT

In pedatric ICU (PICU) patients, nursing assessment and management targets the complications of anemia associated with diminished oxygen carrying capacity, altered tissue perfusion, and altered fluid volume. Depending on the acuity and rapidity of onset, children can present in varying degrees of extremis. If anemia develops gradually, compensatory mechanisms such as expanding plasma volume can blunt hemodynamic compromise. However, if anemia develops more rapidly dyspnea, tachycardia, and hypotension may be more pronounced. Restoring oxygen carrying capacity is crucial and depends on adequate Hgb and oxygen availability in the bloodstream. Decreasing physiologic oxygen demand by reducing fear and anxiety can be helpful. The semi-Fowlers position is optimal as it minimizes ventilation-perfusion mismatch (Spruit, 2019).

Administering blood products and oxygen as ordered is key. Blood transfusions aren't without risks, as studies utilizing liberal transfusion protocols have shown increased morbidity and mortality in PICU patients compared to more judicious controls (Steffen et al., 2017). Nurses should utilize methods preventing iatrogenic anemia caused by phlebotomy and large amounts of blood required for diagnostic procedures. Evaluation of G6PD, Hgb electrophoresis, and iron studies should be considered. In certain situations, such as end-stage renal disease (ESRD), administering erythropoietin 1 to 3 times a week to stimulate endogenous RBC production is needed (Spruit, 2019). Descriptions of blood products, their components, indications, and administration implications are provided in Table 5.4.

Table 5.4 Blood Product Components, Indications, and Administration Implications

Blood Product	Components	Indications	Administration

Whole blood	RBCs, WBCs, platelets,
	  plasma
		Massive blood loss,
		  hypovolemic shock
			Not frequently given
			Dose is 20 mL/kg
			Given as fast as tolerated
			Can be warmed, irradiated, and
			  leukocyte-reduced
			Platelets, WBCs, and clotting factors aren't
			  functional

PRBCs	RBC concentrate
	  separated from
	  plasma
	Small amounts
	  of leukocytes,
	  platelets, and
	  clotting factors
	  present
		Anemia, hypovolemia	Dose is 10–20 mL/kg
			Multiple transfusions can result in dilution
			  of clotting factors and hypocalcemia
			Can be leukocyte-reduced and irradiated
			Wait 4–6 hrs to recheck HCT

(*continued*)

Table 5.4 Blood Product Components, Indications, and Administration Implications (*continued*)

Blood Product	Components	Indications	Administration
Platelets	Platelet concentrate separated from RBCs and plasma	Thrombocytopenia, active bleeding, abnormal platelet function	Random platelets indicate units collected from multiple donors, which increases antigen exposure Pheresed platelets indicate units collected from a single donor Reactions include fever, rash, puritis and bleeding With limited RBC component, blood type (ABO) incompatibility is often well tolerated
FFP	Plasma portion of blood separated from blood cell components Contains all clotting factors in near normal concentrations	Deficiency in clotting factors such as DIC, liver failure, dilution from massive PRBC transfusions Should only be used for volume expansion if coagulopathy is present	Maximal infusion rate of 1 mL/kg/min Must be ABO compatible Can cause hypocalcemia
WBCs	Concentrated leukocytes	Augment current infection fighting measures Questionable benefit	Dose 10–15 mL/kg Infused over 2–4 hrs G-CSF administered prior Reaction includes chills, rash, dyspnea Considered most frequently for immunocompromised patient populations
Cryoprecipitate	Prepared from plasma and contains fibrinogen, factor VIII, VWF, factor XIII and fibronectin	Active bleeding, low fibrinogen, DIC	Dose is 1 unit/10 kg of body weight Units are smaller volume compared to other blood products, can be administered IV push over a few minutes
Albumin	Liquid preparation of albumin derived from pools of human plasma Available in 5% and 25% preparations	Hypovolemia, hypoproteinemia	Dose 5%—10–20 mL/kg can be given as fast as tolerated Dose 25%—2–4 mL/kg given over 2–4 hrs, often followed by diuretics No infectious risks Must use within 6 hrs of spiking container
IVIG	Concentrate of the pooled immunoglobulins derived from 1,000 to 100,000 healthy donors Composition closely corresponds with normal immunoglobulin levels human plasma—primarily IgG (90%), IgA, other Igs, cytokines, and soluble receptors	Immunodeficiencies, immunomodulation for autoimmune and inflammatory conditions, hyperimmune therapy for specific infections agents	Given slowly over several hrs with the rate upward titrated over 15–30 minutes Typically, a large volume infusion, so can cause hypervolemia Side effects typically mild such as headache Anaphylaxis can occur

(continued)

Table 5.4 Blood Product Components, Indications, and Administration Implications (*continued*)

Blood Product	Components	Indications	Administration
Exchange transfusion	RBCs and/or platelets are removed and then replaced with transfused cells	Sickle cell disease, hyperbilirubinemia	Can be done manually or by pheresis
Plasmapheresis	Plasma is separated from blood cell components and either treated then returned to circulation or replaced with albumin or FFP	Autoimmune antibody removal, inflammatory cytokine removal, and many other acute self-limiting disease processes	Side effects include hypotension, bradycardia, hypocalcemia, chills, nausea, fever, uticaria, and bleeding

DIC, disseminated intravascular coagulation; FFP, fresh flozen plasma; G-CSF, granulocyte colony stimulating factor; HCT, hemocrit; IVIG, intravenous immunoglobin; PRBCs, packed red blood cells; RBCs, red blood cells; WBCs, white blood cells.
Source: Slota, M. (Ed.). (2019). *AACN core curriculum for pediatric high acuity, progressive, and critical care nursing* (3rd ed.). Springer Publishing Company.

▶ NEUTROPENIA

Neutropenia is a specific type of leukopenia affecting granulocytes. It is characterized by an absolute neutrophil count of 1,000 per mm^3 or less, severe neutropenia is 500 per mm^3 or less.

Clinical Pearl

Absolute neutrophil count (ANC) = (% neutrophils + % bands) × (total WBC)/100
WBC: 4,300/μL
Neutrophil/granulocyte: 35%
Neutrophilic bands: 3%
((35 + 3) × (4,300))/100
(38 × 4,300)/100
163,400/100
ANC = 1,634 (not neutropenic)
A normal ANC is over 1,000.

Febrile neutropenia is often discovered incidentally during the investigation of febrile illnesses amongst immunocompetent children. This type of neutropenia is usually transient, without serious complications, and follows typical viral and bacterial illness timelines. Patients at particular risk for life-threatening infection from neutropenic fever include those using chemotherapeutic agents or other medications that alter immune function, patients with certain infections, such as HIV, or individuals with congenital or acquired immune-deficiency states (Wittmann et al., 2018). Common pathogens include viruses, fungi, and gram-positive bacteria such as *Staphylococcus*, *Streptococcus*, and *Enterococcus* species. Drug-resistant organisms, including *Pseudomonas aeruginosa*, *Acinetobacter* species, *Stenotrophomonas maltophilia*, *Escherichia coli*, and *Klebsiella* species, have also been identified as infectious agents. Infections with gram negative organisms have higher mortality rates than all other causes of infection (Grace, 2015).

SIGNS AND SYMPTOMS

Neutropenic patients at risk for life-threatening infections often have a limited ability to counter an effective immune response. Children present atypically with pain, altered temperature (hypo- or hyperthermia), and subtle changes in vital signs being the only symptoms. Other systemic clinical signs are tachycardia, tachypnea, confusion, irritability, rigors, chills, decreased level of activity, and malaise. CBC reveals a decreased total WBC count with differential revealing abnormally low neutrophils and increased monocytes. Neutropenia's are defects within the myeloid cell lines, so lymphocytes aren't always affected. Site specific tests reveal positive abnormalities such as infiltration on chest x-ray (CXR; Spruit, 2019).

NURSING IMPLICATIONS AND TREATMENT

After ensuring a clean and safe environment for the neutropenic patient, promoting optimal skin and mucosal integrity is the goal of preventative nursing care. Critically ill children are at higher risk for altered skin integrity related to decreased oxygenation/tissue perfusion, inadequate nutrition, immunosuppression, immobility, and the use of invasive procedures and technology (Spruit, 2019). Nurses should observe patients closely for signs and symptoms of septic shock by monitoring vital signs, peripheral perfusion, and intake and output. The patient's neurologic status is also monitored closely because lethargy, irritability, or a change in consciousness can indicate sepsis. Antimicrobial medications should be administered as ordered within 60 minutes of presentation.

Collaborate with physician colleagues and explore whether enteral nutrition is appropriate to decrease likelihood of bacterial translocation. Rectal temperatures and suppositories are avoided in all neutropenic patients based on the risk for tearing the anal mucosa and introducing bacteria (Dinauer et al., 2015).

Antipyretics can decrease fever and increase comfort, both of which decrease physiologic oxygen and metabolic demands. Discuss with provider if these are appropriate.

Administer **granulocyte colony stimulating factor (G-CSF)** if indicated. G-CSF is a naturally occurring cytokine/glycoprotein that guides hematopoiesis by stimulating the bone marrow to produce granulocytes and stem cells to be released into the blood stream. In patients with primary and acquired neutropenias, a recombinant form of G-CSF is administered to augment granulocyte production and differentiation. Daily administration of G-CSF is needed lifelong for those affected with congenital neutropenia. In patients at high risk for febrile neutropenia after chemotherapy, G-CSF is commonly administered to decrease the amount of time and severity of neutropenia, thus decreasing infection risks. Filgrastim agents are shorter acting and usually given daily. Pegfilgrastim agents are longer acting and usually given weekly (Mehta et al., 2015).

There are different types of G-CSF, including:

- lenograstim (Granocyte)
- filgrastim (Neupogen, Zarzio, Nivestim, Accofil)
- long acting (pegylated) filgrastim (pegfilgrastim, Neulasta, Pelmeg, Ziextenco) and lipegfilgrastim (Lonquex)

▶ THROMBOCYTOPENIA

The normal circulating platelet count for all ages ranges from 150,000 to 400,000/μL. Circulating platelets constitute two-thirds of total body platelets; the remaining platelets are located within the spleen. The average life span of platelets is 7 to 10 days, although survival of transfused platelets in a thrombocytopenic recipient is reduced proportionately to the severity of the thrombocytopenia. Causes of thrombocytopenia in pediatrics fall into three broad categories:

- platelet sequestration
- increased platelet destruction
- decreased platelet production

Etiologies are further described in Table 5.5 (Wilson, 2015).

Table 5.5 Etiology of Thrombocytopenia Classified by Functional Defect

Functional Defect	Etiology of Thrombocytopenia
Sequestration	Hypersplenism, hypothermia, burns
Increased destruction	Immune thrombocytopenias, HIV, drug induced, posttransfusion, infection, anaphylaxis, thrombotic microangiopathic, Von Willibrand's disease, DIC, HLH
Decreased production	Hereditary thrombocytopenias, aplastic anemia, radiation or drug induced, neonatal hypoxia or placental insufficiency, marrow infiltrative processes

DIC, disseminated intravascular coagulation; HLH, hemophagocytic lymphohistiocytosis.
Source: Brugnara, C., Oski, F. A., & Nathan, D. G. (2015). *Nathan and Oski's hematology and oncology of infancy and childhood* (8th ed.). Saunders, an imprint of Elsevier Inc.

SIGNS AND SYMPTOMS

Clinical signs of thrombocytopenia include:
- petechiae
- ecchymoses
- prolonged bleeding at incision or venipuncture sites
- epistaxis
- gastrointestinal hemorrhage
- hematuria
- menorrhagia
- intracranial hemorrhage may occur but is rare (Wilson, 2015).

There is a lack of direct correlation between the platelet count and the risk of bleeding episodes. The risk of hemorrhage is affected by many factors, such as coexisting coagulation defects, trauma, and surgery. In older children and adults, serious spontaneous bleeding does not occur until the platelet count is less than 20,000/μL. The risk for severe bleeding is more likely in children with a defect in production than those with a destructive platelet problem (Wilson, 2015).

NURSING IMPLICATIONS AND TREATMENT

Nurses regularly assess a thrombocytopenic patient's risk for bleeding and communicate any pertinent laboratory findings or symptoms to the clinical team. Factors that determine platelet administration thresholds are platelet count, risk for bleeding, active bleeding, and underlying physiology. Patients receiving platelets are monitored carefully during and after the transfusion for signs of transfusion reaction (Branowicki et al., 2015).

Pharmacologic treatments to increase platelet production have evolved over the last 10 years. Cloning thrombopoietin, the natural cytokine/hormone that guides megakaryocyte production and maturation, has proven to be difficult. However over the last decade, **two thrombopoietin receptor agonists** (Romiplostim and Eltrombopag) have proven to be effective in increasing platelet numbers and production. These agents are U.S. Food and Drug Administration (FDA) approved for treatment of specific refractory autoimmune platelet disorders and are considered for cases of severe thrombocytopenia in other populations such as hematopoietic stem cell transplant (HSCT) patients (Ghanima et al., 2019).

▶ DISORDERS OF HEMOSTASIS

As stated earlier, proper coagulation depends on a balance between procoagulation factors and anticoagulation factors within the bloodstream. There is a natural predominance toward anticoagulation until vessel or tissue injury triggers the clotting cascade. The blood clotting process requires the presence of platelets, von Willebrand factor (VWF; which is released from platelets and blood vessel endothelium), and clotting factors synthesized in the liver. Inactivated forms of clotting factors are present in the bloodstream at all times. Each procoagulation factor, factors I-XIII, perform a specific step in the coagulation process. The activation of one clotting factor activates the next clotting factor.

Two traditional pathways for clot activation exist: intrinsic and extrinsic. The terminal step in both pathways is the same: activation of factor X, and the conversion of prothrombin → thrombin, which converts fibrinogen → fibrin, which allows stable clot formation. The intrinsic pathway is slower and stimulated when blood comes in contact with collagen from an injured blood vessel wall. The extrinsic pathway activates more quickly in response to tissue factors released during tissue injury or trauma. Clot dissolution, which is fibrinolysis, is the final step in the clotting cascade, which prevents excess clot formation (Gaspard, 2009). Anticoagulation factors inactivate the above procoagualtion factors and inactivate thrombin, thus providing protection against uncontrolled thrombus (Gaspard, 2009). The disorders of hemostasis and the clotting cascade is illustrated in more detail in Figure 5.1. Primary or acquired defects within any pieces of the clotting cascade lead to pathologic hyper or hypocoaguable states.

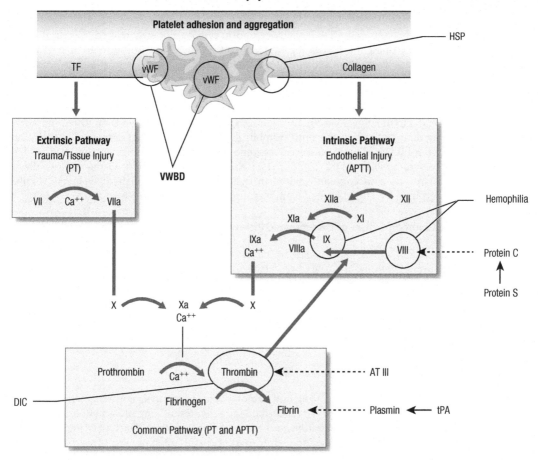

Figure 5.1 Disorders of hemostasis and the clotting cascade
After tissue injury, platelets arrive at the site and adhere to the blood vessel wall with the aid of von Willibrand factor (VWF), which is released from the blood vessel endothelium and platelet granules. Shortly after platelet aggregation, the clotting cascade is activated via two simultaneous pathways both terminating in a common pathway with factor X activation. The intrinsic pathway is stimulated by blood coming in contact with endothelia collagen, while the extrinsic pathway is activated by tissue factors released from the injured tissue. The intrinsic pathway activates factor XII, which then activates factor XI, which then in conjunction with factor VIII activates factor IX. Activated factor IX combines with calcium to form factor X. The activated partial thromboplastin time (APTT) laboratory test reflects the factors in this pathway. After activation by tissue factors, the extrinsic pathway uses calcium to activate factor VII, which then forms factor X. The PT laboratory test reflects the factors in this pathway. With the help of calcium, factor X activation commences the common pathway, reflected in both APTT and PT laboratory tests. Prothrombin is converted into thrombin, which then converts fibrinogen into fibrin. Thrombin also aids in the activation of other clotting factors in the intrinsic pathway, such as factor VIII. The final steps in hemostasis are the fibrinolytic pathway. Antithrombin III deactivates and breaks down thrombin. Tissue plasminogen activators convert plasminogen to plasmin, which breaks down fibrin. Protein C deactivates factor VIII and other clotting factors. Protein S accelerates the effectiveness of protein C. Disorders discussed in the next part of this chapter affect different steps of the clotting cascade. Von Willibrand diseases affect the availability and function of von Willibrand factor, which is crucial for platelet aggregation. Henoch Scholein Purpura is a form of vasculitis, which contributes to blood vessel injury. Hemophilia affects clotting factors VIII and IX. Disseminated intravascular coagulation (DIC) reflects a breakdown of multiple levels of the clotting cascade but begins with a dysregulation of thrombin.

Sources: Norris, T. L. (2019). *Pathophysiology concepts of altered health states* (8th ed.). Wolters Kluwer Health; Slota, M. (Ed.). (2019). *AACN core curriculum for pediatric high acuity, progressive, and critical care nursing* (3rd ed.). Springer Publishing Company.

▶ DISSIMINATED INTRAVASCULAR COAGULATION

Dissiminated intravascular coagulation (DIC) is a severe form of coagulopathy related to critical illness. It is a failure of normal hemostatic mechanisms characterized by widespread and unregulated activation of the coagulation sequence with a subsequent decrease in clotting factors and platelets leading to uncontrolled systemic bleeding. Simultaneous thrombo-embolic complications and bleeding lead to multiorgan dysfunction and failure (Levi & van der Poll, 2017).

Rather than a primary coagulation disorder, DIC is a result of numerous processes affecting critically ill children. In normal circumstances, activation of coagulation is controlled by three important physiological anticoagulant pathways: the antithrombin system, the activated protein C system, and tissue factor pathway inhibitor. These pathways become deranged in conditions that trigger DIC. Neonates are the most vulnerable to DIC compared to older infants and children due to low plasma reserves of procoagulant and anticoagulant factors in their developing hemostatic systems (Veldman et al., 2010). Common causes for DIC classified by age group are listed in Table 5.6.

Table 5.6 Common Causes of Dissiminated Intravascular Coagulation by Age Group

Age Group	Causes of DIC
Neonates	Sepsis, severe hypoxia, single twin demise, hypothermia, acidosis
Older infants and children	Sepsis, trauma, burn, crush injury, severe hypoxia, malignancy, toxins/snake venoms, liver disease, Reyes syndrome, transfusion reaction, transplant rejection, autoimmune disease

Source: Rajagopal, R., Thachil, J., & Monagle, P. (2017). Dissiminated intravascular coagulation in paediatrics. *Archives of Disease in Childhood, 102*(2), 187–193. https://doi.org/10.1136/archdischild-2016-311053.

SIGNS AND SYMPTOMS

Clinical signs of DIC are reflective of the clotting and hemorrhagic components occurring simultaneously. For clotting, the triggering endothelial injury or tissue damage activates inflammatory cytokines leading to increased thrombin generation, platelet activation, and pro-coagulation factors. The typical anticoagulation regulation pathways are also impaired, causing a shift to a procoagulant state. With this, fibrin thrombi rapidly accumulate in the microvascular causing ischemic tissue injury and impaired end-organ function. Clotting symptoms of DIC include bruising, cool mottled skin, pallor, and circulatory collapse.

Thrombosis in the peripheral vasculature can cause diminished pulses, cyanosis of fingers, toes, nose, earlobes, tissue necrosis, and gangrene (Spruit, 2019). Thrombosis within organs such as the brain, liver, kidneys, gastrointestinal (GI), and lungs can cause functional damage including altered mental status, jaundice, decreased urine output, mesenteric infarction, intrabdominal bleeding, and difficulty breathing.

For bleeding, endothelial injury concurrently activates the fibrinolytic pathway via tissue plasminogen activators, which can contribute to the hemorrhagic component of DIC. However, the bleeding seen with DIC is more reflective of a *consumptive coagulopathy*, meaning fibrinogen, platelets, and clotting factors are consumed at too rapid a pace for stable clot formation to occur at injured sites, thus predisposing to systemic bleeding. Bleeding symptoms include prolonged oozing from venipuncture sites and invasive devices such as endotracheal tubes and urinary catheters. Subtle to occult hemorrhage can occur from any orifice.

Nurses should be aware of symptoms of bruising, gingival bleeding, hematuria, hematemesis, melana, headache, loss of consciousness, and shock (Spruit, 2019). *No single laboratory test confirms the diagnosis of DIC.* Common laboratory abnormalities include thrombocytopenia, prolonged prothrombin time (PT) and partial thromboplastin time (PTT), decreased fibrinogen, elevated d-dimer and fibrinogen degradation products, and markedly decreased levels of protein C, S, and antithrombin. This scoring system has a sensitivity and specificity greater than 90%; however, it can only be applied to children with an identified underlying cause for DIC (Spruit, 2019).

NURSING IMPLICATIONS AND TREATMENT

Nursing interventions target treating the underlying cause of DIC and supporting vital organ function. Early detection and prompt management of underlying disorders can prevent complications and death. Treatment begins when children become symptomatic rather than on laboratory values alone. Maintaining mucous membrane integrity, monitoring for internal bleeding, and controlling overt bleeding is standard.

Administering blood products as ordered to replace depleted clotting factors, fibrinogen, and platelets is crucial. In cases of hemorrhagic shock, blood products with an RBC component such as whole blood act as volume expanders while increasing oxygen carrying capacity through increasing Hgb levels. Blood product administration with goal laboratory values are in Table 5.7.

Table 5.7 Goals for Blood Product Replacement in Dissiminated Intravascular Coagulation

Blood Product	Goal Range
Platelets	Platelets >50,000/mm^3
Cryoprecipitate	Fibrinogen >1.5 g/L
FFP	PT values < double normal range
PRBCs	Hgb >10 g/dL

FFP, fresh frozen plasma; Hgb, hemoglobin; PRBCs, packed red blood cells; PT, prothrombin time.
Source: Slota, M. (Ed.). (2019). *AACN core curriculum for pediatric high acuity, progressive, and critical care nursing* (3rd ed.). Springer Publishing Company.

Complications related to end-organ hypoxic and ischemic changes result from thromboembolic infarction, impaired gas exchange, and impaired cardiac output secondary to bleeding. Nurses should be prepared to support end-organ compromise including brain infarcts, renal failure, pulmonary embolism (PE), acute respiratory distress syndrome (ARDS), GI bleeding, mesenteric thrombosis, and intrahepatic hemorrhage. Improvement is reflected by increases in fibrinogen and platelet counts as these indicate an interruption in the consumptive process and that bleeding is controlled.

▶ VON WILLEBRAND DISEASE

Von Willebrand Factor (WVF) is glycoprotein that contributes to the adherence of platelets to damaged endothelium and serves as a carrier protein for plasma factor VIII (Di Paola et al., 2015). It is one of the earliest elements needed for primary hemostasis. Disorders of VWF cause primary platelet dysfunction and secondary factor VIII deficiencies, both of which predispose to bleeding. Three different types of von Willebrand disease (VWD) have been identified:

TYPE 1

- most common and mildest form
- lower than normal levels of VWF and factor VIII

TYPE 2

- The body makes normal amounts of VWF, but it doesn't work as it should.
- subdivided into four different types each with a different dysfunctional mechanism

TYPE 3

- most severe form
- The body makes little to no VWF causing low levels of factor VIII.

SIGNS AND SYMPTOMS

Signs and symptoms include epistaxis, ecchymoses, menorrhagia, and unusual postpartum and postoperative bleeding. Since severity is typically mild and nose bleeds and bruising are common complaints throughout childhood, initial manifestations of VWD may be delayed until adolescences when menorrhagia is apparent or after an elective surgery.

It is important to determine whether the size and distribution of ecchymoses and amount of bleeding are proportional to the severity of the initiating trauma. Epistaxis in an older child should warrant further investigation. Many typical screening labs will be normal in those with VWD, especially if the disease is mild.

Unless there is an acute hemorrhage, anemia isn't present. Clotting times will also be in normal range unless there is a severe deficiency in factor VIII, which will result in a prolonged activated partial thromboplastin clotting time (APTT). Confirmatory laboratory testing for the VWD requires assessment of both VWF level and VWF activity, the latter requiring multiple assays because of the many functions carried out by VWF to help prevent bleeding.

NURSING IMPLICATIONS

Appropriate treatment of VWD requires a specific diagnostic laboratory workup and correct classification of the type of VWF deficiency. Nursing implications in VWD are to restore normal circulating levels of VWF and factor VIII in critical situations such as surgery, child birth, acute bleeding, and trauma. If the patient produces normal VWF but its concentration is reduced (Type 1 and mild forms of Type 3), the plasma level can usually be increased by administering desmopressin, which induces release of VWF from endothelial storage sites into plasma (Di Paola et al., 2015). This is a more concentrated form of desmopressin (DDVAP) than used for diabetes insipidus. Intravenous (IV) and intranasal formulations are available.

COMPLICATIONS

Hyponatremia, syndrome of inappropriate antidiuretic hormone secretion (SIADH), and seizures can occur as a result of treatment. Close monitoring of neurologic status and electrolytes is necessary. If the VWF protein that is present is abnormal, mild bleeding episodes might still be resolved with increased concentrations of the "abnormal" VWF (induced by desmopressin), but severe bleeding episodes may require the administration of normal VWF from plasma-derived products such as Humate-P, Alphanate, and Wilate (Di Paola et al., 2015). Cryoprecipitate contains substantial levels of VWF but is not used regularly because of the lack of viral attenuation treatment. The use of cryoprecipitate is reserved for areas of the world where VWF-containing concentrates are not available.

▶ HEMOPHILIA

Children affected by hemophilia have a deficiency in one or more clotting factors. It follows an X-linked recessive inheritance pattern and occurs almost exclusively in males, 1 in every 5,000 males. Hemophilia A and hemophilia B are the two most common types with type A accounting for 80% to 85% of cases (Di Paola et al., 2015).

- hemophilia A (classic hemophilia): deficient in VIII
- hemophilia B (Christmas Disease): deficient in factor IX

Adequate factor X production is dependent on factors VIII and IX, so children affected by hemophilia have a compromised ability to form thrombin and fibrin. Severity of disease is related to degree of factor VIII or IX deficiency. It is typically expressed in percentages of factor activity within 1 mL of normal plasma, so 100% equates to full or normal factor activity (Di Paola et al, 2015; Spruit, 2019).

- **mild**: factor level of greater than 5 U/dL (>5%)
- **moderate**: factor level between 1 and 5 U/dL (1%–5%)
- **severe**: factor level of less than 1 U/dL (<1%)

Those with severe hemophilia often have bleeding episodes after minimal or unknown trauma, with children experiencing unprovoked muscle and joint bleeding between one and six times per month. Children with moderate hemophilia will have bleeding after mild to moderate injuries, whereas children with mild hemophilia may only have bleeding after significant trauma or at the time of surgery (Di Paola et al., 2015).

SIGNS AND SYMPTOMS

Bleeding can occur anywhere in the body secondary to trauma, normal activity, and even spontaneously depending on disease severity (Spruit, 2019).

- bleeding after circumcision (30% of males)
- bleeding into joint spaces (hemarthrosis) → painful, swollen, and bruised ankles, knees, elbows; can cause joint deformity and permanent disability
- bleeding into deep muscles → muscle pain, weakness, iliopsoas bleeding; can be life-threatening
- central nervous system (CNS) bleeding → altered mental status, hemiplegia, nerve compression
- exsanguinating hemorrhage particularly around the airway and GI tract
- slow persistent bleeding from minor cuts and injuries, including gum irritation
- severe bleeding after dental extractions

- epistaxis after facial injury
- easy bruising, petechiae rare
- hematuria

The majority of children are diagnosed at birth related to family history. Bleeding with circumcision is another common finding. Hemophilia presents as a new mutation in 30% of cases, so those children are often diagnosed in infancy and toddlerhood as hemarthrosis becomes apparent.

Clinical Pearl

Hematoma formation can induce an inflammatory response with fever, leukocytosis, and hyperbilirubinemia secondary to RBC destruction.

Diagnostic labs are presented in Table 5.8.

Table 5.8 Diagnostic Labs for Hemophilia A and B

	CBC	PT, PTT, Fibrinogen	Factor Assays
Hemophilia A	Normal	PT—normal PTT—markedly prolonged Fibrinogen—normal	VIII—decreased VWF testing must be done to differentiate cause of mild-mod factor VIII deficiency
Hemophilia B	Normal	PT—normal PTT—markedly prolonged Fibrinogen—normal	IX—decreased

CBC, complete blood count; PT, prothrombin time; PTT, partial thromboplastin time; VWF, von Willebrand factor.
Source: Slota, M. (Ed.). (2019). *AACN core curriculum for pediatric high acuity, progressive, and critical care nursing* (3rd ed.). Springer Publishing Company.

NURSING IMPLICATIONS

Nursing interventions are aimed at restoring normal clotting activity, minimizing pain, tissue, and joint damage, and prepping the critically ill child with hemophilia for a procedure or surgery. Nurses work closely with the PICU and hematology teams to determine immediate and prophylactic treatment of bleeding episodes.

Recombinant factor replacement is the gold standard and preferred over plasma concentrates. For active bleeding, repeat doses of factor replacement are necessary. The half-life of factor VIII is 10 to 12 hours, and the half-life of factor IX is 18 to 24 hours. DDAVP is first-line treatment for mild to moderate hemorrhage. Factor replacement treatments for different types of hemorrhages in both A and B types are described in Table 5.9.

Table 5.9 Treatment of Specific Hemorrhages in Hemophilia A and B

Type of Hemorrhage	Hemophilia A (Factor VIII)	Hemophilia B (Factor IX)
Major surgery or life-threatening hemorrhage	Bolus 50–75 unit/kg, then initiate continuous infusion of 3 unit/kg/hr to maintain factor VIII >100 unit/dL for 24 hr, then give 2–3 unit/kg/hr for 5–7 days to maintain the level >50 unit/dL, then continue bolus dosing to maintain level >30 unit/dL for an additional 5–7 days, monitor factor VIII levels	Bolus 80–100 unit/kg, then bolus 20–40 unit/kg every 12–24 hrs to maintain factor IX >40 unit/dL for 5–7 days, then >30 unit/dL for 5–7 days, monitor factor IX levels
Hemarthrosis	50 unit/kg initially, 20 unit/kg the following day; consider additional treatment every other day, goal factor VIII levels are 30–50 unit/dL	80 unit/kg initially, 40 unit/kg the following day; consider additional treatment every other day, goal factor IX levels are 25–30 unit/dL

(continued)

Table 5.9 Treatment of Specific Hemorrhages in Hemophilia A and B (*continued*)

Type of Hemorrhage	Hemophilia A (Factor VIII)	Hemophilia B (Factor IX)
Muscle or significant subcutaneous hematoma	50 unit/kg initially, may need 20 unit/kg every other day until well resolved	80 unit/kg initally, may need 40 unit/kg every other day until well resolved
Epistaxis	Apply pressure for 15–20 min, pack with petrolatum gauze, antifibrinolytic therapy (amicar, TXA); 20 unit/kg factor VIII concentrate if preceding measure fails	Apply pressure for 15–20 min, pack with petrolatum gauze, antifibrinolytic therapy (amicar, TXA), 30 unit/kg factor IX concentrate if preceding measure fails
Mouth, tooth extraction	20 unit/kg or 40 unit/kg if molar extraction, antifibrinolytic therapy; remove loose deciduous tooth	40 unit/kg or 80 unit/kg if molar extraction, antifibrinolytic therapy; remove loose deciduous tooth
Iliopsoas	50 unit/kg initially, 25 unit/kg every 12 hrs until asymptomatic, and then 20 unit/kg every other day for a total of 10–14 days	80 unit/kg initially, 20–40 unit/kg every 12–24 hrs to maintain factor IX >40 IU/dL until asymptomatic, and then 30 unit/kg every other day for a total of 10–14 days
Hematuria	Bed rest, 1.5 × maintenance fluids; if not controlled in 1–2 days, 20 unit/kg bolus; if not controlled, prednisone if human immunodeficiency virus negative	Bed rest, 1.5 × maintenance fluids; if not controlled in 1–2 days, 30 unit/kg bolus; if not controlled, prednisone if human immunodeficiency virus negative

TXA, tranexamic acid.
Source: Brugnara, C., Oski, F. A., & Nathan, D. G. (2015). *Nathan and Oski's hematology and oncology of infancy and childhood* (8th ed.). Saunders, an imprint of Elsevier Inc.

Affected children can develop inhibitors or antibodies to recombinant factor treatments, necessitating a different agent to be used with future bleeding episodes. Interventions for hemarthosis include compression wraps, cooling therapies, elevation and decreased use of affected limb, and pain control. Minimizing tissue injury is crucial, so venipunctures should be limited and done only in superficial vein sites. Medications such a nonsteroidal anti-inflammatory drugs (NSAIDs) and aspirin should be avoided (Spruit, 2019).

▶ IMMUNE THROMBOCYTOPENIC PURPURA

Immune thrombocytopenic purpura (ITP) is the most common autoimmune disorder affecting a blood element and has both acute and chronic forms (Wilson, 2015). Acute ITP is usually a benign, self-limited condition that occurs in young children, most commonly between 2 and 6 years old. Viral infection or vaccination often precedes the onset of acute ITP. In most of these patients, the thrombocytopenia resolves within weeks or a few months from the time of symptom manifestation.

Chronic ITP is seen more commonly in children older than 10 years old, in females, and is insidious in onset. Chronic ITP is controversially defined as persistent thrombocytopenia, platelet count <150,000/mm^3, for more than 6 months. Hematologist struggle with this definition, as a large fraction of children with acute ITP recover in 6 to 12 months, making persistent thrombocytopenia >12 months a more accurate definition (Wilson, 2015).

In children diagnosed with acute ITP, the platelet count returns to normal in 1 to 2 months after diagnosis for approximately half of patients and by 3 months in two thirds of the remaining children. Chronic ITP is rare in pediatrics and accounts for 20% of cases (Wilson, 2015).

SIGNS AND SYMPTOMS

ITP is caused by autoantibodies that interact with glycoprotein antigens on the surface of platelets and megakaryocytes resulting in their accelerated destruction. Because of these antibodies, the immune system recognizes the platelet as foreign and inappropriately targets platelets for phagocytosis in the spleen. These antibodies are also thought to impair platelet production in the bone marrow (Wilson, 2015). With this, platelet counts decrease rapidly resulting in bleeding. Although purpura, bruises caused by bleeding into the skin, are a classic sign of ITP, platelet counts <50,000/mm³ can lead to bleeding anywhere in the body. Viral illnesses precede symptom onset in most children.

Clinical Pearl

Intercranial hemorrhage is the most serious complication occurring in less than 1% of those affected by ITP.

The exact cause of ITP is often unknown, so other causes of primary thrombocytopenia such as inherited platelet disorders, as well as secondary causes such as sepsis, meningococcemia, systemic lupus erythematosus, DIC, toxins, and drug exposures need to be ruled out (Grace & Lambert, 2022).

Clinical Pearl

Symptoms such as malaise, bone pain, and adenopathy should alert the clinician to consider alternative diagnosis such as leukemia.

Clinical signs and symptoms include abrupt onset of bruising and bleeding in an otherwise healthy child. Platelet counts are quite low, typically <20,000/mm³, while RBCs, WBCs, and coagulation studies remain within normal limits. Petechiae and ecchymosis are seen in most while epistaxis and oral mucosal bleeding are seen in less than one-third of patients. Hematuria, hematochezia, and melena is rare. Menorrhagia may be observed in adolescents (Wilson, 2015).

NURSING IMPLICATIONS AND TREATMENT

The majority of children affected by ITP recover quickly with minimal or no therapy. PICU admission is rare, usually only necessary for acute and life-threatening hemorrhage. Nursing implications are aimed at controlling bleeding, maintaining skin integrity, and creating an individualized treatment plan. The American Society of Hematology guidelines for ITP recommend first-line treatment with glucocorticoids, typically prednisone, or intravenous immunoglobulin (IVIG) in patients with platelets <20,000/mm³ plus significant mucosal bleeding or platelets <10,000/mm³ plus minor purpura (Spruit, 2019). These and other treatments for ITP are described in Table 5.10.

Table 5.10 Treatments, Mechanism of Action, and Side Effects for Acute and
Chronic Immune Thrombocytopenic Purpura

Treatment	Mechanism	Side Effects	Condition
Glucocorticoids	Inhibition of phagocytosis and antibody synthesis, improved platelet production, improved endothelial stability	Cushingoid facies, weight gain, fluid retention, growth retardation, hyperglycemia, hypertension, avascular necrosis, and osteoporosis	Acute and chronic
IVIG	Inhibition of phagocytosis, produces a more rapid increase in platelets than glucocorticoids	Flu-like symptoms such as headache, nausea, lightheadedness, and fever; consider pretreatment with antihistamines and analgesics	Acute and chronic
Splenectomy	Removal of major site of antibody production and platelet destruction	Bleeding and sepsis, particularly related to encapsulated microorganisms; not recommended in children less than 5 years old	Chronic

(continued)

Table 5.10 Treatments, Mechanism of Action, and Side Effects for Acute and Chronic Immune Thrombocytopenic Purpura (*continued*)

Treatment	Mechanism	Side Effects	Condition
Immunosuppressive agents	Interfere with B cell and T cell activity; typical agents include rituximab, alemtuzumab, azathioprine, cyclophosphamide, cyclosporine, tacrolimus, and vinca alkaloids	Opportunistic infections, renal and liver toxicity, hypertension, tremor, headache, myelosuppression	Chronic
RH$_o$(D) immunoglobulin	In RH$_o$(D)+ individuals, this coats circulating RBCs with antibodies cleared by spleen, occupying the reticuloendothelial system allowing antibody coated platelets to survive	Anemia	Chronic

IVIG, intravenous immunoglobin.
Source: Brugnara, C., Oski, F. A., & Nathan, D. G. (2015). Nathan and Oski's hematology and oncology of infancy and childhood (8th ed.). Saunders, an imprint of Elsevier Inc.

While thrombocytopenic, patients should be educated about protection from sources of trauma such as hard or sharp toys and contact sports. Medications that affect platelets such as aspirin and cox inhibitors should also be avoided.

▶ HENOCH-SCHÖNLEIN PURPURA

Henoch-Schönlein purpura (HSP) is an autoimmune vasculitis that often presents after respiratory infections, especially with *Streptococcal* origin (Wilkenson, 2019). HSP affects smaller blood vessels, such as capillaries and arterioles, that supply blood flow to organ systems. The skin, GI, and renal systems are most commonly affected.

The mechanism of HSP is not fully understood; however, there is a defect in the breakdown of IgA complexes in the bloodstream, so these larger complexes cause endothelial injury, thus triggering an immune response and complement activation. Once the complement cascade is activated, membrane attack complexes form, which rupture capillary and blood vessel walls. This furthers the inflammatory response resulting in a characteristic purpuric rash, which typically occurs on lower extremities, but can be seen anywhere on the body.

HSP is the most common vasculitis in childhood with the median age at onset being 5 years old. HSP is seen in predominantly in Asian and White ethnicities. Males are affected more than females at a ratio of three to two. The process is typically self-limiting; however, permanent renal and joint damage can ensue with relapsing disease (Wilson, 2015).

SIGNS AND SYMPTOMS

Signs and symptoms of HSP are described in Table 5.11. In addition to the classic triad of rash, joint pain, and GI symptoms, a history of recent febrile illness is typically present. Depending on degree of skin and joint involvement, a child can present in moderate to severe pain. The bruising is in response to blood vessel and capillary wall injury rather than platelet destruction, so platelet counts are normal in children with HSP. Although not often indicated, deposition of IgA complexes are present on biopsy (Wilson, 2015). Although lung involvement is rare, diffuse alveolar hemorrhage is the most common pulmonary complication. Development of chronic kidney disease cannot be predicted based upon initial clinical and histological presentation (Daven, 2014).

Table 5.11 Signs and Symptoms of Henoch-Schönlein Purpura Classified by Organ System

Organ System	Clinical Manifestation
Skin	Petechiae or larger purpuric rash primarily affecting extensor surfaces of lower extremities and buttocks but can occur anywhere on the body and in pressure dependent areas
Renal	Proteinuria, hematuria, hypertension

Table 5.11 Signs and Symptoms of Henoch-Schönlein Purpura Classified by Organ System (*continued*)

Organ System	Clinical Manifestation
Gastrointestinal	Pain, hematemesis, melena, intussusception occurs in 4% of patients
Musculoskeletal	Arthralgia, warm and swollen joints, present in 80% of patients
Pulmonary	Diffuse alveolar hemorrhage, hemoptysis, tachypnea

NURSING IMPLICATIONS AND TREATMENT

Treatment for HSP is typically supportive with rehydration and analgesics if needed. Glucocorticoid therapy can resolve joint, renal, and dermatologic manifestations of the disease but should be reserved for those with severe symptoms. There is little evidence that glucocorticoids prevent renal involvement or intussusception (Wilson, 2015). With severe nephritis and pulmonary complications pulse, methylprednisolone, cyclophosphamide, and plasma exchange are aggressive treatments to consider. Affected children should be followed by nephrology long term for early treatment of chronic kidney disease if it develops.

▶ HEPARIN-INDUCED THROMBOCYTOPENIA

Heparin induced thrombocytopenia (HIT) is an immune phenomenon caused by the formation of antibodies against heparin complexes bound to platelet factor 4 (PF4), a protein found in platelet granules. The subsequent immune-mediated complexes cause platelet activation resulting in thrombus formation and thrombocytopenia (Chok et al., 2021).

Clinical Pearl

Approximately 0.5% to 5% of adults on heparin therapy develop HIT. The incidence is less in pediatrics and almost nonexistent in neonates.

SIGNS AND SYMPTOMS

Clinical signs include unexplained thrombocytopenia within 5 to 10 days of starting heparin, arterial or venous thrombosis, bruising, and bleeding if platelet counts are extremely low. Antibodies can remain in circulation for 100 days, allowing for immediate manifestation of symptoms upon reexposure to heparin (Chok et al., 2021).

NURSING IMPLICATIONS AND TREATMENT

In addition to clinical criteria, HIT is confirmed through laboratory testing when heparin-PF4 antibodies are detected in the blood (Spruit, 2019). With this, immediate discontinuation of heparin therapy is necessary. Nurses should administer an alternative anticoagulant as ordered, such as antithrombin argatraban or fondaparinux. Common complications include deep vein thrombosis, PE, and skin necrosis. The risk of complications are the highest within the first 10 days, but the procoagulant state can remain for 30 days post discontinuation of heparin (Nicolas et al., 2021). In pediatrics, standards methodology and diagnostic criteria for HIT vary considerably between institutions.

COMPLICATIONS

Since the management of HIT requires immediate substitution of heparin with an alternative anticoagulant drug, many of which pose significant bleeding risks in children, over-diagnosis of HIT has serious consequences for patient safety and outcomes. Additionally, the implications of lifelong heparin avoidance are particularly significant in children with complex congenital heart disease (Chok et al., 2021).

▶ IMMUNE DEFICIENCIES

Pediatric immune deficiencies are disorders primarily of WBCs. They are characterized by inadequate numbers or inadequate function of one or more components of the immune system. Disorders are classified by the involvement of either B lymphocytes, T lymphocytes, phagocytes, complement, or a combination of these. Although there are over 200 known congenital immune deficiencies, incidences are relatively rare to the general population. See Table 5.12 for general descriptions of primary congenital immune disorders and common examples.

Table 5.12 General Descriptions of Primary Congenital Immune Disorders

Disorder Type	Manifestations	Common Examples
B lymphocyte—diminishes immunoglobulin production	Deficiency in a single class of immunoglobulin Deficiency in all classes of immunoglobulins Deficiencies in some classes of immunoglobulins and overproduction in others Predisposes to infection with *S. pneumoniae, S. aureus, H. influenzae*, gram-negative bacteria, and enteroviruses Does not predispose to fungus	IgA deficiency X-linked agammaglobulinemia Combined variable immunodeficiency
T lymphocyte—inadequate number or function of T lymphocytes	Deficiency in number of mature T lymphocytes Inability to assist in activation of immune response Survival and replication of pathologic organisms inside host immune cells Predisposes to opportunistic fungal infections, herpes viruses, Salmonella typhi, and mycobacteria	DiGeorge syndrome X-linked immunodeficiency with hyper-IgM
Phagocyte dysfunction	*Extrinsic Factors* Deficiency in opsonization related to decrease in antibody or complement Suppression of neutrophils related to alterations in complement Decreased circulating lymphokines Medications with immunosuppressive effect on phagocyte function or number *Intrinsic Factors* Defects in the metabolic pathways of phagocytes Increased incidence of staphylococcal, gram-negative, and fungal infections even with a "normal WBC count"	Chronic granulomatous disease Leukocyte adhesion deficiency Secondary disorders can be drug or disease induced such as corticosteroids, immunosuppressive agents, and diabetes mellitus
Complement	Deficiency in any of the key components of the complement system Deficiencies in C1q, C3, and C4 are most commonly associated with increased susceptibility to infection Increased risk of encapsulated bacterial infection, *S. pneumoniae*, Increased risk for development of autoimmune disease such as vasculitis or Systemic lupus erythematosus (SLE)	Hereditary deficiency of compliment proteins Acquired disorders that consume complement
Combined B and T lymphocyte—humoral and cell-mediated immunity (CMI)	Unable to form antibody, orchestrate a cell mediated response, or destroy virally infected cells or infected cells with intracellular organisms Increased susceptibility to infections from all microorganisms Infections are often recurrent and severe	Severe combined immunodeficiency disorder Wiskott-Aldrich syndrome Ataxia-telangiectasia Combined immunodeficiency syndrome *may result from exposure to radiation, cytoxic, and immunosuppressive pharmacologic agents

CMI, cell-mediated immunity; SLE, systemic lupus erythematosus; WBC, white blood cell.
Source: Slota, M. (Ed.). (2019). *AACN core curriculum for pediatric high acuity, progressive, and critical care nursing* (3rd ed.). Springer Publishing Company.

A large number of children admitted to ICUs have impaired immune function related to a variety of stressors such as anesthesia, tissue injury, medications, malignancy, and malnutrition. These immune deficiencies are acquired and considered secondary immune deficiencies. These patients are at risk for infection related to WBC hyporeactivity (Spruit, 2019).

▶ SEVERE COMBINED IMMUNODEFICIENCY

The term severe combined immunodeficiency (SCID) reflects a genetically heterogeneous group of primary immune deficiencies characterized by impaired development and function of lymphocytes (Bonilla & Notarangelo, 2015). SCID has been linked to 14 different genetic mutations with a slight majority (55%) following an autosomal recessive inheritance pattern. The remaining 45% are X-linked defects in the common gamma chain (Kobrynski, 2021).

All forms of SCID affect T lymphocytes, and some forms also affect B cell and natural killer cell development (Bonilla & Notarangelo, 2015). The most common form of autosomal recessive SCID is adenosine deaminase deficiency (ADA); and the most common form of X-linked SCID is related to a mutation in the ; interleukin 2 receptor subunit gamma (*IL2R*) gene.

Clinical Pearl

Because T cells play a critical role in most B cell responses, serious T cell dysfunction impedes effective humoral immunity regardless of whether the form of SCID directly affects B cell development. This causes a complete absence of specific cellular and humoral immunity in patients with SCID, leading to an extreme infectious diathesis early in life.

SIGNS AND SYMPTOMS

Since 2018, all 50 states in the United States include SCID as part of universal newborn screening. The newborn screening process reveals infants with T cell lymphopenia at birth; however, this is not diagnostic for SCID. Confirmatory testing includes flow cytometry of peripheral blood lymphocytes. A CXR may reveal a small or absent thymus. SCID is characterized by an unusual and increased frequency of common infections, chronic diarrhea, and failure to thrive (Bonilla & Notarangelo, 2015). Due to the presence of protective maternal antibodies, infants typically appear healthy at birth then develop severe infections within the first few months of life. Affected infants experience significant recurrent illness with common viral and bacterial pathogens as well as opportunistic infections with *Pneumocystis jirovecii*, cytomegalovirus, and *Candida* species (Kobrynski, 2021). In children with SCID, oral thrush is resistant to pharmacologic therapy. Additionally, dietary changes minimally impact the chronic diarrhea, as it's infectious in origin. Dehydration is common and can be life-threatening.

NURSING IMPLICATIONS AND TREATMENT

Identification of a child with SCID should be considered a pediatric emergency. For affected infants, the most immediate life-threatening complication is sepsis; therefore, nursing implications target monitoring of infection and preventing septic shock. Specific nursing interventions are described in Box 5.1.

Box 5.1 Preventative Nursing Interventions for Severe Combined Immunodeficiency

Nursing Interventions
Isolation
Diligent hand hygiene
Diligent skincare and mucosal hygiene
Monitor for signs of infection
Monitor for signs of septic and/or hypovolemic shock
Volume resuscitate as indicated
Administer antimicrobials (prophylactic and therapeutic) as ordered
Optimize nutritional status
Avoid live virus immunization

Source: Slota, M. (Ed.). (2019). *AACN core curriculum for pediatric high acuity, progressive, and critical care nursing* (3rd ed.). Springer Publishing Company.

Transfusion of blood products containing viable lymphocytes may lead to fatal graft-versus-host disease in children affected by SCID, so all administered blood products should be irradiated (Bonilla & Notarangelo, 2015).

First line and definitive therapy for children affected by SCID is bone marrow transplant (BMT). When transplantation is performed in infants younger than 3.5 months of age, survival is greater than 95%, emphasizing the importance of newborn screening. Treatment with IVIG should start immediately after immunologic evaluation and continue every 1 to 4 weeks until definitive therapy is achieved with BMT. Enzyme replacement therapy is indicated in ADA, weekly injections of **polyethylene glycol-modified bovine adenosine deaminase (PEG-ADA)** have shown to improve immune function, although immune reconstitution is incomplete. **Gene therapy** is also a possibility. With this, a functional copy of the defective gene is placed in a retroviral vector and transduced into populations of mature T cells or bone marrow cells. The new cells are able to reestablish T cell mediated immunity in the host. Although findings are encouraging for those without suitable bone marrow transplant options, an increased incidence of leukemia has been seen with this method.

▶ AIDS

AIDS represents the most advanced stage of disease progression in those infected with HIV. With recent advances in antiretroviral therapies, HIV infection, which was a presumed lethal diagnosis a few decades ago, is now considered a chronic disease in the United States (Spruit, 2019).

Characteristically, HIV causes a slowly progressive disease with an incubation period of months to years before clinical symptoms appear. This incubation period appears to be shorter for children perinatally infected compared to those that acquire the virus through other modes of transmission. For children less than 13 years old, transmission from mother to infant is the most common method of viral contraction, either through the birthing process or ingestion of breastmilk. In children older than 13, sexual intercourse and IV drug use is the most common. Adolescents and young adults account for 20% new HIV infections each year (Grace, 2015).

SIGNS AND SYMPTOMS

HIV is an RNA retrovirus that attacks cluster of differentiation 4 (CD4) helper T lymphocytes, which influence and orchestrate cell mediated and humoral immunity. The death of these lymphocytes causes severe immunodeficiency in the host, leading to life-threatening opportunistic infections and malignancy. Clinical signs include thrombocytopenia, anemia, lymphopenia as CD4 count decreases, hypoalbuminemia, nephropathy (urinalysis), hyperglycemia, hepatic transaminitis, and renal insufficiency. With congenital infections, constitutional symptoms occur within the first few months of life including unexplained diarrhea, fever, night sweats, rashes, lymphadenopathy (specifically epitrochlear nodes), hepatosplenomegaly, tone abnormalities, and ankle clonus. Other prominent early manifestations include failure to thrive, CNS abnormalities, and developmental delays. Recurrent susceptibility to common bacterial and viral pathogens, as well as to opportunistic infections, should increase the index of suspicion for AIDS as an underlying disorder (Grace, 2015).

NURSING IMPLICATIONS AND TREATMENT

Early diagnosis of HIV infection and early initiation of antiretroviral therapy (ART) reduces morbidity and mortality in neonates, infants, and children. Tests available for making the diagnosis of HIV infection are divided into two groups:
1. Those that detect HIV antibodies produced in response to the virus (enzyme linked immunosorbent assays and rapid diagnostic tests)
2. Those that detect the genetic material of HIV, indicating the presence of the virus, and referred to as nucleic acid tests or virological assays (qualitative assay/HIV-PCR and quantitative assay/-VL test)

Complexities exists when considering HIV testing in the pediatric population. Antibody tests are not recommended in children less than 18 months old with perinatal exposure as maternal HIV antibodies cross the placenta and their presence does not always indicate infection in the child. Secondly, HIV-PCR and HIV-VL becomes undetectable in an HIV affected person on ART. With the increased number of drugs and longer duration of maternal ART during pregnancy, HIV-infected infants have demonstrated significantly reduced VLs in the first month of life (Sherman & Mazanderani, 2020).

Physical assessment varies with age and level of immunodeficiency. Actively infected children are small for their age; growth retardation is secondary to poor appetite, oral candidiasis, persistent diarrhea, anemia, and/or poor maternal health. Increased work of breathing can be seen with pneumonias related to Pneumocystis pneumonia or other bacteria, causing respiratory compromise and failure. Acquired microcephaly, dementia, abnormal tone, spastic diplegia, and other motor deficits are consistent with encephalopathy (Grace, 2015). HIV-associated cardiomyopathy, pericardial effusion, and conduction abnormalities generally manifest later in childhood.

Children who are initiated on ART from birth do not present with the classical signs and symptoms of HIV infection. Studies have shown that early access to ART impacts favorably on growth and neurodevelopment and leads to fewer opportunistic infections (Sherman & Mazanderani, 2020).

For children infected with HIV, nursing priorities are aimed at initiating ART as early as possible and supporting adequate hemodynamics during hospitalization for opportunistic infections. Respiratory failure from Pneumocystis pneumonia is the leading cause of early mortality in this population. It primarily affects infants 3 to 6 months old and poses the most risk when CD4 counts and percentages are markedly low (Spruit, 2019).

Clinical Pearl

The following clinical signs have been independently correlated with Pneumocystis pneumonia: age younger than 6 months, respiratory rate >59 breaths/minute, arterial oxygen saturation <92, and lack of emesis (Spruit, 2019).

TMP-SMX is the first line agent for Pneumocystis pneumonia treatment and prophylaxis. If administered within 72 hours of symptom onset, a short course of steroids might suppress enough of the inflammatory response caused by Pneumocystis pneumonia to decrease subsequent pulmonary edema (Spruit, 2019).

As stated previously, early initiation of ART is imperative in preventing morbidity and mortality associated with HIV infection. A combination of antiretroviral drugs acting at different sites in the HIV lifecycle is standard treatment. The number of drugs in the regimen is balanced against the cumulative toxicity of the drug combination, pill burden and the cost. Most clinical guidelines recommend a three-drug ART regimen as the ideal compromise between prevention of resistance and limiting toxicity for newly diagnosed patients starting ART (Sherman & Mazanderani, 2020). See Table 5.13 for more information regarding ART.

Table 5.13 Site and Mechanism of Action of Antiretroviral Therapy in HIV

Site of Action in HIV Life Cycle	ART Class	Mechanism of Action
Attachment	CCR5 antagonists	Prevents the HIV from entering uninfected cells by blocking the CCR5 coreceptor needed for entry into CD4 cells
Fusion	Fusion inhibitors	Blocks entrance and fusion of HIV with CD4 cells, blocking the entrance of viral genetic material
Reverse transcription	RTIs	Interferes with enzyme reverse transcriptase which reverse transcribes viral RNA into DNA for insertion into the host DNA sequence
Integration	Integrase inhibitors	Prevents HIV genome from integrating into host's genome by blocking integration step of viral cycle
Replication	Protease inhibitors	Binds to protease enzyme, preventing cleavage into individual proteins

RTIs, reverse transcriptase inhibitors.
Source: Slota, M. (Ed.). (2019). *AACN core curriculum for pediatric high acuity, progressive, and critical care nursing* (3rd ed.). Springer Publishing Company.

▶ PLASMAPHERESIS

Plasmapheresis or therapeutic plasma exchange (TPE) is a procedure that extracorporeally removes and separates the plasma from a patient's blood while simultaneously giving back a replacement fluid. Clinical indications include a variety of pathologies where antibodies, immune complexes, cytokines, and toxins circulate through the plasma portion of the blood and attack healthy cells and tissues. Approximately 63% of harmful circulating substances are removed with the first treatment (Main, 2017). Treatments can be one time only or sequential for a specific number of days. TPE filters protein bound substances from the plasma, including medications and total parenteral nutrition (TPN). With this, nurses should administer important medications after the TPE session is complete. ACE inhibitors should be held for 24 to 48 hours prior to TPE as they can cause hypotension, bradycardia, dyspnea and vasodilation due to a buildup of bradykinin (Main, 2017). Other complications include citrate toxicity leading to hypocalcemia, metabolic alkalosis, anaphylaxis and infection. Liver and renal insufficiency increases the likelihood of citrate toxicity (Main, 2017). In addition to hypocalcemia, hypomagnesemia and hypokalemia can also occur during TPE. Electrolytes should be corrected prior to next TPE session. Fibrinogen levels will be lower for up to 72 hours after treatment; therefore, nurses should monitor for bleeding. Administering fresh frozen plasma (FFP) as ordered after TPE can decrease bleeding risks. Pediatric patients are twice as likely to develop complications secondary to their smaller body size and intravascular volume. Hypocalcemia can be difficult to monitor and can manifest as irritability, pallor, emesis, abdominal pain, bradycardia and hypotension (Main, 2017).

▶ ONCOLOGIC COMPLICATIONS

Oncology patients admitted to the PICU have unique medical and nursing needs. Oncologic emergencies can present throughout all stages of treatment. Emergencies upon presentation and early in treatment include the management of tumor lysis syndrome, hyperleukocytosis, superior mediastinal mass syndrome, and spinal cord compression. HSCT patients form another unique group of patients with distinctive risk factors such as graft-versus-host disease and veno-occlusive disease. Mortality remains increased in those with multiorgan failure, sepsis, and on multiple PICU therapies (Praven et al., 2020).

▶ TUMOR LYSIS SYNDROME

Tumor lysis syndrome (TLS) is the most common pediatric oncologic emergency causing life threatening metabolic derangements as intracellular contents of cancer cells, which are typically excreted in the urine, spill into the bloodstream. This leads to hyperuricemia, hyperkalemia, and hyperphosphatemia, which if left unmanaged, will cause acute kidney injury (AKI), cardiac arrhythmias, seizures, and even death. TLS occurs most frequently in children with hyperproliferating malignancies such as acute leukemia and non-Hodgkin lymphoma, as there is rapid cellular destruction after administration of cytotoxic agents (Russell & Kram, 2020).

> ## Clinical Pearl
>
> *Predictors of TLS include bulky disease, adenopathy, hepatosplenomegaly, leukocytosis, elevated lactate dehydrogenase (LDH), and renal impairment (Spruit, 2019).*

SIGNS AND SYMPTOMS

Clinical signs include diarrhea, vomiting, edema, fluid overload, and tetany. Symptoms include lethargy, nausea, anorexia, and muscle cramps (Spruit, 2019). Laboratory TLS is defined as two or more of the following serum values, when compared to normal reference values for age (Russell & Kram, 2020):

- elevated uric acid, potassium, or phosphorus and decreased calcium
- These abnormalities must also be present during the same 24-hour period and within 3 days before or up to 7 days after the initiation of chemotherapy.

  Clinical TLS requires the presence of laboratory TLS plus one of the following clinical sequelae:
- increased creatinine level, seizures, cardiac dysrhythmia, or death

NURSING IMPLICATIONS AND TREATMENT

Nursing interventions target preventing AKI and renal failure by diligently monitoring electrolytes, LDH, uric acid, and blood urea nitrogen (BUN)/creatinine. Management strategies for TLS are described in Table 5.14.

Table 5.14 Management Strategies for Tumor Lysis Syndrome

Problem	Treatment Strategy
Decreased renal tubular flow	2 x maintenance IVF with 5% dextrose with age appropriate sodium content Hydration is presumed to be adequate with appropriate urine output and urine specific gravity <1.010
Hyperkalemia	For K + >6 meq/L and asymptomatic: sodium polystyrene sulfonate For K + >7 meq/L and/or symptomatic: albuterol nebulization, bolus insulin and glucose With increased risk of Ca precipitation in the setting of hyperphos, only administer Ca if lethal arrythmia is present Consider dialysis if hyperkalemia refractory to above strategies
Hyperphosphatemia (>6 mmol/L)	Oral phosphate binders Dialysis should be considered in cases of impaired renal function
Elevated uric acid (>8 mg/dL)	Allopurinol—this impedes production of uric acid, does not break it down Recombinant urase oxidase, directly breaks down uric acid, expensive

IVF, intravenous fluids.

Source: Slota, M. (Ed.). (2019). *AACN core curriculum for pediatric high acuity, progressive, and critical care nursing* (3rd ed.). Springer Publishing Company.

▶ HYPERLEUKOCYTOSIS

Hyperleukocytosis, defined as a WBC count >100,000/µL is a complication seen in 5% to 20% of patients with acute leukemia.It can be associated with early morbidity and mortality because of pulmonary, neurological, and metabolic complications.These can be due to severe leukostasis caused by the hyperviscosity in the microcirculation. Clinical leukostasis occurs most commonly in acute myeloid leukemia , likely related to proinflammatory cytokine release with cell lysis (Abla, 2016; Spruit, 2019).

SIGNS AND SYMPTOMS

Some children remain asymptomatic in the setting of hyperleukocytosis; however, symptom onset can be tenuous and rapid. Symptoms are dependent on microvasculature involved and include (Spruit, 2019):

- **respiratory**: increased work of breathing, hypoxia, respiratory failure, ARDS
- **neurological**: headache, tinnitus, dizziness, stroke, seizures
- renal failure
- priapism
- cardiac failure
- dactylitis
- CBC with WBC >100,000/µL is diagnostic

NURSING IMPLICATIONS AND TREATMENT

The most effective way to prevent catastrophic multisystem complications of hyperleukocytosis is to rapidly reduce circulating blasts and WBCs through appropriate cytotoxic methods decided by the oncology team (Spruit, 2019). Obtaining adequate vascular access and administering aggressive hydration allows for hemodilution of the hyperleukocytosis and promotes blood flow to vital organs.

Patients should be monitored closely for TLS. Transfusions of RBCs should be minimized until leukocyte count and blood viscosity is reduced. Current evidence does not support leukapheresis as a standard therapy for hyperleukocytosis. Rates of early death appear to be similar in children who undergo leukapheresis compared to those receiving only cytotoxic agents. Nursing implications for patients undergoing leukapheresis are similar to other plasma exchanges; however, there is a higher incidence of CNS complications related to thrombosis and hemorrhage. Thrombocytopenia increases these risks factors (Abla, 2016).

▶ SPACE OCCUPYING LESIONS

Space occupying lesions are typically masses or solid tumors that compress vital structures and vasculature anywhere in the body. When these lesions occur in the mediastinum and spinal cord they require emergent interventions.

▶ SUPERIOR MEDIASTINAL SYNDROME

Superior mediastinal syndrome (SMS) is a complication of an anterior mediastinal mass compressing the heart, great blood vessels, tracheobronchial tree. Most common malignancies associated with mediastinal masses are Hodgkin and non-Hodgkin lymphomas, acute lymphocytic leukemia, and neuroblastoma (Spruit, 2019).

SIGNS AND SYMPTOMS

Clinical signs include cough, wheeze, varying degrees of respiratory distress that worsen in the supine position, facial/neck/upper airway edema, altered mental status, and shock secondary to cardiopulmonary compromise.

NURSING IMPLICATIONS AND TREATMENT

Physical assessment reveals evidence of:
- **airway obstruction**: cough, orthopnea, anxiety, hoarseness, cyanosis
- **cardiovascular compromise**: engorgement of superior vena cava (SVC), face, neck, upper extremities, syncope and altered mental status

Initial diagnostic testing is determined by clinical stability. A simple CXR is first line as it is easy to obtain and reveals general size of mass and degree of surrounding structure compression. Chest CT is a valuable tool for differentiation, origin, and location of mass; however, hemodynamic stability might not allow for supine positioning and traveling off unit. Echocardiogram confirms SVC compression and pericardial effusions. Biopsy, pathology, and bone marrow aspiration are needed for diagnosis of malignancy. Empiric life-saving therapy, such as steroids, chemo, and radiation, might be needed prior to formal diagnosis. Once diagnosis is established, a more formalized treatment plan should be followed per the oncology team.

COMPLICATIONS

Patients with SMS pose a high anesthetic risk. All efforts to support spontaneous respirations should be taken to maintain chest wall and airway tone. Neuromuscular blockade should be avoided. If anesthesia is required, all caregivers should be informed of the risk of a difficult airway (Spruit, 2019).

▶ SPINAL CORD COMPRESSION

Spinal cord compression affects a small amount of the pediatric cancer population, 3% to 5%.

> ### Clinical Pearl
>
> *4 types of tumors account for 50% of SCS cases: neuroblastoma, soft tissue sarcomas, Ewings sarcoma, and rhabdomyosarcoma.*

SIGNS AND SYMPTOMS

Clinical signs and symptoms depend upon degree of compression and include back pain, gait disturbances, ataxia, incontinence, decreased strength, reflexes, and sensation (Spruit, 2019). Depending on lesion size and location, physical assessment can also reveal vital signs consistent with increased intracranial pressure. MRI of the brain and spinal cord is the preferred method of imaging.

NURSING IMPLICATIONS AND TREATMENT

Relieving compression and restoring neurologic function are the goals of treatment. Nurses should rapidly administer dexamethasone as ordered if the child is showing signs of neurologic impairment. Monitor vital signs to optimize brain and spinal cord perfusion before and after surgical decompression and laminectomy.

Sometimes adjunctive chemotherapy and radiation is indicated to decrease tumor burden, especially in highly proliferative tumors such as atypical teratoid rhabdoid tumor. Risks of radiotherapy include stunted growth, secondary malignancies, and repeat anesthetics for sequential session (Spruit, 2019).

▶ HEMATOPOIETIC STEM CELL TRANSPLANT

Hematopoietic stem cell transplants (HSCTs) involve the transplantation of multipotent stem cells that are capable of complete differentiation and renewal as to completely replace an existing disordered or failing bone marrow. This gives rise to an entirely new hematopoietic system for the recipient (Spruit, 2019). Two types of HSCTs exist:

- **autologous**: uses stem cells from patient's own marrow or peripheral blood
- **allogenic**: transplantation of cells from a nonself donor

The scope of pediatric diseases treatable by HSCT includes high-risk acute leukemias and solid tumors, a wide range of hereditary conditions, including storage and metabolic disorders, hemoglobinopathies, osteopetrosis, and immune deficiencies (Fraint et al., 2020). Success of treatment is dependent upon elimination of underlying problem, prevention of rejection, prevention of graft-versus-host disease (GVHD), and management of acute multisystem complications that often require pediatric critical care resources (Spruit, 2019). Description of acute complications is listed in Table 5.15.

Table 5.15 Complications of Veno-Occlusive Disease Classified by Organ System

Organ System	Complication	Description
Hepatic	VOD	Endothelial and hepatocyte damage leads to microemboli in portal circulation, progresses to obstruction and hepatocyte necrosis, reversal of portal flow, hepatorenal syndrome can lead to Multiple organ system failure (MOSF)
GI	Mucositis	Denuding of epithelial lining of entire GI mucosa, provides portal of entry for infection
Renal	Secondary injury	Injury caused by chemo and other pharmacologic agents, aggravated by pre-renal problems such as hypovolemia or hypoperfusion, or obstructive uropathy such as clots from hemorrhagic cystitis
Pulmonary	Idiopathic pneumonia syndrome	Acute respiratory compromise, often fatal, infiltrative process on x-ray independent of fluid overload, infection, cardiac or renal failure, often inflammatory in origin
	Diffuse alveolar hemorrhage	Presents with cough, SOB, hypoxia, increasingly bloody bronchoalveolar fluids
	BOS	Obstructive syndrome that leads to obliteration of small airways
	Bronchiolitis obliterans organizing pneumonia	Late complication indicating presence of granulation tissue in alveolar ducts and alveoli
Cardiac	Cardiomyopathy	Complication caused by pre-transplant cancer therapy
GU	Hemorrhagic cystitis	Metabolite from chemo produces ulceration of bladder mucosal tissue, small vessels in the underlying tissue hemorrhage into the bladder, can also be caused by BK virus

BOS, bronchiolitis obliterans syndrome; GI, gastrointestinal; GU, genitourinary; MOSF, multiple organ system failure; SOB, shortness of breath.
Source: Slota, M. (Ed.). (2019). *AACN core curriculum for pediatric high acuity, progressive, and critical care nursing* (3rd ed.). Springer Publishing Company.

SIGNS AND SYMPTOMS

- **Veno-occlusive disease (VOD)**: fluid retention, tender hepatosplenomegaly, ascites, hyperbilirubinemia, pulmonary edema or infiltrates, and renal insufficiency, reversal of portal flow on ultrasound
- **Mucositis**: painful inflammation of all mucous membranes, nausea, vomiting, diarrhea, mucosal bleeding, focal GI hemorrhage, anorexia, dysphagia, even if mucosal exam appears unremarkable.

Endoscopy procedures with biopsy can evaluate origin, tissue biopsies should be sent to rule out GVHD, course should improve upon engraftment.

- **AKI**: renal dysfunction differences in children s/p HSCT include hyperkalemia is rare; hypokalemia is common, increased BUN is difficult to interpret as steroids and blood in the GI tract can increase BUN independent of GFR; otherwise signs and symptoms are the same as described in renal chapter.
- **Pulmonary complications**: fever, cough, dyspnea, hypoxia, hemoptysis, increased work of breathing, and diminished pulmonary function tests
- **Cardiomyopathy**: weight gain, peripheral edema, tachycardia, dyspnea on exertion, orthopnea, rales and crackles in lungs; echocardiogram is used to assess ventricular dysfunction.
- **Hemorrhagic cystitis**: red-tinged urine and clots, dysuria, urethral obstruction, and signs of postrenal failure; urinalysis, bladder ultrasound, and infectious studies are helpful in identifying degree of clot burden and microbial causes.

NURSING IMPLICATIONS AND TREATMENT

- **VOD**: supportive care including aggressive fluid management, continuous renal replacement therapy (CRRT) may be necessary; supporting adequate oxygenation and tissue perfusion, mechanical ventilation may be necessary; transfusion support as indicated; administer thrombolytic medications, such as defibrotide, as ordered. Mild to moderate VOD is usually self-limiting, severe VOD is associated with high mortality.
- **mucositis**: peaks 10 to 14 days post-transplant, administer antibiotics as ordered, diligent oral care, explore with medical team options for adequate pain control
  - antiemetics as ordered for nausea and vomiting
  - Monitor fluid balance and electrolytes with diarrhea and apply barrier cream to protect skin
  - Monitor for infectious etiologies
  - hemorrhage: maintain hemodynamic stability and treat source
  - Angiography or surgery may be indicated.
- **AKI**: CRRT is sometimes needed to correct life-threatening electrolyte imbalances, remove waste products, restore and maintain fluid balance.
- **Pulmonary complications**: Treatment is dependent on underlying physiology and requires supportive care in the way of appropriate antimicrobials, supplemental oxygen, invasive and noninvasive positive pressure, assessment of fluids status; other pharmacologic adjuncts include azithromycin for its antiinflammatory properties, corticosteroids (not effective for Bronchiolitis obliterans syndrome [BOS]), and immunomodulators such as etanercept.
- **Cardiomyopathy**: Changes are typically irreversible, so patients will show continued decline; precise fluid management, diuretics, ionotropic agents, pharmacologic agents to promote contractility, maintain comfort, and decrease myocardial oxygen demand.
- **Hemorrhagic cystitis**: Mild cases respond to aggressive hydration; severe cases require continuous bladder irrigation; maintain platelets >20,000/mm^3 if not actively bleeding, >50,000/mm^3 for active bleeding.

▶ SICKLE CELL CRISIS

Sickle cell disease (SCD) is a group of inherited disorders characterized by mutations in the Hgb gene. These mutations result in sickling of RBCs in response to deoxygenation. The sickled RBCs increase blood viscosity, lead to erythrostasis, and occlude microvasculature (Spruit, 2019). Hypoxia, dehydration, hyper- and hypothermia reinforce this vicious sickling cycle leading to thrombosis, ischemia, and infarction of vital organs if circulation is not restored.

The term "sickle cell crisis" is used to describe several acute conditions such as the vaso-occlusive crisis (acute painful crisis), aplastic crisis, splenic sequestration crisis, hyperhemolytic crisis and acute chest syndrome. Vaso-occlusive crisis is the most common presentation of SCD.

SIGNS AND SYMPTOMS

The microocclusion tissue ischemia cascade activates nociceptors causing moderate to severe pain. Reperfusion intensifies the inflammation and resultant pain. Pain typically presents in the long bones, back, pelvis, chest, and abdomen. Microvasculature within any organ can be affected, some having more life-threatening consequences than others: spleen, lungs, brain.

Symptoms may start as early as 6 months of age with pain and swelling in both hands and feet (dactylitis). Patient report is the only reliable method of evaluating presence or absence of pain (Bornhade & Kondamudi, 2021). If chest pain is present, obtain a CXR to rule out acute chest syndrome. If fever is present, blood cultures should be drawn. Other helpful labs include CBC, reticulocyte count, and urinalysis. In severe cases, Hgb electrophoresis is helpful in determining the percentage of red cells that are sickled (Hgb S). Patients with percentages higher than 30% will likely need some form of blood transfusion to augment oxygen carrying capacity. Anemia is present at baseline in children with SCD and is not a worrisome finding in isolation. However, anemia combined with symptoms of hypoxia and tissue ischemia warrants further management.

NURSING IMPLICATIONS AND TREATMENT

Vaso-occlusive crisis can only be relieved by interrupting the cycle of hypoxemia and sickling. With this, providing adequate hydration, oxygenation, rapid pain assessment, and relief are the backbones of nursing interventions. Administer IV fluids at 1.5 times maintenance and provide supplemental oxygen if ordered. Frequent monitoring of vital signs during fluid administration is essential to prevent pulmonary complications or cardiac compromise. Analgesia must be sufficient to control the pain. IV opioids will likely be needed for patients needing PICU admission.

▶ RED CELL EXCHANGE TRANSFUSIONS

Over the last 15 years, transfusion support has become a larger part of SCD management. RBC transfusions can increase Hgb and decrease the percentage of Hgb S and are used for acute and long-term needs. General blood transfusions increase Hgb but also increase blood viscosity. This can be problematic in some circumstance, such as in children with acute chest syndrome at high risk for cerebrovascular accident (CVA), because increasing blood viscosity has catastrophic neurologic implications. In these circumstances, the best way to increase Hgb without increasing blood viscosity is through a red cell exchange transfusion. Red cell exchange transfusion can be done manually or with an automated pheresis machine. In both methods, a portion of the patient's blood is phlebotomized and replaced with donor packed red blood cells (PRBCs). Goals for exchange transfusions are typically to achieve a Hgb >9 and Hgb S <30% (Inati et al., 2017). Acute reasons for exchange transfusions include anemia, stroke, acute chest syndrome, hepatic sequestration, refractory VOD and multisystem organ failure (Inati et al., 2017). Achieving adequate vascular access can be a challenge for these types of transfusions, as arterial lines, large gauge IV, central venous, and pheresis catheters are needed. Nurses caring for children undergoing exchange transfusions need to be knowledgeable of the signs, symptoms, and management of transfusion reactions.

▶ TRANSFUSION REACTIONS

Children experience double the rate of transfusion reactions compared to adults (Vossoughi et al., 2018). Prevention of reactions includes diligent verification of patient information with specific unit crossmatching. Nurses should adhere to strict monitoring procedures at the beginning of the transfusion and increase infusion rates gradually over time (Spruit, 2019). Common transfusion reactions and management are described in Table 5.16.

Table 5.16 Common Transfusion Reactions and Management

Reaction and Cause	Signs and Symptoms	Management
Hemolytic Hemolysis of RBCs from transfusion of ABO incompatible cells	Lumbar pain Impending sense of doom Fever, chills, hypotension, shock, chest pain, DIC	Stop transfusion, notify physician (MD) or advanced practice provider (APP), KVO, treat shock and respiratory distress, osmotic diuresis to prevent ATN, correct DIC
Febrile nonhemolytic Recipient's antibodies reacting to transfused leukocytes or plasma proteins	Fever (>1°C baseline) Chills, headaches, palpitations, hives	Stop transfusion, notify MD or APP, KVO, treat symptoms with antipyretics and antihistamines, may continue transfusion if symptoms were mild, consider premedication and leukapheresed products for future transfusions

(continued)

Table 5.16 Common Transfusion Reactions and Management (*continued*)

Reaction and Cause	Signs and Symptoms	Management
Anaphylactic Caused by antigen-antibody complexes to IgA; occurs in patients who are IgA or haptoglobin deficient	Bronchospasm, cough, urticaria, hives, hypotension, vomiting	Stop transfusion, notify MD or APP, give epinephrine and steroids, treat hypotension, support respiratory status, consider washed blood products for future transfusions
Alloimmunization Recipient creates antibodies to alloantigens on donor cells; antibodies then destroy future transfused cells with targeted antigens	Immunization takes place days to weeks after initial transfusion and is asymptomatic, minimal increase in cells/effectiveness of future transfusions.	To make future transfusions more effective, preemptive antibody testing can be done in recipient to allow for better matched future blood products, leukodepleted blood products reduce risk of alloimmunization
Transfusion associated circulatory overload Transfused volume exceeds capacity of circulatory system	Respiratory distress, hypoxia, rales, hypertension	Monitor fluid status closely, transfuse smaller alloquats as indicated, acute treatment of pulmonary edema may include diuretics and colloid infusions
Transfusion related lung injury Granulocyte activation and alveolar capillary membrane injury related to WBC antibodies and proinflammatory proteins	Onset within 6 hours of transfusion, acute hypoxia, noncardiac pulmonary edema	Immediate respiratory support, often mechanical ventilation, notify blood bank immediately, a leading cause of infusion related mortality
Citrate toxicity Used as an anticoagulant in stored blood, causes decrease in ionized calcium	Hypocalcemia, ventricular arrythmias, associated with multiple transfusions over a short period of time and those with existing hepatic and renal failure	Replace calcium as ordered, replace clotting factors in addition to PRBCs, give 1 unit of FFP for every 3 units of PRBCs

ATN, acute tubular necrosis; DIC, disseminated intravascular coagulation; FFP, fresh frozen plasma; KVO, keep vein open; PRBCs, packed red blood cells; WBC, white blood cell.

Source: Slota, M. (Ed.). (2019). *AACN core curriculum for pediatric high acuity, progressive, and critical care nursing* (3rd ed.). Springer Publishing Company.

Clinical Pearl

Within the pediatric population, allergic reactions to platelets and RBCs were the most frequently reported reaction types.

CASE STUDY

A 3-month-old presents to the ED with lethargy, decreased oral intake, and hypothermia. The infant has a history of recurrent otitis media. The infant's parents report an increase in diarrhea-like stools over the past week. On physical exam, the infant's skin is cool, 2+ pulses, capillary refill is 2 to 3 seconds. Other than mild tachycardia, their vital signs are normal for age. The infant will wake to tactile stimulation and moves all extremities.

1. What other exam finding would be significant in diagnosis and management?
   A. Macrocephaly
   B. Oral thrush
   C. Still murmur
   D. Polydactyly

2. In the ED, the infant becomes mottled and hypotensive. They administer 20 mL/kg of normal saline (NS) and admit the infant to the pediatric ICU (PICU). Which intervention should be the nurse's next priority?
   A. Obtain an arterial blood gas, basic electrolytes, and lactate
   B. Assist physician with lumbar puncture
   C. Administer broad spectrum antibiotics as ordered
   D. Orient the anxious parents to the PICU environment

3. Based on the following lab data, what tests should be made a priority for further investigation to confirm underlying diagnosis? Select all that apply.

Complete blood count (CBC) with differential results as follows:

White blood cell (WBC; cells/µL)	3,600/µL
Red blood cell (RBC; M/mm³)	5.2
Hemoglobin (Hgb; g/dL)	13.2
Hemocrit (HCT) %	39.6
Platelets (K/mm³)	200

A. Newborn screen
B. Lymphocyte subsets and flow cytometry
C. Chest x-ray (CXR)
D. Hemoglobin (Hgb) electrophoresis

White Blood Cell Diff:

Neutrophil %:	60
Neutrophil #:	10
Lymphocyte %:	0
Lymphocyte #:	0
Monocyte %:	15
Monocyte #:	2
Eosinophil %:	5
Eosinophil #:	0.7
Basophil %:	1
Basophil #:	0.05

(See answers next page.)

ANSWERS TO CASE STUDY QUESTIONS

1. B) Oral thrush

As maternal antibodies decline during the first months of life, infants affected by unrecognized immunodeficiencies will begin to present with recurrent infections. Oral thrush within the context of an unwell appearing infant is a common sign of an underlying immunodeficiency.

2. C) Administer broad spectrum antibiotics as ordered

Sepsis is the most life-threatening risk for these children, so broad spectrum antimicrobials should urgently be administered as part of initial stabilization and management.

3. A) Newborn screen; B) Lymphocyte subsets and flow cytometry

Severe combined immunodeficiency (SCID) is a serious congenital immunodeficiency that is now part of routine newborn screening. Confirmative diagnosis of SCID requires an immunology workup with T cell subset flow cytometry. Sometimes a CXR will reveal a small or absent thymus, but it's not considered a confirmatory finding.

● KNOWLEDGE CHECK: CHAPTER 5

1. Which of the of the following statements are true concerning disseminated intravascular coagulation (DIC)?
   A. DIC is often seen during bone marrow engraftment after hematopoietic stem cell transplantation (HSCT) due to a systemic pro-inflammatory state.
   B. Because of their developed hemostatic systems, older children and adolescents are at higher risk for DIC than neonates.
   C. The hemorrhagic component of DIC is most attributed to unregulated activation of tissue plasminogen activator (tPA) resulting from endothelial injury.
   D. Improvement is reflected by increases in fibrinogen and platelet counts as these indicate an interruption in the consumptive process.

2. Which is the priority nursing action when caring for a patient with severe veno-occlusive disease (VOD)?
   A. Aggressive fluid and electrolyte management
   B. Administer defibrotide injection as ordered
   C. Advocate of an escalation of oxygen therapy to noninvasive positive pressure ventilation (NIPPV)
   D. Administer platelets for persistent thrombocytopenia

3. An absolute reticulocyte count of 4% would coincide with _____.
   A. Splenectomy
   B. G6PD deficiency
   C. Parvovirus B19 infection
   D. End-stage kidney disease

4. The following are preventative nursing interventions in the neutropenic patient EXCEPT:
   A. Ensure a clean and safe environment
   B. Diligent skin and mucosal hygiene
   C. Administer live virus vaccines
   D. Optimize nutritional state

5. A 16-year-old girl presents to the pediatric ICU (PICU) with a 2-day history of cough, orthopnea, and increasing anxiety. Her physical exam is remarkable for jugular venous distention, hoarseness, and head and neck swelling. She is tachycardic with blood pressures in the 5th percentile for age. As the bedside nurse, you are most concerned about:
   A. Dilated cardiomyopathy
   B. Superior mediastinal syndrome
   C. Angioedema
   D. Acute chest syndrome

6. You are caring for a boy with a new diagnosis of acute lymphocytic leukemia (ALL). Prior to the initiation of cytotoxic therapy his labs reveal a potassium of 4.9 mEq/L, phosphate of 5.2 mg/dL, and uric acid level of 9.2 mg/dL. Which of the following therapies is most beneficial in decreasing the likelihood of this child needing continuous renal replacement therapy?
   A. Hyperhydration with 1.5 x maintenance intravenous (IV) fluids
   B. Allopurinol
   C. Oral phosphate binders
   D. Rasburicase

(See answers next page.)

1. D) Improvement is reflected by increases in fibrinogen and platelet counts as these indicate an interruption in the consumptive process.

Since DIC is a consumptive coagulopathy, consistently higher levels of fibrinogen and platelets in the bloodstream means they are no longer being consumed in a thrombotic process. The pro-inflammatory state associated with bone marrow engraftment manifests as a capillary leak syndrome, rather than DIC. Neonates are most vulnerable to DIC because of their immature hemostatic systems. The hemorrhagic component of DIC is more reflective of the body's coagulant factors being consumed in thrombotic processes faster than they can be replaced, rather than the fibrinolytic pathway being activated.

2. A) Aggressive fluids and electrolyte management

Aggressive fluid and electrolyte management is critical in prevention as well as supportive therapy for patients with VOD. Defibrotide injection is used to treat children with hepatic VOD but is not always indicated in severe cases due to complications with hemorrhage. Although respiratory compromise is also common, not all patients require NIPPV or mechanical ventilation. Due to the need for aggressive fluid management and risks associated with transfusions, platelet replacement should not be prophylactic but follow goal parameters and whether there is active bleeding.

3. B) G6PD deficiency

G6PD deficiency is a type of hemolytic anemia that results in an increased absolute reticulocyte count. Those with splenectomy should have a reticulocyte count within normal range (0.5%–2%). Parvovirus B19 infection and end-stage kidney disease result in bone marrow suppression, so a low reticulocyte percentage would be expected.

4. C) Administer live virus vaccines

Live virus vaccines should not be given to children who are actively neutropenic, as they could result in infection. A clean environment, diligent skin and mucosal hygiene, and optimized nutrition are all preventative strategies to decrease infection risks in the neutropenic child.

5. B) Superior mediastinal syndrome

All of the signs and symptoms in the case scenario are associated with a space occupying lesion in the anterior mediastinum causing cardiopulmonary compromise. Hoarseness, facial, and neck swelling aren't associated with dilated cardiomyopathy. Angioedema does cause facial swelling; however, it has an acute onset within hours. Acute chest syndrome is associated with pulmonary infiltrate and sickle cell disease, none of which were present in the previous scenario.

6. D) Rasburicase

Specifically for tumor lysis syndrome (TLS), elevated uric acid levels are the leading cause of acute kidney injury (AKI), as they cause crystal precipitation and deposition in the renal tubules; therefore, decreasing uric acid levels should be priorized. Allopurinol is preventative and does not decrease existing uric acid levels, so rasburicase is the appropriate pharmacologic treatment. Hyperhydration should be 2 x maintenance intravenous fluids. Phosphorous level is marginally high, so oral phosphate binders might not be indicated.

7. The primary site of hematopoiesis in a preschool child is:
   A. Thymus
   B. Red marrow present in all bones
   C. Red marrow only present in cranium, vertebrae, pelvis, and sternum
   D. Spleen

8. A patient with a hemoglobin (Hgb) of 6.3 is ordered to receive an aliquoted type and crossmatched packed red blood cells (PRBCs) transfusion. Which of the following reactions is most likely?
   A. Febrile nonhemolytic
   B. Transfusion associated circulatory overload (TACO)
   C. Alloimmunization
   D. Hemolytic

9. You are caring for a child in the pediatric ICU (PICU) with tachypnea, dyspnea, and a new noninvasive positive pressure ventilation (NIPPV) requirement. She is day +20 from her hematopoietic stem cell transplantation (HSCT). Her weight and abdominal girth have been increasing over the last 3 days and urine output has dropped to <0.5 mL/kg/hr. Her heart rate (HR) is 140, respiratory rate (RR) 45, blood pressure (BP) 80/34(50). Her SpO2 is 94% on 60% oxygen via 20L/min heated HFNC. She is febrile and pancytopenic. Her abdomen is tender and assessment reveals hepatomegaly. What is the most likely contributor to her decreased urine output?
   A. Intrabdominal hemorrhage
   B. Hypoperfusion secondary to septic shock
   C. Acute kidney injury (AKI) secondary to bone marrow transplant (BMT) nephrotoxic medications (chemo prep)
   D. Hepatorenal syndrome

10. A 5-month-old girl is admitted to the pediatric ICU (PICU) with HIV. Her respiratory rate (RR) is 66 beats/min, SpO2 is 88% on room air. Parents report a decrease in oral intake over the last 3 days, no vomiting or diarrhea. The most likely cause of her respiratory distress is:
    A. *Streptococcus (S.) pneumoniae* bacteremia
    B. Cytomegalovirus (CMV) pneumonia
    C. Pneumocystis pneumonia
    D. Dehydration

(See answers next page.)

7. B) Red marrow only present in cranium, vertebrae, pelvis, and sternum

During fetal development, hematopoiesis occurs in many places such as the yolk sac, lymph nodes, liver, spleen, and thymus. Shortly after birth these transition to the red marrow located in all bones throughout the body. Over decades, yellow marrow replaces the red marrow in long bones, so the main sites of hematopoiesis in adults are the cranium, vertebrae, pelvis, and sternum.

8. A) Febrile nonhemolytic

In pediatrics, allergic reactions are the most common reaction to PRBCs; however, of the answer choices febrile nonhemolytic is the most appropriate. The unit is appropriately typed and crossmatched so a hemolytic reaction would be surprising. The patient is receiving an aliquoted amount, making TACO less likely. It is not stated whether the patient in the scenario has had a PRBC transfusion before, which would make alloimmunization more of a possibility. With the information provided in the question and the choices available, febrile nonhemolytic would be the most expected.

9. D) Hepatorenal syndrome

This patient is showing classic signs of veno-occlusive disease (VOD), making hepatorenal syndrome the most likely reason for the declining urine output.

10. C) Pneumocystis pneumonia

S. pneumoniae, CMV, and pneumocystis pneumonia are all associated with pneumonia in a child with HIV. Infection with pneumocystis pneumonia is a leading cause of early mortality in children infected with HIV. The four clinical findings presented in the case have been independently associated with pneumocystis pneumonia infection.

REFERENCES

Abla, O., Angelini, P., Di Giuseppe, G., Kanani, M. F., Lau, W., Hitzler, J., Sung, L., & Naqvi, A., (2016). Early complications of hyperleukocytosis and leukapheresis in childhood acute leukemias. *Journal of Pediatric Hematology/ Oncology, 38*(2), 111–117. https://doi.org/10.1097/MPH.0000000000000490

Bonilla, F.A., & Notarangelo, L. (2015). Primary immunodeficiency diseases. In S. H. Orkin, D. E. Fisher, A. T. Look, S. E. Lux, IV, D. Ginsburg, & D. G. Nathan (Eds.), *Nathan and Oski's hematology and oncology of infancy and childhood* (8th ed., pp. 886–921). Saunders, an imprint of Elsevier Inc.

Borhade, M. B., & Kondamudi, N. P. (2021). Sickle cell crisis. In B. Abai, A. Amal Abu-Ghosh, A. B. Acharya, U. Acharya, S. G. Adhia, R. Adigun, T. C. Aeby, N. R. Aeddula, A. Agarwal, M. Agarwal, S. Aggarwal, R. Ahlawat, R. A. Ahmed, F. Akhtar, A. M. Al Aboud, Y. Al Khalili, E. Al Zaabi, G. Alexander, M. Saleh Alhajjaj, . . . K. J. Allen (Eds.), *StatPearls* [Internet]. StatPearls Publishing. https://www.ncbi.nlm.nih.gov/books/NBK526064/

Branowicki, P. A., Houlahan, K. E., Conley, S, B, & Kline, N. E. (2015). Nursing care of patients with childhood cancer. In S. H. Orkin, D. E. Fisher, A. T. Look, S. E. Lux, IV, D. Ginsburg, & D. G. Nathan (Eds.), *Nathan and Oski's hematology and oncology of infancy and childhood* (8th ed., pp. 2292–2320). Saunders, an imprint of Elsevier Inc.

Brugnara, C., Oski, F. A., & Nathan, D. G. (2015). Diagnostic approach to the patient with Anemia. In S. H. Orkin, D. E. Fisher, A. T. Look, S. E. Lux, IV, D. Ginsburg, & D. G. Nathan (Eds.), *Nathan and Oski's hematology and oncology of infancy and childhood* (8th ed., pp. 293–307). Saunders, an imprint of Elsevier Inc.

Chok, R., Turley, E., & Bruce, A. (2021). Screening and diagnosis of heparin-induced thrombocytopenia in the pediatric population: A tertiary centre experience. *Thrombosis Research, 207*, 1–6. https://doi.org/10.1016/j.thromres.2021.08.020

Di Paola, J., Montgomery, R. R., Gill, J. C., & Flood, V. (2015). Hemophilia and von Willibrand disease. In S. H. Orkin, D. E. Fisher, A. T. Look, S. E. Lux, IV, D. Ginsburg, & D. G. Nathan (Eds.), *Nathan and Oski's hematology and oncology of infancy and childhood* (8th ed., pp. 1028–1054). Saunders, an imprint of Elsevier Inc.

Dinauer, M. C., Newberger, P. E., & Booregaard, N. (2015). Phagocyte systems and disorders of granulopoiesis and granyloctye function. In S. H. Orkin, D. E. Fisher, A. T. Look, S. E. Lux, IV, D. Ginsburg, & D. G. Nathan (Eds.), *Nathan and Oski's hematology and oncology of infancy and childhood* (8th ed., pp. 773–847). Saunders, an imprint of Elsevier Inc.

Fraint, E., Holuba, M. J., & Wray, L. (2020). Pediatric hematopoietic stem cell transplant. *Pediatrics in Review, 41*(11), 609–611. https://doi.org/10.1542/pir.2020-0130 PMID: 33139417.

Gaspard, K. J. (2009) Disorders of hemostasis. In C. M. Porth & G. Matfin (Eds.), *Pathophysiology concepts of altered health states* (8th ed., pp. 262–277). Wolters Kluwer Health, Lippincott Williams & Wilkens.

Ghanima, W., Cooper, N., Rodeghiero, F., Godeau, B., & Bussel, J. B. (2019). Thrombopoetin receptor agonists: 10 years later. *Hematologica, 104*(6). https://doi.org/10.3324/haematol.2018.212845

Grace, R. F. (2015). Hematologic manifestations of systemic disease. In S. H. Orkin, D. E. Fisher, A. T. Look, S. E. Lux, IV, D. Ginsburg, W., & D. G. Nathan (Eds.), *Nathan and Oski's hematology and oncology of infancy and childhood* (8th ed., pp. 1167–1202). Saunders, an imprint of Elsevier Inc.

Grace, R. F., & Lambert, M. P. (2017). An update on pediatric immune thrombocytopenia (ITP): Differentiating primary ITP, IPD, and PID. *Blood, 140*, 542–555. https://doi.org/10.1182/blood.2020006480

Inati, A., Mansour, A. G., Sabbouh, T., Amhez, G., Hachmen, A., & Abbas, H. A. (2017). Transfusion therapy in children with sickle cell disease. *Journal of Pediatric Hematology/Oncology, 39*(2), 126–132. https://doi.org/10.1097/MPH.0000000000000645

Kobrynski, L. J. (2022). Newborn screening in the diagnosis of primary immunodeficiency. *Clinical Reviews in Allergy & Immunology, 63*, 9–21. https://doi.org/10.1007/s12016-021-08876-z

Levi, M., & van der Poll, T. (2017). Coagulation and Sepsis. *Thrombosis Research, 149*, 38–44. https://doi.org/10.1016/j.thromres.2016.11.007

Main, S. (2017). Expanding nursing knowledge for therapeutic plasma exchange a literature review paper. *Transfusion and Apheresis Science, 56*(5), 774–777. https://doi.org/10.1016/j.transci.2017.08.022

Mehta, H. M., Malandra, M., & Corey, S. J. (2015). G-CSF and GM-CSF in neutropenia. *Journal of Immunology, 195*(4), 1341–1349. https://doi.org/10.4049/jimmunol.1500861

Nicolas, D., Nicolas, S., Hodgens, A., & Reed, M. (2021). Heparin induced thrombocytopenia. In B. Abai, A. Amal Abu-Ghosh, A. B. Acharya, U. Acharya, S. G. Adhia, R. Adigun, T. C. Aeby, N. R. Aeddula, A. Agarwal, M. Agarwal, S. Aggarwal, R. Ahlawat, R. A. Ahmed, F. Akhtar, A. M. Al Aboud, Y. Al Khalili, E. Al Zaabi, G. Alexander, M. Saleh Alhajjaj, . . . K. J. Allen (Eds.), *StatPearls* [Internet]. StatPearls Publishing. https://www.ncbi.nlm.nih.gov/books/NBK482330/

Norris, T. L. (2019). *Pathophysiology concepts of altered health states* (8th ed.). Wolters Kluwer Health.

Praven, R., Tan, E. E. K., Sultana, R., Thoon, K. C., Chan, M. Y., Lee, J. H., & Wong, J. J. (2020). Critical illness epidemiology and mortality risk in pediatric oncology. *Pediatric Blood & Cancer, 67*(6), e28242. https://doi.org/10.1002/pbc.28242 PMID: 32187445.

Russell, T. B., & Kram, D. E. (2020). Tumor lysis syndrome. *Pediatrics in Review, 41*(1), 20–26. https://doi.org/10.1542/pir.2018-0243

Sherman, G., & Mazanderani, A. H. (2020). Diagnosis of HIV infection in children and adolescents. In R. Bobat (Ed.), *HIV infection in children and adolescents* (1st ed., pp. 15–22). Springer Nature Switzerland AG.

Slota, M. (Ed.). (2019). *AACN core curriculum for pediatric high acuity, progressive, and critical care nursing* (3rd ed.). Springer Publishing Company.

Spruit, J. L. (2019). Hematology and immunology systems. In M. C. Slota (Ed.), *AACN core curriculum for pediatric high acuity, progressive, and critical care nursing* (3rd ed., pp. 583–665). Springer Publishing Company.

Steffen, K., Doctor, A., Hoerr, J., Gill, J., Markham, C., Brown, S. M., Cohen, D., Hansen, R., Kryzer, E., Richards, J., Small, S., Valentine, S., York, J. L., Proctor, E. K., & Spinella, P. C. (2017). Controlling phlebotomy volume diminishes PICU transfusion: Implementation processes and impact. *Pediatrics,140*(2), e20162480. https://doi.org/10.1542/peds.2016-2480

Veldman., A., Fischer, D., Nold, M. F., & Wong, F. Y. (2010). Intravascular coagulation in term and preterm neonates. *Seminars in Thrombosis and Hemostasis, 36*(4), 419–428. https://doi.org/10.1055/s-0030-1254050

Vossoughi, S., Perez, G., Whitaker, B. I., Fung, M. K., & Stotler, B. (2018). Analysis of pediatric adverse reactions to transfusions. *Transfusion, 58*(1), 60–69. https://doi.org/10.1111/trf.14359

Warner, M. J., & Kamran, M. T. (2021). Iron deficiency anemia. In B. Abai, A. Amal Abu-Ghosh, A. B. Acharya, U. Acharya, S. G. Adhia, R. Adigun, T. C. Aeby, N. R. Aeddula, A. Agarwal, M. Agarwal, S. Aggarwal, R. Ahlawat, R. A. Ahmed, F. Akhtar, A. M. Al Aboud, Y. Al Khalili, E. Al Zaabi, G. Alexander, M. Saleh Alhajjaj, . . . K. J. Allen (Eds.), *StatPearls* [Internet]. StatPearls Publishing. https://www.ncbi.nlm.nih.gov/books/NBK448065/

Wilkenson, A. (2019). Early recognition and treatment of Henoch-Schönlein purpura in children. *Nursing Children and Young People, 31*(5), 36–40. https://doi.org/10.7748/ncyp.2019.e1118

Wilson, D. B. (2015). Acquired platelet defects. In S. H. Orkin, D. E. Fisher, A. T. Look, S. E. Lux, IV, D. Ginsburg, & D. G. Nathan (Eds.), *Nathan and Oski's hematology and oncology of infancy and childhood* (8th ed., pp. 1076–1102). Saunders, an imprint of Elsevier Inc.

Wittmann, O., Rimon, A., Scolnik, D., & Glatstein, M. (2018). Outcomes of immunocompetent children presenting with fever and neutropenia. *The Journal of Emergency Medicine, 54*(3), https://doi.org/10.1016/j.jemermed.2017.10.022

Gastrointestinal System Review

David Jack and Maureen Fitzgerald

The gastrointestinal (GI) system functions in digestion, nutrient absorption, and waste elimination. GI trauma can result in injuries to a number of gastrointestinal organs including: the stomach, small bowel, colon, or rectum resulting in serious acute or long-term sequela. Due to the potentially life-threatening nature of these injuries, nurses need to be able to identify, monitor, and prevent pediatric patients for GI complications (Martin, 2019).

▶ ABDOMINAL COMPARTMENT SYNDROME

Intra-abdominal pressure (IAP) is pressure within the abdominal cavity and is measured in mmHg. Normal IAP in a well child is zero. Abdominal pressure is commonly measured by bladder pressures via a transduced foley catheter after the injection of 25 to 30 mL of sterile saline. In a sick ventilated child, a normal IAP is 5 to 7 mmHg. Intra-abdominal hypertension (IAH) is defined as a pressure >12 mmHg. Abdominal compartment syndrome (ACS) occurs when there is end-organ dysfunction as a result of sustained elevated IAP (Urden et al., 2022).

Increased pressure within the abdomen can impinge on diaphragmatic excursion. This may be exhibited by increased peak pressures in ventilated children and can affect the ability to properly ventilate children. IAH is graded as follows:

- **grade I:** IAP (12–15 mmHg)
- **grade II:** IAP (16–20 mmHg)
- **grade III:** IAP (21–25 mmHg)
- **grade IV:** IAP (>25 mmHg; Urden et al., 2022)

Surgical decompression of the abdomen may be required for abdominal pressures >20 to 25 mmHg accompanied by a tense, taunt abdomen with signs of organ dysfunction with the heart, lungs, or kidneys (Urden et al., 2022).

ACS is associated with organ dysfunction and failure and may be classified as primary or secondary abdominal compartment syndrome.

- **primary:** results from direct injury to the abdomen or pelvic region such as in the cases of blunt or penetrating trauma or ruptured abdominal aortic aneurysm
- **secondary:** does not originate from the abdominopelvic region but associated with severe shock (requiring massive fluid resuscitation) hemorrhage, sepsis, capillary leak syndrome or major burns, severe gut edema, pancreatitis, ischemia reperfusion injury, interperitoneal or retroperitoneal bleeding and/or ascites

ACS can be seen in conditions where there is both vascular leakage and high-volume fluid resuscitation, such as:

- status post laparotomy
- severe abdominal injury
- severe burns
- sepsis
- pancreatitis

Clinical Pearl

Patient groups that are high risk for ACS include trauma, burns, septic shock, and post-abdominal surgery, particularly those requiring large volumes of fluid resuscitation.

Elevated intra-abdominal pressure causes decreased perfusion to the intra-abdominal organs due to elevated pressure on the vena cava and eventually progresses to increased pressure on the aorta and arterial vessels. Clinical manifestations include:
- decreased cardiac output
- decreased tidal volume
- increased pulmonary peak pressure
- decrease urine output
- hypoxia

Elevated IAP impacts other body organ systems outside the abdominal cavity (Ballman et al., 2021).
- **Respiratory:** Upward movement of the diaphragm results in bibasilar compressive pulmonary atelectasis and ventilation-perfusion mismatch. Reduced functional residual capacity and low lung volumes with decreased chest wall compliance may result in increased work of breathing.
- **Cardiac:** Elevated IAP may affect cardiovascular function by having a negative effect on preload, afterload, and contractility.
- **Renal:** Decreased renal perfusion leads to secretion of catecholamines, angiotensin II, and aldosterone with subsequent vasoconstriction that may result in increased systemic vascular resistance.
- **Central nervous system (CNS):** Elevated IAP causes an increase in intracranial pressure (ICP) and reduction of cerebral perfusion pressure (CPP) leading to reduced Glasgow Coma Scale (GCS) scores and blood flow to the brain (Divarci et al., 2016).

The most common multisystem effects occurring along with organ failure include (Chedly & Chiaka-Ejike, 2017):
- metabolic acidosis despite resuscitation
- oliguria despite volume repletion
- elevated peak airway pressures
- hypercarbia refractory to increased ventilation
- hypoxemia refractory to oxygen and positive end expiratory pressure (PEEP)
- intracranial hypertension ($\uparrow$ ICP)

NURSING IMPLICATIONS AND TREATMENT

- Due to the tissue necrosis and possible surgical decompression associated with ACS, these children are at high risk for infection.
- Obtain baseline IAP measurements for children at risk for IAP/ACS.
  - Measure IAP at end of expiration.
  - Zero the transducer at the level of the iliac crest at the mid-axillary line.
- Obtain serial IAP measurements.
- Monitor the child's vital signs and surgical wound closely for infection and report to provider if assessment findings consistent with infection are identified.
- Assess the child's pain using a valid and reliable (developmentally appropriate) pain rating scale. Notify provider if more analgesia is required to achieve comfort.
- Perform a focused GI assessment every shift or more frequently as needed. Make particular note of abdominal distention, discoloration, firmness, and bowel sounds.
- Strict intake and output (I&O) should be undertaken and maintained.

ASSESSMENT

Failure to recognize symptoms of ACS may result in a critical delay in management, which can contribute to the high morbidity and mortality of this clinical disorder. Early detection of IAP is essential to the prevention of ACS and requires close monitoring of IAP with frequent measurements and monitoring by the pediatric critical care nurse. According to the World Society of the Abdominal Compartment Syndrome (WSACS; 2021), the bladder method is the most accurate indirect method for measuring IAP in children. Figure 6.1 depicts the setup system.

Assessment findings of ACS include:
- increased abdominal girth, with a tensely distended abdomen
- difficulty breathing with progressive hypoxia
- increased ventilatory requirements
- decreased urine output with progressive oliguria
- nausea and vomiting
- inability to palpate femoral pulses, with lower extremity cyanosis
- hypotension, tachycardia, elevated jugular venous pressure and venous distention, peripheral edema

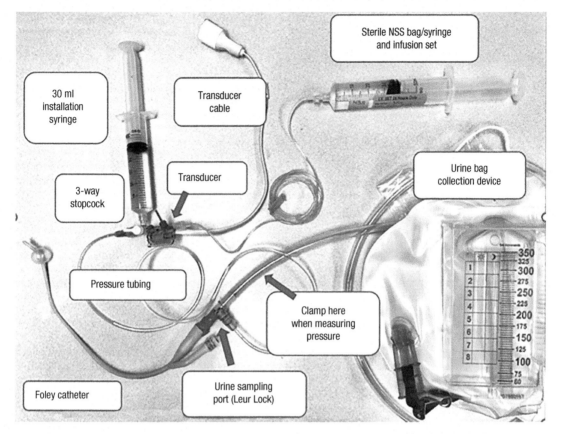

Figure 6.1 Closed system to measure bladder (abdominal) pressure constructed with readily available ICU equipment

NSS, normal sterile saline.

- presence of agitation
- **subjective signs include** malaise, weakness, lightheadedness, dyspnea, or abdominal pain

For children in the postoperative phase of surgery, assessment remains the same as for presurgical children with the addition of possible wound management. Wound care may involve the maintenance of dressings and drainage systems (e.g., vacuum-assisted closure system), and use of skin grafts for abdominal wound closure if needed.

LABS AND DIAGNOSTICS

Diagnostic criteria for ACS include:
- elevated IAP (>12 mmHg–15 mmHg)
- new onset end organ compromise including hypotension
- increased ventilatory requirement
- decreased urine output of <0.5 mL/kg per hour
- increase in lactic acid

TREATMENT AND MANAGEMENT

Avoiding elevated IAP is a critical element in the prevention of ACS. In the case of overt ACS (>20 mmHg–25 mmHg), emergent surgical decompression (opening the abdomen) is performed with the aims of improved respiratory mechanics, restoring venous return to the heart, and restoring abdominal organ perfusion. Note that while opening the abdomen may solve ventilation difficulties, it will also affect afterload and blood pressure may suddenly drop significantly. Having vasopressors ready is most important. Surgical decompression can be performed via laparotomy or through surgical midline incision. The abdominal muscle fascia may be left open, and an alternative dressing closure may be used (like a Wittman patch with vac-system) for days until the pressure decreases enough to return the abdominal contents to the abdomen and close the abdominal skin. Daily redresses of the open abdomen may be required. The drains from the abdomen will be connected to suction for best abdominal decompression (Kirkpatrick et al., 2013; WSACS, 2021).

COMPLICATIONS
- urinary tract infections with IAP monitoring
- organ system dysfunction and failure with elevated abdominal pressures and ACS
- high mortality if IAP is not reduced

▶ ABDOMINAL TRAUMA

Abdominal trauma is defined as any injury to the abdomen, which includes both blunt and penetrating injuries sustained by various mechanisms of force or penetration. Developmentally, children are at greater risk for intra-abdominal injuries after blunt trauma due to (Shaw & Bachur, 2020):
- immature musculoskeletal system (rib cage not yet protecting their abdominal organs)
- higher abdominal organ-to-body mass ratio, which results in a force delivered to the abdomen over a smaller body surface area, increasing the likelihood of injury to the underlying structures
- abdominal organs more anterior with less subcutaneous (SC) fat for organ protection
- smaller blood volume compared to adults resulting in hypovolemia with relatively smaller volume losses
  Based on their developmental age, children are at high risk for different mechanism of injuries that lead to blunt or penetrating abdominal trauma.

BLUNT TRAUMA

Blunt trauma involves a **direct blow** to the abdomen (such as being kicked or struck by a baseball ball or bat, sports injuries, assault) or impact with an object (as in falling off a bicycle or impact with handlebars of the bicycle, sports injuries).
- Direct trauma to the abdomen will result in local injury and damage to the overlying skin and subcutaneous blood vessels. The depth of the injury is directly related to the force of the blow.
- **Waddell's triad** comprises three distinct features seen in pediatric pedestrian patients with blunt force trauma from a direct impact with a motor vehicle: Ipsilateral femoral shaft fracture, ipsilateral intrathoracic or intra-abdominal injury, and contralateral head injury.
- Although any abdominal organ can be injured, blunt trauma is the most common cause of acute **pancreatitis** in children due to compression of the pancreas against the spine.
- The spleen is the organ most commonly damaged, followed by the liver and hallow viscus (typically small intestines).
- Blunt injury may result in a hematoma in solid organ or the wall of a hollow viscus.
  Sudden **acceleration/deceleration** (such as restrain by a lap belt in a motor vehicle accident, when a skier hits a barricade, or falling from a height) injury occurs when a moving child is abruptly brought to a stop.
- This type of injury may cause complete disruption of deep organs and very few superficial signs.
- Children involved in deceleration injuries often may have injuries to other parts of the body, including the thoracic aorta.

PENETRATING TRAUMA

Penetrating abdominal trauma may be the result of stab, gunshot wound, or sharp object (impalement). Penetrating injuries may or may not penetrate the peritoneum and, if they do, may not cause organ injury. Gunshot wounds are more likely to cause intra-abdominal damage than stab wounds.
- Penetrating trauma to the chest (below the 4th intercostal space) should be evaluated as a potential abdominal wound because of the location of the abdominal organs within the chest during a respiratory cycle.
- Gunshot wounds frequently involve multiple organs while stab wounds are often isolated, especially if the wound is limited to the back or flank.
- Penetrating trauma may result in laceration, followed by hemorrhage. Minor vascular laceration or hallow viscus laceration is often associated with low volume blood loss.
- More severe penetrating injury can result in massive hemorrhage with symptoms of shock, acidosis, and coagulopathy.
  - Internal hemorrhage may be intraperitoneal or retroperitoneal.
  - Rupture/laceration of hollow viscus can allow contents (gastric, intestinal, and urinary) to enter the peritoneal cavity, leading to peritonitis.

NURSING IMPLICATIONS AND TREATMENT

INJURY CATEGORIZATION

In addition to the mechanism of injury (blunt or penetrating), injuries are often categorized by the type of structure that is damaged:

- abdominal wall
- solid organ (liver, spleen, pancreas, kidneys)
- hallow viscus (stomach, small intestine, colon, ureters, bladder): range from hematomas to full thickness injury. Accounts for 1% of all blunt abdominal trauma injuries.
- vasculature

Injury scales have been developed to classify severity of abdominal organ injury ranging from grade I (minimal) to grade VI (maximum, severe). Mortality and need for operative intervention increase as grade increases.

Spleen Injury

The American Association for the Surgery of Trauma (AAST) developed a grading system used for spleen trauma that ranges from grade I (less severe) to grade V (severe; Table 6.1). The grading system provides guidelines for the providers regarding treatment decisions and management of the injury ranging from observation to surgical intervention.

Table 6.1 Spleen Injury Scale

Grade	Injury Description
I	
Hematoma	Subcapsular, nonexpanding, <10% of surface area
Laceration	Capsular tear, nonbleeding, <1 cm of parenchymal depth
II	
Hematoma	Subcapsular, non-expanding, 10%–50% of surface area, intraparenchymal, non-expanding <5 cm diameter
Laceration	Capsular tear, 1–3 cm of parenchymal depth that does not involve a trabecular vessel
III	
Hematoma	Subcapsular, >50% of surface area or expanding, ruptured subcapsular or hematoma, intraparenchymal hematoma, >5 cm expanding
Laceration	>3 cm of parenchymal depth or involving the trabecular vessels
IV	
Hematoma	Ruptured intraparenchymal hematoma with active bleeding
Laceration	Laceration involving segmental or hilar vessel production major devascularization (>25% of spleen)
V	
Hematoma	Completely shattered spleen
Laceration	Hilar vascular injury that devascularizes the spleen

Source: Slota, M. (Ed.). (2019). *AACN core curriculum for pediatric high acuity, progressive, and critical care nursing* (3rd ed.). Springer Publishing Company.

Liver Injuries

- Severity graded I to VI (Table 6.2)

Table 6.2 Liver Injury Scale

Grade	Injury Description
I	
Hematoma Laceration	Subcapsular, <10% of surface area Capsular tear, <1 cm of parenchymal depth
II	

(continued)

Table 6.2 Liver Injury Scale (*continued*)

Grade	Injury Description
Hematoma Laceration	Subcapsular, 10%–50% of surface area, intraparenchymal, <10 cm in diameter 1–3 cm parenchymal depth, <10 cm in length
IV	
Laceration	Parenchymal destruction involving 25%–75% of hepatic lobe or 1–3 Couinaud's segments within a single lobe
V	
Laceration	Parenchymal destruction involving >75% of hepatic lobe or >3 Couinaud's segment within a single lobe
Vascular	Juxtahepatic venous injuries, i.e., retrohepatic vena cava/central major hepatic veins
VI	
Vascular	Hepatic evulsion

Source: Slota, M. (Ed.). (2019). *AACN core curriculum for pediatric high acuity, progressive, and critical care nursing* (3rd ed.). Springer Publishing Company.

Clinical Pearl

Physiologically, children can maintain normal vital signs even in the setting of significant blood loss. As much as one quarter of the blood volume can be lost prior to the onset of hypotension.

NURSING IMPLICATIONS AND MANAGEMENT

Nursing care is directed toward maintaining perfusion of organ systems, decreasing complications (infection, sepsis, inflammation), fluid and electrolyte balance, nutritional needs, and any potential body image disturbances (Wolters Kluwer, 2021).

- Obtain history of injury, mechanism of injury, onset, and progression of symptoms.
- Assess vital signs for adequate organ perfusion, hemodynamic stability, signs of inflammation and infection.
- Assess central venous pressures (CVP), abdominal pressures (when indicated), fluid balance, and urinary output.
- Assess oxygen level using pulse oximetry and administer supplemental oxygen as prescribed by provider.
- Assess pain. Instruct patient on methods to splint the abdomen.
- Administer intravenous (IV) fluids, transfusions, hyperalimentation, and antibiotic therapy as prescribed by the provider.
- Vaccination with *S. pneumoniae*, *Haemophilus influenzae* type b, and *Neisseria meningitides*, if splenectomy was required.
  - Penicillin prophylaxis is recommended in children younger than 5 years and for 2 years following splenectomy.
- Monitor for infection.
- Encourage coughing, deep breathing, incentive spirometry and turning every 2 to 4 hours.
- Contact child protective services if child maltreatment is suspected.
- Children who sustain an isolated spleen injury are restricted from contact sports and strenuous physical activity for a period **consisting of the grade of injury** (i.e., grade 5 = 5 weeks) **plus 2 weeks** (5 weeks + 2 weeks = 7 weeks total).

ASSESSMENTS

Examination of the abdomen does not reliably indicate the severity of the abdominal injury. Initial symptoms may be vague. If the child experienced trauma, pain associated with extra-abdominal injuries may obscure abdominal findings. Assessment findings of abdominal trauma include:

- **Abdominal pain and tenderness**: Pain from spleen injury (left upper quadrant [LUQ]) with *radiation to the left shoulder* is **Kehr's sign**; note any guarding or rebound tenderness, which could indicate the presence of intraperitoneal blood.

- Signs of retroperitoneal bleeding include **Cullen's sign** (ecchymosis around the umbilicus) and **Grey Turner's sign** (ecchymosis over the flank).
- Vital signs may demonstrate tachycardia first (compensation), followed by hypovolemia and proceed to shock if not detected. Hypotension may be a late sign in children.
- **abdominal ecchymosis:** reveal marks from a lap belt (although an unreliable sign)
- **abdominal distention:** may indicate severe hemorrhage as in a hemoperitoneum
- absent bowel sounds
- nausea and vomiting
- abdominal rigidity, guarding, and rebound tenderness is often associated with peritonitis.
- bleeding from the rectum or urethra if there is a colonic lesion or perineal hematoma due to urinary tract injury

Attention should be paid to the anterior and posterior abdomen and to both flanks, as well as to the lower thorax, when considering abdominal injuries.

Clinical Pearl

Abdominal distension	Suggests blood, fluid, intestinal perforation, or acute gastric distension
Generalized guarding	Suggests peritonitis, usually a sign of massive bleeding or perforation
Blood at the urethral meatus	Suggests urethral trauma

LABS AND DIAGNOSTICS

- **Lab testing:** If an intra-abdominal injury is suspected, hemoglobin measurement and typing and cross-matching should be undertaken.
  - Complete blood count (CBC) or hemoglobin (Hgb) and hematocrit (HCT) may be repeated every 4 to 6 hours.
  - serum liver transaminase levels: expect to be elevated
  - amylase/Lipase
  - serum lactate level
  - arterial blood gas analysis
  - occult blood analysis from gastric content, stool, or urine
  - urine analysis: to detect any bleeding (gross or microscopic)
- **Imaging studies:**
  - **CT scan/ultrasonography of the abdomen**
  - chest x-ray (CXR; looking for presence of free air under the diaphragm as in diaphragmic rupture or perforation of a hollow viscus)
  - **extended focused assessment with sonography for trauma (EFAST)**
- **Procedural:**
  - exploratory laparotomy
  - diagnostic peritoneal lavage
  - In a **diagnostic peritoneal lavage**, aspiration of blood is considered a positive tap.
    - ❏ A tap positive for blood indicates hemoperitoneum but provides no information on the bleeding source. If no blood is obtained, then 10 mL/kg of normal saline solution (NSS) or Ringer's lactate solution (RL) is infused through the catheter and the effluent is drained by gravity.
    - ❏ Cell count and chemistries are obtained.

TREATMENT AND MANAGEMENT

The American Pediatric Surgical Association (APSA) guidelines for the treatment of isolated solid organ injury in children were published in 2000 and have been widely adopted among clinicians. These guidelines can be found at https://apsapedsurg.org/wp-content/uploads/2020/10/APSA_Solid-Organ-Injury-Guidelines-2019.pdf.

Current management of pediatric blunt liver and spleen injury is based on hemodynamic status, not grade.

- **spleen injury**
  - **Nonoperative management** of spleen injuries includes observation, bedrest, monitoring of serial Hgb and HCT, vital sign (hemodynamic) stability, intravenous fluids (IVF), and interventional radiology with angioembolization.
  - **Surgical traditional treatment** includes splenectomy or splenorrhaphy.

■ **liver injuries**
  ● major source of hemorrhage, but most stop bleeding on their own
  ● often occur with rib and pelvic fractures
  ● right upper quadrant tenderness
  ● increasing abdominal girth and tenderness
  ● signs of shock (hypovolemic)
  ● diagnosed with CT
  ● Monitor liver transaminases AST and ALT for liver.
    ❑ **aspartate transaminase (AST;** normal <40) **elevated >200 U/L**
    ❑ **alanine transaminase (ALT;** normal <35) **elevated >100 U/L**
  ● Usually does not require surgery unless hemodynamically unstable and severe.
  Treatment of **hollow viscera and viscus** is primarily operative with the main challenge surrounding identification of injury and the subsequent timing of intervention.
  Management of abdominal trauma includes:
■ airway and C-spine stabilization
■ oxygen
■ Intravenous/intraosseous large bore access should be established. If hemodynamically unstable, administer a rapid fluid bolus of 20 mL/kg of an isotonic crystalloid solution (Lactated Ringer's [LR] or normal sterile saline [NSS]), and repeat if vital signs do not improve.
  ● If hemodynamic instability persists after 40 mL per kg of crystalloid, ongoing bleeding should be suspected, and administration of blood may be required.
■ observation and monitoring for noncritical blunt intra-abdominal injuries with abdominal trauma
  ● Any gunshot wound to the abdomen mandates immediate exploration.
■ **laparoscopy/laparotomy:** especially for eviscerations, pneumoperitoneum, organ repair, or hemodynamic instability
■ **angioembolization:** used in children and adolescents with blunt trauma to control bleeding
■ **Transfusions as needed:** Children suspected of ongoing hemorrhage should be considered for angiography with embolization (as previously stated) or immediate laparotomy.
■ nasogastric (NG)/orogastric (OG) decompression with a nasogastric tube/orogastric to facilitate bowel rest.
■ surgical intervention
■ **Impalement injury** is an uncommon, but possible, type of penetrating injury in children. Principles of impalement injury include the following:
  ● The impaled object should be left in place by first responders to provide a tamponade effect.
  ● The child should be rapidly stabilized at the scene and transported, preferably, to a trauma center.
  ● After evaluation in the ED, transport to the operating room (OR) for definitive intervention (Shimizu et al., 2019).

▶ BOWEL INFARCTION, OBSTRUCTION, AND PERFORATION

Bowel infarction is rare in children. This area of the bowel has decreased blood flow, lacking oxygen, causing ischemia to the area. Bowel infarction can be mild or severe, and sudden or gradual depending on the cause, for example, with atherosclerosis, hypotension, or bowel obstruction.

Bowel obstruction can be acute or chronic. There are three types of obstructions: **complete, partial,** and **intermittent**.

Causes of obstruction:
■ **mechanical obstruction** (physical obstruction)
■ **functional obstruction** (impaired peristalsis)
■ **GI perforation**

Clinical Pearl

Hirschsprung's (congenital aganglionic megacolon) is a condition where a section of bowel is not innervated with ganglionic cells (needed for peristalsis), so stool gets caught up and the proximal portion of the bowel dilates. They cannot move bowels. If they do it is ribbon-like. They have bilious emesis. Surgical correction with possible temporary colostomy with further reanastomosis. Low residue, high calorie, high protein diet.

SIGNS AND SYMPTOMS

Children with GI tract injuries or abnormalities usually show signs of decreased motility. Signs and symptoms are dependent on the cause.

NURSING IMPLICATIONS AND TREATMENT

Nurses caring for these patients need to:
- monitor vital signs continuously as ordered
- assess and monitor NG tube with gastric decompression
- monitor I&O
- assess for pain
- administer nothing by mouth (NPO)

ASSESSMENT

Assess the child's stooling pattern. If an NG tube was placed, assess output for bilious drainage, which is indicative of these conditions. Also monitor for complications such as peritonitis. Assessment findings include:
- sudden abdominal pain (unrelenting, persistent abdominal pain may indicate perforation), irritability in infants
- tense, rigid (board-like) abdomen
- tenderness and guarding with palpation
- assess for redness on the abdomen, which may indicate localized peritonitis
- distention or scaphoid abdomen
- diminished or absent bowel sounds, except for certain instances such as in bowel obstruction, which can have high-pitched or hyperactive bowel sounds depending on location
- nausea, vomiting (can be bilious emesis) and/or diarrhea, persistent vomiting noted with bowel obstruction
- fever
- weight loss; feeding intolerance; feeling full after eating minimal amount
- frequent urge to have bowel movement
- constipation
- respiratory distress
- hematemesis (bloody vomitus) and/or hematochezia (bright, red blood from rectum)
- melena (black, tarry stools)
- GI hemorrhage
- shock or death

TREATMENT AND MANAGEMENT

Treatment includes:
- gastric decompression
- rigorous intravenous fluid resuscitation (IVF) using isotonic LR solution to replace fluid losses
- administration of pain medications such as IV opioids
- Give broad-spectrum antibiotics for peritonitis or necrosis as needed.

▶ GASTROESOPHAGEAL REFLUX

Gastrointestinal reflux (GER) is the retrograde movement of gastric contents passing through the lower esophageal sphincter (LES) and into the esophagus with or without vomiting. Anatomically, this reflux is normally prevented by the correct function of the gastroesophageal junction (cardiac sphincter), also known as the antireflux barrier. Gastroesophageal reflux disease (GERD) can cause complications such as irritability, respiratory problems, poor feeding, and possibly poor growth leading to failure to thrive (FTT). Although GERD can occur throughout the lifespan, infancy is the most prevalent time with an estimated 85% of infants occurring slightly more frequently in male children as opposed to female children.
- GER starts to decrease after 7 months of age and the incidence of GER drops significantly after 18 months of age due to growth and maturation of the GI system—often resolves spontaneously as the newborn matures.

▥ The most common cause of GERD in infants is similar to that of GERD in older children and adults in that the lower esophageal sphincter (LES) fails to prevent reflux of gastric contents into the esophagus (Garcia et al., 2013).

PATHOPHYSIOLOGY

Opening of the gastroesophageal junction depends on the relaxation of the LES.

There are three basic mechanisms that can lead to GER: **transient relaxation of the LES, a transient increase in abdominal pressure that momentarily exceeds the competence of the sphincter, and a low LES tone.**

Other factors can cause GER such as:
▥ NG/OG tube placement
▥ delayed gastric emptying
▥ neuromuscular disorders
▥ medications (such as adrenergic agonists, bronchodilators, and opiates)
▥ hormone-induced dysmotility
▥ intubation and increased risk in the mechanically ventilated child

Transient episodes of LES relaxation can occur due to stomach distention related to fluid or air, being overfeed (excessive food causes a higher gastric pressure) or being ventilated.

▥ Positioning has also been implicated with GER, with the right lateral position being associated with more episodes of reflux then the left lateral position even though gastric emptying was faster in the right lateral position. Sitting increases gastric pressure and increases reflux.
▥ A **gastric pH above 4** is needed to prevent the complications of esophagitis.

NURSING IMPLICATIONS AND TREATMENT

▥ Smaller more frequent feedings will help to keep the pressure in the stomach down making reflux less likely.
▥ Burp infant after every 1 to 2 ounces to express swallowed air during feedings.
▥ Provide emotional and psychological support and determine the effectiveness of coping strategies. Reassure care takers as needed.
▥ Assist the child identify foods, lifestyle modifications that may be associated with reflux and encourage these modifications.
▥ Encourage the child to maintain an upright position for 2 to 3 hours after eating or elevate the head of bed.
▥ Assess for decreased pulse oximetry level when feeding a neonate or infant (Wolters Kluwer, 2021).

ASSESSMENT

The chief symptom of gastroesophageal reflux is frequent regurgitation (spitting up). In obtaining subjective historic data, caregivers often refer to this spitting up as vomiting, but it is not actually vomiting because it is not due to gastric peristaltic contractions. These episodes of spit-ups are effortless and not forceful.

Additional GERD symptoms include:
▥ irritability, which may include episodes of arching the back and/or turning head to one side, crying, and grimace
▥ respiratory symptoms such as chronic recurrent coughing, stridor, or wheezing
▥ possible episodes of periodic breathing or apnea, desaturations
▥ cardiorespiratory (bradycardia, tachycardia, tachypnea, increased respiratory effort)

Older children's manifestations may include:
▥ heartburn, dysphagia, and retrosternal pain
▥ asthma, chronic cough

Clinical Pearl

▥ *A validated questionnaire to measure GERD symptoms is the Infant Gastroesophageal Reflux Questionnaire Revised (I-GERQ-R). This 12-item questionnaire is completed by both caregiver and provider, and a score >16 is suggestive of acid GERD.*

LABS AND DIAGNOSTICS

- Hgb level may be reduced if esophageal erosion leads to bleeding.
- **Imaging studies with contrast:** Upper GI series may be initially ordered; it may help diagnose reflux and also identify any anatomic GI disorders that cause regurgitation. Finding barium reflux into the mid or upper esophagus is much more significant than seeing reflux into only the distal esophagus.
  - A gastric emptying study demonstrates reflux or delayed emptying.
  - A gastric scintiscan can diagnose gastric emptying and GERD but is used mainly to detect aspiration.
- **Esophagogastroduodenoscopy (with/without biopsy)** can determine the state of the esophagus and degree of esophagitis, assist with diagnosing infection or food allergy.
- Esophageal manometry reveals abnormal LES pressure and sphincter incompetence.
- Laryngotracheobronchoscopy may be done to detect laryngeal inflammation or vocal cord nodules.
- Endoscopy is only indicated if there is a suspicion of complications of GER.
- **Esophageal pH or multichannel intraluminal impedance (MII) probes:** Esophageal pH-metry (24 hours) was initially introduced in 1969 and it was considered the gold standard for the diagnosis of GERD since the 1980s. MII is a newer technique that, in combination with pH-metry, increases the sensitivity and specificity of the detection of GER as it detects both episodes of acid and of alkaline reflux.
  - *An episode of acid reflux is defined as a fall in the esophageal pH to below 4 for at least 5 seconds.*
  - According to several pediatric gastroenterologists, the presence of more than nine episodes of acid GER per day is believed to be pathological in children.
  - Caregivers record the occurrence of symptoms and are then correlated with reflux events detected by the probe.
  - A pH probe can also assess the effectiveness of acid-suppression therapy; however, pH-metry is limited in detecting detect episodes of alkaline reflux.
  - An MII probe has the ability to detect nonacid reflux as well as acid reflux.

TREATMENT AND MANAGEMENT

For infants that experience reflux, maturation of systems will correct the issue and they will outgrow the reflux. Conservative treatment strategies may include:

- dietary/lifestyle modifications
  - Utilize thickened feedings by adding 1/2 to 1 tbsp of rice cereal to 30 mL of formula—enlarging or crisscross cutting the bottle nipple will enhance flow of the formula but use cautiously. Burp infant frequently.
  - If food allergies are expected, a hypoallergenic formula should be used in formula-fed infants for 2 to 4 weeks. For breastfed infants, having the mother avoid cow-milk protein may mitigate the reflux.
- positioning
  - Despite being associated with a lower incidence of GER, placement in the prone position is not recommended for infants due the association with sudden infant death syndrome (SIDS).
  - After feeding, infants are kept in an upright position or held for 20 to 30 minutes. Do not use an infant seat/car seat/carrier as this increases abdominal pressure.
  - **For critical care children, elevation of the head of the bed and the use of transpyloric tubes also helps to reduce GER.**
- pharmacologic
  - **histamine-2 receptor antagonists (H2RAs)**
    - ❏ famotidine (Pepcid)
    - ❏ cimetidine (Tagamet)
    - ❏ nizatidine (Axid)
  - **proton pump inhibitors (PPIs)**
    - ❏ lansoprazole (Pepcid)
    - ❏ pantoprazole (Protonix)
    - ❏ omeprazole (Prilosec)
  - **prokinetics**
    - ❏ metoclopramide (Reglan)
    - ❏ erythromycin

■ surgery
  ● **Nissen Fundoplication:** For cases that do not respond to medication therapy and severe cases, surgical Nissen fundoplication is the treatment option (fundus of stomach is wrapped around the esophagus in varying degrees; Pearl et al., 2017).

COMPLICATIONS

Hematemesis, esophagitis, esophageal stricture and/or ulceration, aspiration pneumonia leading to chronic pulmonary disease, ventilator-associated pneumonia (VAP) in intubated children, anemia from esophageal bleeding, poor weight gain, and possible dental abnormalities secondary to acid effects on tooth enamel.

▶ GASTROINTESTINAL HEMORRHAGE

GI hemorrhage in children is usually acute, self-limiting, and uncommon. GI bleeding can be idiopathic or occur from several conditions such as infection, allergy, drugs, or stress.
■ **upper GI bleeding** (proximal to the ligament of Treitz)
  ● gastritis, varices, irritating ingestion
■ **lower GI bleeding** (distal to the ligament of Treitz)
  ● necrotizing enterocolitis (NEC), volvulus, milk allergy
Clinical presentation of pediatric patients with sudden massive blood loss includes decreased blood pressure and metabolic acidosis. Pediatric critical care nurses must monitor for hemodynamic instability, respiratory distress, and prevent complications such as rebleeding, shock, sepsis, and/or death (Slater et al., 2017).

SIGNS AND SYMPTOMS

■ vomiting blood: bright red or coffee ground (**hematemesis**)
■ bloody/tarry stools (**hematochezia**); foul smelling stools (**melena**)
■ abdominal pain, tenderness, distention
■ increased abdominal girth
■ diminished or absent bowel sounds
■ metabolic acidosis
■ signs and symptoms of hypovolemic shock

> ### Clinical Pearl
>
> *Twenty percent to 25% of circulating blood loss leads to decreased systolic blood pressure and acidosis. It takes **15%** to **20%** of circulating blood loss to stimulate the autonomic nervous system to maintain blood pressure and perfusion.*

NURSING IMPLICATIONS AND TREATMENT

ASSESSMENT

When patients with GI bleeding/hemorrhage present, it is important to ask caregivers about the amount of blood loss and to describe it. Some descriptions may include a few drops smaller than the size of coins, a spoonful, a cupful, and so on. A thorough perfusion assessment by the nurse is a priority.

LABS AND DIAGNOSTICS

Laboratory specimens include:
■ stool culture and fecal leukocytes
■ CBC
■ prothrombin time (PT)/partial thromboplastin time (PTT)
■ fibrinogen and fibrin split products to monitor for disseminated intravascular coagulation (DIC)
■ liver function tests (LFTs)
■ electrolytes
■ blood, urea, nitrogen (BUN) and creatinine
Monitor laboratory results for anemia, thrombocytopenia, DIC, and metabolic acidosis.
Diagnostic tests include:

- abdominal x-rays
- endoscopy to determine the level (upper or lower) and the source of the bleeding

TREATMENT AND MANAGEMENT

Management depends on the source of the bleeding, which can occur in the upper or lower GI tract. Nursing care consists of:
- vital signs as ordered
- placing a NG tube for saline lavage (room temperature, iced will cause necrosis of the tissue)
- I&O

Treatment of GI hemorrhage includes:
- rapid volume resuscitation with IVF
- blood transfusions
- platelets and/or fresh frozen plasma (FFP) as necessary
- medications
  - H2RAs, PPIs, and sucralfate are indicated to stop or prevent the reoccurrence of bleeding.
  - Vasopressin (a potent vasoconstrictor) may be ordered for acute massive GI hemorrhage.

COMPLICATIONS

- rebleeding
- shock
- DIC
- sepsis (if child may have perforated)

Depending on diagnosis, GI surgery may be required.

▶ GASTROINTESTINAL SURGERY

GI surgery may be required for different GI disorders. There are two types of surgical drains.
1. active drains (closed or closed suction drains)—usually have an expandable chamber that creates suction to remove fluid from the wound.
   - Jackson-Pratt
   - Hemovac
2. passive drains (relies on gravity)
   - Penrose drain—usually sutured in place

NURSING IMPLICATIONS AND TREATMENT

- Monitor vital signs pre- and postsurgery as ordered.
- Administer pain medication as ordered.
- Administer broad-spectrum antibiotics if ordered.
- Document intake and output; monitor wound drainage.
  - Note amount, color, odor of drainage.
- **Assess skin around drains and ostomies for skin breakdown:** Redness, warmth, pain, purulent drainage, odor; ensure that the drains are functioning appropriately.
- Perform wound care as ordered.
- Provide ostomy care (if present).

▶ LIVER DISEASE AND FAILURE

The liver performs essential functions that include detoxifying poisonous chemicals, including alcohol and drugs (prescribed and over-the-counter drugs as well as illegal substances), bile formation to aid in digestion, storage of energy (carbohydrates, glucose, and fat), storage of iron, vitamins, and minerals, manufactures new proteins (especially those needed for blood coagulation), and serves as a location for hematopoiesis during fetal development. Liver failure is the inability of the liver to function properly and is commonly seen due to injury or dysfunction of liver cells (Bhatt & Rao, 2018).

This can lead to:
- encephalopathy
- cerebral edema

- coagulopathy
- renal failure
- hemodynamic instability

Hepatic failure can occur as:

- chronic
- "decompensated" chronic
- acute-chronic liver failure
- acute liver failure (ALF)

Most children have a chronic presentation of hepatic failure versus an acute presentation.

- *Chronic hepatic failure* occurs when a long-lasting liver disease becomes much worse, either slowly or suddenly.
- *Decompensated chronic hepatic failure (cirrhosis)* refers the loss of the liver's normal synthetic capacity over time accompanied by the development of jaundice and complications of portal hypertension, including ascites, variceal bleeding, and hepatic encephalopathy.
- *ALF*
  - ALF is characterized by a rapid deterioration in liver functions, including mainly a coagulopathy and changes in the mental status, leading to an encephalopathy. The characteristics of ALF include the following four elements:
    - ❑ hepatic-based coagulopathy defined as a PT ≥15 seconds or international normalized ratio (INR) ≥1.5 not correctable with vitamin K in the presence of hepatic encephalopathy
    - ❑ PT ≥20 seconds or INR ≥2 regardless of hepatic encephalopathy
    - ❑ biochemical evidence of acute liver injury
    - ❑ no known evidence of chronic liver disease
  - This severe liver injury can be reversible, and substantial advances in the treatment have remarkably improved survival in recent years.
  - ALF can further be sub-classified as (1) *hyper-acute liver failure* that is fulminant hepatic failure (FHF) with the time from jaundice to encephalopathy of fewer than 7 days; (2) *ALF* with the time from jaundice to encephalopathy between 7 and 28 days; and (3) *subacute liver failure* from the time from jaundice to encephalopathy more than 28 days.

PATHOPHYSIOLOGY

Once the liver can no longer perform its function to detoxify the blood, liver dysfunction occurs. Collateral vessels that shunt blood around the liver to the systemic circulation allow toxins to be absorbed from the GI tract to circulate freely to the brain leading to hepatic encephalopathy. The normal liver converts ammonia (a byproduct of protein metabolism) to urea, which the kidneys excrete. When the liver is no longer able to convert ammonia to urea, ammonia blood levels rise and the ammonia is delivered to the brain. Additionally, short-chain fatty acids, serotonin, tryptophan, and false neurotransmitters may also accumulate in the blood. The kidneys may then cease to function appropriately, which may cause the accumulation of vasoactive substances that trigger inappropriate constriction of renal arterioles, leading to decreased glomerular filtration and oliguria; a condition referred to as **hepatorenal syndrome.** Vasoconstriction acts as a compensatory response to portal hypertension and the pooling of blood in the spleen circulation. Blood volume expands, hydrogen ions accumulate, and electrolyte disturbances occur. Chronic liver disease differs from acute in that the presentation of chronic disease relates to the rate of parenchymal (organ-specific tissue) injury. Fibrosis leads to cirrhosis with development of portal hypertension evident by the presence of hepatosplenomegaly, varices, and ascites. A variety of disease and illness states have been associated with liver failure and liver dysfunction (D'Agata & Balistreri, 1999).

- Some examples of acute dysfunction/failure include (list is not exhaustive) include:
  - acetaminophen overdose and/or use of other hepatotoxic medications
  - hepatitis due to viruses. Primarily hepatitis A, B, and C.
  - toxins
  - mushroom poisoning
- Examples of chronic dysfunction/failure include:
  - liver cancer
  - biliary atresia (obstruction or lack of formation of bile ducts)
  - nonalcoholic fatty liver disease or cirrhosis

- nonviral or viral hepatitis
- metabolic disorders (galactosemia, glycogen storage disease, etc.)
- hemochromatosis
- cytomegalovirus
- heatstroke

NURSING IMPLICATIONS AND TREATMENT

ASSESSMENT

It is important to obtain a thorough history, which may give the clinician insight in determining the presence and type of liver dysfunction. Specifically inquire about any dietary changes as this may be associated with inborn error of carbohydrate metabolism. Obtain a family history noting any genetic disorder. A birth history of idiopathic neonatal hepatitis or biliary atresia would be significant. For a *diagnosis of ALF*, hepatic encephalopathy must be present, and the manifestations are graded on a scale of I to IV with increasing severity of symptoms. Additional manifestations include:

- initially normal appetite and weight gain (early)
- jaundice
- acholic (pale, clay colored) stools
- weight loss, anorexia, fever, vomiting, abdominal pain (later)
- darkening of the urine (bile present), presence of foamy urine
- confusion, altered mental status, and even coma (hepatic encephalopathy)
  - signs of cerebral edema or increased ICP
  - decreased level of consciousness (LOC), papilledema
- fatigue
- scleral icterus (yellowing of the sclera)
- complaints of pruritus (itchiness)
- hepatomegaly (may be the only sign of liver disease), splenomegaly/hepatosplenomegaly
- ascites, abdominal tenderness, right upper quadrant pain
- hypotension (secondary to intravascular volume depletion), tachycardia, peripheral edema
- bleeding: esophageal varices, hematemesis, melena
- signs of liver disease in the first year of life:
  - ascites, poor growth, rickets, hypoproteinemia, edema, petechiae

Clinical Pearl

- *Jaundice in any infant after 2 weeks of age should raise the suspicion of liver disease and promptly be evaluated.*
- *Teenagers who become jaundiced always should be questioned privately about IV drug abuse.*

Effects of Liver Failure

- decreased filtration of blood
  - increased risk of infection
- decreased bile salt synthesis
  - malabsorption of fats and fat-soluble vitamins (A, D, E, K)
- bile salt accumulation
  - pruritus from skin deposition
- cholestasis (biliary obstruction)
  - hyperbilirubinemia and jaundice
- altered carbohydrate metabolism
  - hypoglycemia follows initial hyperglycemia r/t liver stress
- altered protein metabolism
  - edema and ascites
- hepatorenal syndrome
  - rapid deterioration in kidney function due to blood flow changes
  - oliguria and Na retention

LABS AND DIAGNOSTICS

Laboratory

- ▨ **LFTs**
- ▨ **CBC, coagulation studies, ammonia level,** which may reveal:
  - ● anemia
  - ● impaired red blood cell production
  - ● prolonged bleeding and clotting times
  - ● thrombocytopenia
  - ● increased INR ratio
  - ● low blood glucose levels
  - ● increased ammonia levels
- ▨ Serum electrolyte levels reveal **hypokalemia** or **hyperkalemia** (with kidney failure), hypomagnesemia, and altered calcium levels.
- ▨ Creatinine level may be elevated.
- ▨ Phosphate level may be low and arterial blood gases (ABGs) may reveal hypoxemia.
  - ● Serum **lactate** levels may be elevated (with acetaminophen poisoning).
  - ● **Hypoprothrombinemia** may lead to spontaneous bleeding and intracranial hemorrhage.
- ▨ Urine osmolality is increased.

Imaging

- ▨ **Ultrasonography** (liver), CT scanning (liver and biliary tract), or MRI help determine if cancer or metastasis is present and helps to identify portal hypertension, hepatic congestion, and underlying cirrhosis.
- ▨ **Cholescintigraphy** detects abnormal liver uptake of radionuclide providing information on the liver's excretory abilities.
- ▨ **Electroencephalography** assists in ruling out other causes of encephalopathy.

Surgical

- ▨ Percutaneous liver biopsy can be used to determine the underlying liver disease/ dysfunction (Bhaduri & Mieli-Vergani, 1996).

TREATMENT AND MANAGEMENT

It is important to promote oxygenation and perhaps even hyperventilation to treat life-threatening ICP that is not responsive to osmotic diuretics. Hemodynamic monitoring in the intensive care environment should be initiated along with venous thromboembolism (VTE) prophylaxis.

Management of **hepatic encephalopathy** should be undertaken with the monitoring of elevation of increased ICP, neurological impairment. The use of osmotic diuretics, such as mannitol for cerebral edema should be initiated if warranted. Additional treatment strategies include:

- ▨ **diet**
  - ● NPO (in acute stages), enteral or total parenteral nutrition
  - ● Restrict protein to 60 g/day and provide a high-carbohydrate diet.
  - ● sodium restriction if ascites and/or peripheral edema is present
  - ● Monitor fluid and electrolyte status—correct as needed—dialysis may be indicated.
- ▨ **medications**
  - ● **lactulose** to prevent intestinal bacteria from creating ammonia and as a laxative to remove blood and ammonia from the intestines
  - ● Neomycin may be given to decrease GI tract ammonia formation (monitor by counting the number of stools per day).
  - ● mannitol if increased ICP present
  - ● cholestyramine to remove bile salts from enterohepatic circulation (helps with pruritus)
  - ● antacids, H2RAs; or PPIs; or sucralfate to prevent GI bleeding
  - ● analgesics (avoid the use of acetaminophen) or acetylcysteine for acetaminophen overdose
  - ● hepatitis B immune globulin, for patients with ALF from acute hepatitis B virus infection
  - ● activated charcoal for mushroom poisoning
  - ● potassium-sparing diuretics (for ascites), and potassium supplements
  - ● FFP to address coagulopathies
  - ● cryoprecipitate if fibrinogen is <100 mg/dL (Table 6.3)

Table 6.3 Comparing Fresh Frozen Plasma and Cryoprecipitate

	FFP	Cryoprecipitate
Volume	250–300 mL	10–20 mL
Fibrinogen	700–800 mg	150–250 mg
Other coagulation factors	All, including factors II, VII, VIII, IX, X, XI, and VWF	Factors VII, XII, and VWF

FFP, fresh frozen plasma; VWF, von Willebrand factor.
Source: Shaw, K., & Bachur, R. (Eds.). (2020). *Fleisher and Ludwig's textbook of pediatric emergency medicine* (8th ed.). Wolters Kluwer.

- platelets if <50,000
- vitamin K if PT is prolonged
- rifaximin to treat hepatic encephalopathy
- IVF such as NSS if hypotensive. **Must be administered with care. Overhydration can lead to cerebral edema, ascites, and pulmonary edema.**
- vasopressors such as norepinephrine (drug of choice) to maintain mean arterial pressure at 75 mmHg or greater or cerebral perfusion pressure and vasopressin if the patient is unresponsive to norepinephrine
- anticonvulsants for seizures
- **procedures**
  - paracentesis to remove ascitic fluid especially when respiratory compromise occurs
    - ❏ It may precipitate fluid shifts.
    - ❏ Complications include infection and hemorrhage.
  - balloon tamponade to control bleeding varices—endoscopic band ligation of varices
  - placement of ICP catheter for ICP monitoring possibly
  - hemodialysis or liver transplantation
  - plasmapheresis or exchange transfusions

Clinical Pearl

Sedatives should not be used in the presence of hepatic encephalopathy, as these medications are broken down in the liver. In addition, sedatives can mask the signs of worsening encephalopathy or neurological decline. However, if severe agitation is present, low doses of a short-acting benzodiazepines can be utilized.

TREATMENT AND MANAGEMENT

Nursing actions are directed toward maintaining the patient's safety and monitoring, preventing complications associated with the illness.

- Perform a thorough neurological assessment and monitor the patient for signs and symptoms of cerebral edema and worsening hepatic encephalopathy.
  - Initiate seizure precautions if needed, and decrease the sensory stimuli by promoting a quiet and calm environment.
  - Position the patient with the head of the bed elevated 30° to reduce the risk of increased ICP.
- Prevent VTE. Apply antiembolism stockings or sequential compression device (SCD).
- Assess for pain, and treat pain as needed and ordered; provide emotional support.
- Low-protein, high-calorie diet with small, frequent meals and snacks; if the patient's LOC deteriorates, provide parenteral or enteral nutrition as ordered.
- Perform meticulous skin care: If patient's condition allows, turn and reposition the patient regularly and frequently.
- Perform a daily weight and report any significant weight gain.
- Implement measures to relieve pruritus.
- Measure abdominal girth, noting any changes in size.
- Administer medications as ordered. Give lactulose syrup to decrease ammonia levels.
- Assess emesis for evidence of frank or occult bleeding and assist with measures to address variceal bleeding. Institute bleeding precautions as indicated.
- Obtain specimens for laboratory testing, such as liver function studies, electrolyte levels, and ABG analysis.

- Administer supplemental oxygen, as necessary per oxygen saturation levels and ABG results.
- Monitor for signs and symptoms of complications, such as bleeding or infection.
- Prepare the patient and family for surgery, if indicated.

▶ MALABSORPTION AND MALNUTRITION

Malabsorption is defined as failure of the mucosa of the small intestine to absorb or normally digest single or multiple nutrients, and meet hydration needs, thus necessitating the need for parenteral nutrition (PN) delivery. Additionally, intestinal failure, (also referred to as "short gut" but it is not dependent on intestinal length) describes the loss of the absorptive function of the intestine, resulting in malabsorption and malnutrition states.

PATHOPHYSIOLOGY

There are multiple causes that can contribute to malabsorption and malnutrition. The mechanism of malabsorption depends on the cause.

- In **celiac disease**, dietary gluten with the protein gliadin—a product of wheat, barley, rye, and oats—causes injury to the mucosal villi and results in a diminished absorptive surface.
- **Lactase deficiency** is a disaccharide deficiency syndrome. Lactase is an intestinal enzyme that splits nonabsorbable lactose (a disaccharide) into the absorbable monosaccharides, glucose and galactose. Production of lactase may be deficient, or another intestinal disease may inhibit the enzyme.
- **Zollinger–Ellison syndrome** causes increased acid production in the duodenum, which inhibits the release of cholecystokinin, which is required for pancreatic enzyme release and subsequent absorption of nutrients.
- **Cystic fibrosis** can cause blockage to pancreatic enzyme release leading to malabsorption and malnutrition
- **Other conditions can include** hepatobiliary disease, intestinal parasites, certain medications (neomycin, calcium carbonate), cancers (radiation therapy can cause damage to the GI tract), short-gut syndrome, AIDS and HIV, chronic heart failure, and travel to underdeveloped countries.

NURSING IMPLICATIONS AND TREATMENT

ASSESSMENTS

A comprehensive medical history should be taken and any abnormal findings noted:
Manifestations of malabsorption/malnutrition include:

- diarrhea, frequently watery (**most common symptom**), steatorrhea, flatulence; abdominal bloating and cramping
- dry hair or hair loss, dry skin pallor, peripheral edema
- growth failure
- orthostatic hypotension
- fatigue
- muscle wasting
- abdominal distention
- positive Chvostek or Trousseau sign (from electrolyte disturbance)

LABS AND DIAGNOSTICS

Laboratory

- Analysis of **stool specimen for fat** content reveals the excretion of >6 g of fat per day.
- Results of **D-xylose absorption test** (oral dose of 25 g of D-xylose) show <4 g of D-xylose in the urine after 5 hours (reflects disorders of the proximal bowel).
- **Schilling test** results reveal a deficiency of vitamin B12 absorption.
- **Hydrogen breath test** results may be elevated, suggesting lactase deficiency.
- **Culture of duodenal and jejunal contents** confirms a bacterial overgrowth in the proximal bowel.
- **CBC with differential** may reveal microcytic anemia due to iron deficiency or macrocytic anemia due to vitamin B12 or folate deficiency.
- **Tissue transglutaminase IgA** (tTG-IgA) ELISA may be used to diagnose celiac disease.
- **Serum protein levels** may reveal hypoproteinemia and hypoalbuminemia with protein malabsorption.

- **PT** may be prolonged due to inadequate vitamin K absorption.
- **Serum electrolyte** levels may be altered, resulting in hypokalemia, hypocalcemia, or hypomagnesemia.

Imaging
- GI barium studies show the characteristic features of malabsorption in the small intestine.
- CT scanning (abdomen and pelvis) or MRI of the abdomen may reveal structural abnormalities.

Diagnostic Procedures
- Results of upper GI endoscopy and biopsy of the small intestine reveal the atrophy of mucosal villi.
- Endoscopic retrograde cholangiopancreatography may show pancreatic or biliary structural abnormalities.

TREATMENT AND MANAGEMENT
Nursing care is directed toward restoring nutritional deficiencies and identifying and mitigating any complications associated with malabsorption and malnutrition states.
- Administer prescribed diet therapy via the enteral or parental route, perform calorie count.
- Institute measures to prevent bleeding, such as using a soft toothbrush and electric razor (for adolescent boys).
- Assess bowel sounds, obtain and monitor abdominal girth, obtain daily weight.
- Utilize therapeutic communication and provide child/family with coping strategies for potential stressful and chronic issues. Refer child/family to support groups.
- Teach parent/child to prevent infection, **signs of infection, and at discharge, when to see their provider.**

Treatment is focused on the determining the cause and correcting the malabsorption/malnutrition state, which includes replenishing missing nutrients and restoring bowel functioning. Diet changes may be implemented, which can include, recommendations for a gluten-free diet to stop progression of celiac disease and malabsorption, or a lactose-free diet to treat lactase deficiency. A high-calorie, high-protein diet where caloric intake is individualized. Specific guidelines for nutrition include (Mehta et al., 2013):
- PN may be source in which the child receives the needed macronutrients (carbohydrates [dextrose or glucose], protein, and fat), and micronutrients (electrolytes, minerals, vitamins, and trace elements). PN can be infused and administered through a peripheral or central line. However, PN formulations with a **dextrose concentration >12.5% must be administered centrally.**
- Dextrose provides 3.4 kcal/g and constitutes 60% to 70% of the total PN caloric composition.
- Fat emulsions (intralipids) may be administered as a separate solution to provide a major source of calories (20% solution provides 2 kcal/mL) and should constitute 30% to 50% of the total PN caloric intake. Providing 0.5 g/kg/d prevents essential fatty acid deficiency states.
- Certain medications may also be added to PN such as heparin, if central access is being used, and/or famotidine (Pepcid), if GI prophylaxis is indicated.
  - Possible alternatives to PN are to augment the child's nutrition by using dextrose 10% in water (D10W) and intralipids.
- Total parenteral nutrition (TPN) may be considered if malabsorption is severe.

Medications may also be used and include:
- prescribed supplements, such as calcium, iron, vitamins including B_{12}
- protease and lipase supplements for pancreatic insufficiency
- lactacid for lactose deficiency
- antibiotics for bacterial overgrowth
- corticosteroids and anti-inflammatory agents for regional enteritis

COMPLICATIONS
- anemias
- bleeding disorders
- tetany
- malnutrition
- vitamin deficiencies
- cholelithiasis
- failure to thrive
- cognitive alterations

▶ NECROTIZING ENTEROCOLITIS

Necrotizing enterocolitis, often referred to as NEC, is an acute GI infection causing bowel inflammation with necrosis or death of the GI tissues. This is a medical emergency. The illness process occurs as: intestinal inflammation → ischemia → necrosis → septic shock → impending death. Pediatric patients at risk for NEC are premature infants and newborns who experience hypoxia in utero and/or asphyxia during delivery. Maternal infections and preeclampsia can predispose newborns to this serious condition. The lower the gestational age of the newborn, the higher the risk of NEC. Gas-forming bacteria grow in the necrotic area of the bowel and can lead to perforation.

Precipitating factors can include bowel ischemia, bacterial colonization of the intestine, and enteral feedings, which provide a media where bacteria thrive (formula). Nurses should be aware of preventative measures such as breastfeeding, antenatal maternal corticosteroids, and gradual initiation of feedings, antibiotics, and probiotics. In general, NEC patients may need surgery to remove any necrotic area of the bowel if their clinical presentation continues to worsen despite medical management (Children's Health, 2022).

SIGNS AND SYMPTOMS

Pediatric critical care nurses should assess patients for GI issues including:
- *three cardinal signs*: **abdominal distention, bilious vomiting, and bloody stools**
- increased abdominal girth
- decreased bowel sounds
- feeding intolerance
- visual "loops of bowel"
- unstable temperature
- thrombocytopenia
- leukopenia
- respiratory distress

NURSING IMPLICATIONS AND TREATMENT

LABS AND DIAGNOSTICS

Diagnosis involves radiography or x-rays, but not both, of abdomen and kidney-ureters-bladder (KUB), which shows dilated "loops of bowel" and gas bubbles made by bacteria. These radiographs are also used to monitor disease progression and evaluate effects of treatment.

Laboratory specimens include blood cultures, C-reactive protein (CRP), and coagulation studies looking for possible DIC. The pediatric critical care nurse should monitor NEC patients for increased white blood cells (WBCs) and metabolic acidosis.

TREATMENT AND MANAGEMENT

If NEC is suspected, the nurse should stop feedings immediately (NPO) and contact the healthcare provider. The infected bowel needs to rest to promote healing.

Nursing implications and treatment are to:
- Maintain the infant's NPO status.
- Start gastric decompression (NG/OG tube).
- Infuse IVFs and TPN as ordered
- Administer
  - intravenous (IV) broad-spectrum antibiotics
  - pain medications
  - blood products (possibly)
- Monitor intake and output and electrolytes.
- Serial abdominal x-rays and serial platelet counts results will evaluate the pediatric patient with NEC for improvement.

Once resolved, begin to feed the infant as ordered. Follow hospital protocol for advancing feedings. Provide emotional support to caregivers, educate them about ostomy care postsurgery if needed, and discuss possible complications of NEC and surgery: short bowel (gut) syndrome and intestinal strictures.

▶ PERITONITIS

Peritonitis, or peritoneal inflammation, is defined as redness and swelling of the abdominal tissues (peritoneum) and is a serious condition that can be fatal (Children's Hospital at Vanderbilt, 2021).

SIGNS AND SYMPTOMS

Pediatric patients with peritonitis may present the following signs and symptoms:
- severe abdominal pain and tenderness; worsening with movement, guarding
- abdominal distention; hard, rigid abdomen
- bowel sounds absent
- nausea and/or vomiting
- difficulty passing gas and stool or diarrhea
- fever
- dehydration
- loss of appetite
- oliguria
- ascites
- hypotension
- shock and sepsis

NURSING IMPLICATIONS AND TREATMENT

Assess for bowel sounds and peristalsis and recognize that bowel sounds will be absent in peritonitis. If the nurse suspects peritonitis, then a paracentesis may be performed by the provider on the child to assess for infected fluid in the peritoneal cavity. This diagnostic procedure includes testing the fluid for glucose, protein, lactic dehydrogenase (LDH), cell count, culture, and Gram stain. Peritonitis in children is most often treated with surgery and perioperative antibiotics (refer to the section on GI surgery; Stanford Children's Health, 2022).

● CASE STUDY

A 13-year-old girl who was previously healthy with no medical history presents to the ED with the complaints of left upper quadrant (LUQ) abdominal pain, left shoulder pain, and nausea. The patient's history reveals that a fall from a tree occurred 4 hours ago and that she struck her abdomen on a rock. The fall was estimated to be approximately 5 feet in height. Physical exam reveals abdominal distention without any abdominal contusions or hypotension. Abdominal ultrasonography (focused assessment with sonography for trauma [FAST]), finding indicated intraperitoneal fluid, and was followed by a CT scan, which yielded a grade 1 spleen injury.

CASE STUDY QUESTIONS

1. What is the significance of the left shoulder pain?
   A. An injury sustained from the fall
   B. Referred pain from the spleen injury
   C. An adverse reaction to the diagnostic contrast
   D. Related to patient positioning on the examination table

2. For this particular patient, a splenectomy is planned. What has become the standard of care for hemodynamically stable patient who have experienced solid-organ abdominal trauma?
   A. Nonoperative management
   B. Laparoscopic splenectomy
   C. Peritoneal lavage with antibiotic fluid
   D. Angiographic embolization

3. According to the American Pediatric Surgical Association (APSA), this child would be restricted from contact sports and strenuous physical activity for a period of what time?
   A. 2 weeks
   B. 3 weeks
   C. 4 weeks
   D. 6 weeks

(See answers next page.)

ANSWERS TO CASE STUDY QUESTIONS

1. B) Referred pain from the spleen injury

The left-sided shoulder pain is indicative of Kehr's sign. The presentation of spleen injury depends upon associated internal hemorrhage. Patients may present with hypovolemic shock manifesting tachycardia, and hypotension. Other findings include tenderness in the LUQ, generalized peritonitis, or referred pain to the left shoulder (Kehr's sign). Left shoulder pain may occur due to diaphragmatic irritation and nausea. This finding should increase the suspicion of spleen injury.

2. A) Nonoperative management

In children, the use of nonoperative management of hemodynamically stable patients has become the standard of care. The majority (up to 80%) of blunt spleen injuries in a stable patient without signs of peritonitis or ongoing bleeding can be managed nonoperatively. However, these patients should be hospitalized and undergo close observation. Consult pediatric surgery should later surgical intervention be required.

3. B) 3 weeks

According to the APSA, activity restrictions are for a period consisting of the grade of injury (in this case, it is 1 week) plus an additional 2 weeks for a total of 3 weeks of strenuous activity. There is a contact sport restriction.

● KNOWLEDGE CHECK: CHAPTER 6

1. What is the most common condition that requires abdominal surgery in children?
   A. Appendicitis
   B. Abdominal compartment syndrome
   C. Gastrointestinal (GI) obstruction
   D. Liver disease

2. A child is admitted to the pediatric ICU (PICU) with gastrointestinal (GI) bleeding. Vital signs are temperature 38.3°C (101°F), heart rate (HR) 130, respiratory rate (RR) 20, blood pressure (BP) 86/60. Which nursing assessment data about the patient is a priority?
   A. Hemoglobin/hematocrit is 11.3/31
   B. Temperature of 38.3°C (101°F)
   C. HR 130 and BP 86/60
   D. Nasogastric tube has coffee ground drainage

3. A pediatric patient is day 3 postoperative abdominal surgery and has an active, closed drainage tube. Which assessment data should alert a nurse that the Jackson-Pratt® (JP) is functioning appropriately?
   A. The JP drain is fully curved and has 50 mL of fluid.
   B. A pin holds the drainage tube in place to the dressing.
   C. The stoma around the drain is pink and has no drainage.
   D. The JP drain has suction and is compressed.

4. A nurse is providing care to a child with suspected peritonitis. What should the nurse expect to find when reviewing the child's laboratory results?
   A. Hypervolemia and hypotension
   B. Decreased C-reactive protein (CRP) and fever
   C. Hypertension and increased urine output
   D. Fever and hypotension

5. A nurse received handoff report from the night shift nurse about their assigned patients. Which patient should the nurse assess first? The child with:
   A. Peritonitis who is on day 2 of intravenous antibiotics
   B. A 6 out of 10 pain who is day 1 postoperative abdominal surgery
   C. Liver failure who is jaundiced and has ascites
   D. Abdominal pain who has an 8-hour urinary total output of 160 mL and weighs 30 kg

6. A child is admitted with extensive burns and is determined to be at high risk for developing abdominal compartment syndrome (ACS). Beside potential organ failure, what other body system malfunction would be most likely to occur along with the acute organ failure?
   A. Hypoxia, hypercapnia, and respiratory failure
   B. Increased renal perfusion, urinary frequency, and polyuria
   C. Hypertension, increased cardiac output, and elevated arterial pressures
   D. Excessive flatulence, increased peristalsis, and diarrhea

7. The pediatric ICU (PICU) nurse is teaching parents about ways to minimize gastrointestinal reflux in their infant. Which statement, made by the parent would require additional teaching? "We will:
   A. "Thicken our baby's feedings by adding 1/2 to 1 tbsp of rice cereal to 30 mL of formula."
   B. "Place our baby in an infant seat after feeding for at least 30 minutes."
   C. "Be sure to crisscross cut the nipple to allow easier ingestion of the formula."
   D. "Burp the baby more frequently."

(See answers next page.)

1. A) Appendicitis

The most common condition requiring surgery is appendicitis. Children who experience GI abnormalities or conditions such as bowel obstruction, GI perforation, intussusception, and Meckel's diverticulum, may need abdominal surgery. Abdominal compartment syndrome, GI obstruction, and liver disease are less likely than appendicitis.

2. C) HR 130 and BP 86/60

The patient's HR is above normal and the BP is low. These are signs of hypovolemic shock and immediate intervention by the nurse is needed. The patient's hemoglobin/hemocrit is low, but this laboratory information does not warrant immediate intervention since there is a more significant priority in the signs of shock. A temperature of 38.3°C (101°F) shows sign of a fever and could indicate peritonitis but it is not the immediate priority. Coffee ground drainage alerts the nurse that this is old blood, which would be expected in the patient who has esophageal bleeding.

3. D) The JP drain has suction and is compressed.

The active, closed drain (JP, Hemovac drain) should be sunken in or depressed, indicating that suction is being applied and shows that the drain is functioning appropriately. If the drain is round with a significant amount of fluid in it, then the drain needs to be emptied and suction reapplied—therefore the JP drain is not functioning appropriately. The nurse must compress the drain and close it to provide suction for it to work. The tube should be pinned to the dressing or patient gown to prevent the drain from being pulled out of the insertion site—this does not show how the active drain works. The insertion site should be pink and without infection (purulent drainage, warmth, and redness), but this does not show how the drain functions.

4. D) Fever and hypotension

Children with peritonitis may experience the following signs and symptoms: severe abdominal pain and tenderness; worsening with movement, abdominal distention, nausea and/or vomiting, difficulty passing gas and stool or diarrhea, fever, dehydration, loss of appetite, oliguria, ascites, hypotension, shock and sepsis. CRP would be increased, not decreased. Children with peritonitis are at risk for hypovolemic shock. They would not have hypertension and increased urine output.

5. D) Abdominal pain who has an 8-hour urinary total output of 160 mL and weighs 30 kg

The child with abdominal pain who has an 8-hour urinary output of 160mL/hr. The pediatric patient has a urinary output of <1 mL/kg/hr. This child should have 240 mL of output in 8 hours (30 kg × 1 ml = 30 mls/hr, 30 mls/hr × 8 hours = 240 mls in 8 hours). The patient has 1/2 that amount, therefore, this patient may be going into renal failure and hypovolemic shock, and should be assessed first. The child with peritonitis is being treated appropriately with IV antibiotics and is considered stable. The child with 6 out of 10 pain who is day 1 postoperative abdominal surgery is not the priority. Jaundice and ascites are expected in a patient with liver failure; therefore, the nurse should not assess this child first.

6. A) Hypoxia, hypercapnia, and respiratory failure

With ACS, there is upward movement of the diaphragm that compresses pulmonary tissue leading to atelectasis, ventilation-perfusion mismatch, and a reduced functional residual capacity with limited chest wall compliance resulting in possible hypoxia, hypercapnia, and respiratory failure. Increased renal perfusion, urinary frequency, and polyuria are incorrect as there is decreased renal perfusion and subsequent diminished urinary output. Hypertension, increased cardiac output, and elevated arterial pressures are incorrect as there is diminished preload, afterload and contractibility leading to tachycardia, and hypotension with a diminished arterial pressure. Excessive flatulence, increased peristalsis, and diarrhea are incorrect, as abdominal activity is usually diminished and flatulence, hyperactive bowel sounds and diarrhea would not be likely.

7. B) "Place our baby in an infant seat after feeding for at least 30 minutes."

Placing the baby in an infant seat causes increased abdominal pressure causing the likelihood of reflux to occur. Although studies have demonstrated the prone position in mitigating reflux, this positioning is not advocated due to sudden infant death syndrome (SIDS). Maintaining the head of the crib so that is it elevated remains a good option for parents to implement at home. Thickening feedings, crisscross cutting the bottle nipple, and burping the baby more frequently are appropriate strategies to minimize or prevent reflux from occurring following feedings.

8. An 8-year-old boy status post motor vehicle crash (s/p MVC) is admitted to the pediatric ICU (PICU) after being ejected from the car where the car landed on top of them. He is intubated and sedated. He has become very difficult to ventilate and oxygen saturations are dropping (65%). Respiratory therapy suctions the patient and obtains a very small amount of secretions. The ventilator keeps beeping high pressure alarm. Noted is a distended abdomen. What might be the source of this change in physical assessment?
   A. Intra-abdominal hypertension (IAH)
   B. Developing appendicitis
   C. Intussusception
   D. Development of a volvulus

9. An 8-year-old boy status post motor vehicle crash (s/p MVC) is admitted to the pediatric ICU (PICU) after being ejected from the car where the car landed on top of him. He is intubated and sedated. He has become very difficult to ventilate and oxygen saturations are dropping (65%). Respiratory therapy suctions the patient and obtains a very small amount of secretions. The ventilator keeps beeping high pressure alarm. Noted is a distended abdomen. What test might be performed to evaluate for the given situation?
   A. A STAT CT scan
   B. Measurement of intra-abdominal hypertension (IAH) with a transduced foley catheter
   C. Re-intubate as the endotracheal tube (ETT) might be obstructed
   D. Immediate surgical decompression

10. The pediatric ICU (PICU) nurse is admitting a child who ingested an excessive amount of acetamino-phen (Tylenol) and her provider is concerned that acute liver failure may occur as a result of this acetaminophen overdose. What medication does the nurse expect to find in the treatment plan?
    A. Naprosyn
    B. Dilantin
    C. Acetylcysteine
    D. Methotrexate

11. Which of the following infants is at most risk to develop necrotizing enterocolitis (NEC)?
    A. A 37-week-old breastfed baby
    B. A 38-week-old formula fed baby
    C. A 5-week-old who is lactose intolerant
    D. A 36-week-old baby who was anoxic at birth

(See answers next page.)

8. A) Intra-abdominal hypertension (IAH)

The difficulty to ventilate, increasing high pressure alarms, and dropping oxygen saturations along with the abdominal distension are indicative of increasing abdominal hypertension. An appendicitis or a volvulus would not be indicative of this clinical scenario. This 8-year-old is too old to have an intussusception. That usually presents at 6 to 36 months old and is very uncommon after 2 years of age. Remember this is a trauma patient.

9. B) Measurement of intra-abdominal hypertension (IAH) with a transduced foley catheter

The physical exam indicates increasing abdominal pressure (hypertension). After the physician is notified, they most likely would like the nurse to obtain a measurement of IAH using a transduced foley catheter. This is not an obstructed ETT. A STAT CT scan would not give you a pressure measurement. You would want to evaluate for increased abdominal pressure and abdominal compartment syndrome before emergently going to the OR for surgical decompression or being done at the bedside.

10. C) Acetylcysteine

Acetylcysteine is a medication that is used to reverse the toxic effects of acetaminophen on the liver. Naprosyn, Dilantin, and methotrexate remaining medications are liver toxic and may exacerbate liver dysfunction or liver failure.

11. D) A 36-week-old baby who was anoxic at birth

Babies at risk for NEC are premature infants and newborns who experience hypoxia in utero and/or asphyxia during delivery or another stressor. The 36-week-old infant who was anoxic at birth is the one most likely of this group to develop NEC. The other items are not high risks for developing NEC.

● REFERENCES

Ballman, E., Bhuller, S., Weaver, J., & Thorne, P. (2021). Severe constipation in a pediatric patient causing abdominal compartment syndrome. *Journal of Pediatric Surgery Case Reports, 70*, 101874. https://doi.org/10.1016/j.epsc.2021.101874

Bhaduri, B., & Mieli-Vergani, G. (1996). Fulminant hepatic failure: Pediatric aspects. *Seminars in Liver Disease, 16*(4), 349–355. https://doi.org/10.1055/s-2007-1007248

Bhatt, H., & Rao, G. (2018). Management of acute liver failure: A pediatric perspective. *Current Pediatrics Reports, 6*, 246–257. https://doi.org/10.1007/s40124-018-0174-7

Chedly, T., & Chiaka-Ejike, J. (2017). Intra-abdominal hypertension and abdominal compartment syndrome in pediatrics. A review. *Journal of Critical Care, 41*, 275–282. https://doi.org/10.1016/j.jcrc.2017.06.004

Children's Health. (2022, April). *Pediatric ischemic bowel disease*. Children's Health. https://www.childrens.com/specialties-services/conditions/ischemic-bowel-disease

Children's Hospital at Vanderbilt. (2021). *Gastrointestinal perforation/rupture*. https://www.childrenshospitalvanderbilt.org/medical-conditions/gastrointestinal-perforationrupture

D'Agata, I., & Balistreri, W. (1999). Evaluation of liver disease in the pediatric patient. *Pediatrics in Review, 20*(11), 376–390. https://doi.org/10.1542/pir.20.11.376

Divarci, E., Karapinar, B., Yalaz, M., & Ergun, O. (2016). Incidence and prognosis of intra-abdominal hypertension and abdominal compartment syndrome in children. *Journal of Pediatric Surgery, 51*(3), 503–507. https://doi.org/10.1016/j.jpedsurg.2014.03.014

Garcia, M., Cid, J., & Sánchez, C. (2013). Gastroesophageal reflux disease in children: A review. *Gastroenterology, 2013* 824320. https://doi.org/10.1155/2013/824320

Kirkpatrick, A., Roberts, D., De Waele, J., Jaeschke, R., Malbrain, M., Keulenaer, B., Duchesne, J., Bjorck, M., Leppaniemi, A., Ejike, J., Sugrue, M., Cheatham, M., Ivatury, R., Ball, C., Blaser, A., Regli, A., Balogh, Z., D'Amours, S., Debergh, D., . . . The Pediatric Guidelines Sub-Committee for the World Society of the Abdominal Compartment Syndrome. (2013). Intra-abdominal hypertension and the abdominal compartment syndrome: Updated consensus definitions and clinical practice guidelines from the World Society of the Abdominal Compartment Syndrome. *Intensive Care Medicine, 39*, 1190–1206. https://doi.org/10.1007/s00134-013-2906-z

Martin, S. (2019). Gastrointestinal system. In M. Slota (Ed.), *AACN core curriculum for pediatric high acuity, progressive, and critical care nursing* (3rd ed.). Springer Publishing Company.

Mehta, N., Corkins, M., Lyman, B., Malone, A., Goday, P., Carney, L., Monczka, J., Plogsted, S., Schwenk, W., & the American Society for Parenteral and Enteral Nutrition (A.S.P.E.N.) Board of Directors. (2013). Defining pediatric malnutrition: A paradigm shift toward etiology-related definitions. *Journal of Parenteral and Enteral Nutrition, 37*(4), 460–481. https://doi.org/10.1177/0148607113479972

Pearl, J., Pauli, E., Dunkin, B., & Stefanidis, D. (2017). SAGES endoluminal treatments for GERD. *Surgical Endoscopy, 31*, 3783–3790. https://doi.org/10.1007/s00464-017-5639-1

Shaw, K., & Bachur, R. (Eds.). (2020). *Fleisher and Ludwig's textbook of pediatric emergency medicine* (8th ed.). Wolters Kluwer.

Shimizu, Y., Umemura, T., Fujiwara, N., & Nakama, T. (2019). Review of pediatric abdominal trauma: Operative and non-operative treatment in combined adult and pediatric trauma center. *Acute Medicine and Surgery, 6*(4), 358–364. https://doi.org/10.1002/ams2.421

Slater, B., Dirks, R., McKinley, S., Ansari, M., Kohn, G., Thosani, N., Qumseya, B., Billmeier, S., Daly, S., Crawford, C., Ehlers, A., Hollands, C., Palazzo, F., Rodriguez, N., Train, A., Wassenaar, E., Walsh, D., Pryor, A., & Stefanidis, D. (2017). SAGES guidelines for the surgical treatment of gastroesophageal reflux (GERD). *Surgical Endoscopy*. https://doi.org/10.1007/s00464-021-08625-5

Stanford Children's Health. (2022). *Peritonitis*. https://www.stanfordchildrens.org/en/topic/default?id=peritonitis-85-P00391

Urden, L., Stacy, K., & Lough, M. (2022). *Critical care nursing diagnosis and management* (9th ed.). Elsevier.

Wolters Kluwer. (2021). *ThePoint®*. https://thepoint.lww.com/gateway

World Society of the Abdominal Compartment Syndrome. (2021). *WSACS consensus guidelines summary*. https://www.wsacs.org/education/436/wsacs-consensus-guidelines-summary/

Renal and Genitourinary Review

Emily Warren and Angie Tsay

The renal system consists of two kidneys that lie within the retroperitoneal space, two ureters, the bladder, and urethra. Each kidney (Figure 7.1) consists of the:

■ **cortex:** nephrons, glomeruli, proximal and distal tubules, first portions of the loop of Henle, and the collecting ducts
■ **medulla:** collecting ducts and loops of Henle
■ **pelvis:** upper end of the ureter

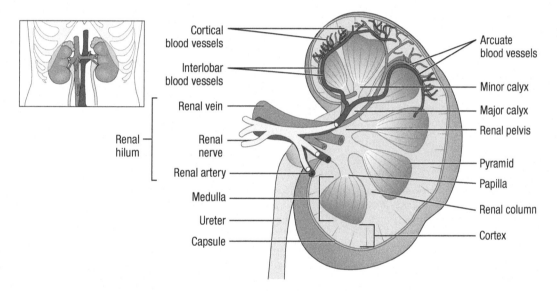

Figure 7.1 Longitudinal section of the kidney
Source: OpenStax College. (2013). Anatomy and physiology, Connexions website.

The nephron is the functional unit of the kidney and the site of urine formation. Urine is formed through a process of filtration through the glomeruli, reabsorption via renal tubules, and secretion from tubular cells to a collecting duct. Fluid, electrolytes, glucose, urea and creatinine are filtered from the blood.

The kidney has several major functions:

■ Regulates plasma osmolarity
■ Maintains acid-base balance
■ Produces the hormone erythropoietin (EPO)
■ Produces renin to regulate blood pressure
■ Converts vitamin D to the active form
■ Produces erythropoietin hormone which stimulates the bone marrow to produce erythrocytes for red blood cell (RBC) production (Ogobuiro & Tuma, 2022)

Clinical Pearl

Glomerular filtration rate (GFR) is a marker of renal function and an estimate of the filtration rate of the nephrons using creatinine levels. Several conditions may affect the GFR such as decreased renal perfusion, shock, glomerular nephritis, or nephrotic syndrome (Dokas, 2019).

Long-term regulation of blood pressure through the renal system involves the renin-angiotensin-aldosterone system. Two hormones released by the renal system in response to a drop or fall in blood pressure aid this.

As the name suggests, the antidiuretic hormone promotes conservation of body water, reducing urine output and resulting in concentrated urine. Aldosterone increases sodium reabsorption, and thus increases sodium and fluid reabsorption to the blood, decreasing urine output. While sodium is being reabsorbed, potassium is being excreted (Fountain & Lappin, 2022).

▶ FLUID COMPARTMENTS

The body's cellular distribution of fluid consist of compartments separated by a semipermeable membrane to create intracellular and extracellular fluid. This membrane selectively allows water and some solutes to move from compartment to compartment (Tobias et al., 2022).

- intracellular fluid
- extracellular fluid
  - interstitial fluid
  - **blood plasma:** intravascular
  - transcellular fluid (Tobias et al., 2022)

The renal systems helps to modulate fluid to maintain fluid balance for the body.

- **antidiuretic hormone:** released by the posterior pituitary
- **aldosterone:** secreted by the adrenal cortex

Clinical Pearl

When cardiac output decreases and renal blood flow is affected, urine output will decrease as an early sign of decreased cardiac output. Normal urine output is 0.5 mL/kg per hour to 1 mL/kg per hour and is considered inadequate when <1 mL/kg per hour (Bradley & McSteen, 2019).

Lab tests specific to testing renal function include:

- **creatinine** (0.5–1.0 mg/dL)
- **blood urea nitrogen (BUN;** 10–30 mg/dL)
- **glomerular filtration rate (GFR;** estimation of filtrate that is cleared by the glomerulus)
- **urine osmolality** (300 mOsm/L; evaluates the ability of the kidney to concentrate urine)
- **urine specific gravity** (1.010–1.015)

Normal values of common renal electrolytes are outlined in Table 7.1.

Table 7.1 Normal Laboratory Values

Laboratory Result	Range
Serum osmolality	272–290 mOsm/L
Urine osmolality	300 mOsm/L
Urine specific gravity	1.010–1.015
Serum sodium	135–145 mEq/L
Serum potassium	3.5–5 mEq/L
Serum magnesium	1.8–2.3 mEq/L
Serum calcium	9–11 mg/dL (total), 1.00–1.4 mmol/dL (ionized)
Serum creatinine	1 mg/dL (≤1 month), <0.5 mg/dL (>1–2 months), <0.6 mg/dL (>2 months–6 years), <1.0 mg/dL (6–15 years old)

(continued)

Table 7.1 Normal Laboratory Values (*continued*)

Laboratory Result	Range
Serum phosphate	4.2–6.5 mg/dL (newborn), 3.5–6.5 mg/dL (children 1–5 years old), 2.5–4.5 mg/dL (children >5 years old)
Blood urea nitrogen (BUN)	10–30 mg/dL
Glomerular filtration rate (GFR)	>90 mL/min per 1.73 m^2 (lower in children and matches expected adult value by 3 years of age)

Source: Dokas, M. A. (2019). Renal system. In M. C. Slota (Ed.), *AACN core curriculum for pediatric high acuity, progressive, and critical care nursing* (3rd ed.). Springer Publishing Company.

Imaging tests to evaluate the kidneys include:
- **renal ultrasounds** to assess for kidney size, position, and obstructions
- **CT scan** to assess structural abnormalities and obstructions
- **kidney biopsy** to evaluate renal function and disease progression
- **urinalysis** to compare waste clearance versus serum lab values
- Cystoscopies allow urologists to directly visualize (with a cystoscope) from the urethra to the bladder for diagnostic purposes including bladder volume and observance of obstructions (Dokas, 2019).

▶ ACUTE KIDNEY INJURY

Acute kidney injury (AKI) is an abrupt loss of renal function that results in reduced GFR, accumulation of urea and waste products, and imbalances in fluid and electrolytes. Early identification and recognition of AKI is important and key to treating and reversing injury. The Kidney Disease: Improving Global Outcomes (KDIGO) defines AKI as any of the following:
- increase in serum creatinine by ≥0.3 mg/dL within 48 hours
- increase in serum creatinine by ≥1.5 times baseline within the prior 7 days
- urine output ≤0.5 mL/kg/hour for 6 hours (KDIGO, 2012)

There are several causes of AKI, which include:
- **prerenal disease**
  - Prerenal causes of AKI are typically a result of poor perfusion to the kidneys secondary to cardiac dysfunction, hypovolemia or medications such as nonsteroidal anti-inflammatories (NSAIDs) or angiotensin-converting enzyme (ACE) inhibitors.
- **intrinsic renal failure** which includes acute tubular necrosis (ATN)
  - Intrinsic renal failure occurs in the setting of decreased blood flow to the renal parenchyma such as in hemolytic uremic syndrome, glomerulonephritis, or interstitial nephritis. Damage to tubular cells may occur from hypoxic/ischemic insults by nephrotoxic drugs, contrast, or solvents.
- **postrenal failure**
  - Postrenal AKI occurs when there is an obstruction in urinary blood flow in children with anatomic abnormalities causing urethral or ureteral obstruction or bladder dysfunction, such as in newborn males with posterior urethral valves.

SIGNS AND SYMPTOMS

Signs and symptoms of AKI occur from changes in kidney function and include:
- edema from fluid overload
- weight gain
- decreased urine output
- hematuria
- hypertension
- elevated serum creatinine and BUN
- urinalysis with sediment, abnormal color, and/or presence of protein and casts

Patients with AKI may exhibit neurologic symptoms of accumulated toxins and waste products which is called **uremia**. These symptoms include:
- insomnia
- itching
- anorexia, nausea and vomiting
- confusion, asterixis, seizures, and coma

Symptoms of ATN will vary as renal injury progresses over four phases:

- **Initial onset** includes the time from the event to renal cell injury. The onset will occur over hours to days and may be reversable.
- **Oliguric phase** occurs over several days and is characterized by **oliguria**, urine output less than 1 mL/kg/hour. Oliguria or **anuria** lasting longer than 3 to 6 weeks is worrisome and may suggest the kidneys are less likely to recover (Gallo, 2021).
- **Diuretic phase** is a period of approximately 7 to 14 days and when renal recovery is beginning. Urine output will increase to large volumes of unconcentrated urine during this phase. Nurses caring for patients during the diuretic phase should anticipate needing to administer urine replacement.
- **Recovery phase** is when renal function slowly begins to return.

Clinical Pearl

Trousseau sign is a clinical sign observed in hypocalcemia. It's characterized by a carpopedal spasm of the hand and wrist. This sign may be noticed while taking a routine blood pressure when the cuff is inflated. The brief ischemia while the brachial artery is occluded will cause a flexion of the wrist, thumb, and metacarpophalangeal joints and hyperextension of the fingers (Patel & Hu, 2021).

NURSING IMPLICATIONS AND TREATMENT

TREATMENT AND MANAGEMENT

Treatment of AKI is tailored to the specific underlying cause but in general will include:
- careful fluid management to correct hypovolemia or hypervolemia and replace fluid losses
- monitoring of electrolytes: avoid administration of potassium or phosphorus, restrict sodium intake, and give electrolyte replacements
- management of hypertension
- avoidance of nephrotoxic drugs, renal dosing medication, and following drug levels closely
- administering inotropes to support cardiac output
- nutritional support with tight glucose control (Devarajan, 2020)

Nurses caring for patients with AKI should monitor vital signs, perfusion, cardiovascular, neurologic and respiratory assessment, and fluid status closely. An indwelling urinary catheter should be placed for close monitoring of urine output and daily weights should be obtained to follow fluid status. Nursing interventions to prevent and avoid infection are important as patients with AKI are at increased risk for infection as macrophages may be suppressed by uremic toxins (Dokas, 2019).

COMPLICATIONS

Complications of AKI include:
- hypertension, congestive heart failure, or pulmonary edema secondary to fluid overload
- anemia and bleeding
- life-threatening electrolyte abnormalities
- uremia

Critically ill infants and children with fluid overload unresponsive to diuretics, severe metabolic acidosis and electrolyte abnormalities, or symptoms of uremia will require renal replacement therapies.

▶ CHRONIC KIDNEY DISEASE

Chronic kidney disease (CKD) is abnormal kidney structure or function lasting for more than 3 months. The criteria for diagnosis with CKD according to KDIGO requires:
- the presence of kidney damage such as with albuminuria, urine sediment abnormalities, electrolyte abnormalities
- structural abnormalities on imaging
- history of kidney transplantation or decreased GFR (KDIGO, 2013)

The severity of CKD is staged according to a patient's GFR and ranges from stage 1 (normal GFR) to stage 5, often called end-stage renal disease or kidney failure, with a GFR of <15 mL/min per 1.73 m^2 (Srivastava & Warady, 2021).

CKD occurs in children due to congenital abnormalities of the kidney or urology track such as kidney hypoplasia, reflux neuropathy, posterior urethral valves, and polycystic kidney disease. Other causes are due to glomerular disorders like focal segmental glomerulosclerosis and hemolytic uremic syndrome, genetic disorders, or interstitial nephritis (Warady & Weidemann, 2021).

SIGNS AND SYMPTOMS

Children with CKD will show signs and symptoms of renal dysfunction including:
- edema and hypertension
- electrolyte abnormalities such as metabolic acidosis, high serum phosphate, low serum calcium, elevated potassium, elevated BUN and creatinine, and high uric acid
- anorexia is common and growth is impaired
- children may be pale and fatigued from anemia that occurs due to decreased erythropoietin production
- bleeding times may be increased because of defective platelet function
- neurologic signs and symptoms such as irritability, lethargy, seizures and coma may result from uremia

NURSING IMPLICATIONS AND TREATMENT

TREATMENT AND MANAGEMENT

Goals of CKD management are to treat causes of underlying kidney disease, slow the progression of disease, and avoid subsequent kidney injury.

Nurses caring for children with CKD should expect to:
- monitor vital signs, especially blood pressure closely. Hypotension may injure kidneys by hypoperfusion and treating hypertension with antihypertensives, such as with ACE inhibitors or angiotensin II receptor blockers, will help slow the progression of CKD
- track height and weights to monitor nutrition and nutrition supplements offered if needed to meet calorie goals
- administer phosphate binders as ordered to avoid hyperphosphatemia and hypocalcemia which may contribute to bone mineral disease
- correct anemia if symptomatic and give iron supplements or erythropoietin stimulating agents
- perform meticulous hand hygiene and other infection prevention best practices as children with CKD are at increased risk for infection

Children with severe CKD will require renal replacement therapy when the GFR is <30 mL/min per 1.73 m^2 or to manage complication such as hypervolemia, severe electrolyte abnormalities, or neurologic signs and symptoms due to uremia (Srivastava & Warady, 2021). Once a child is stable, dialysis can be spaced to an intermittent basis for long-term management. However, dialysis is associated with increased mortality when compared to kidney transplantation and whenever possible, children should be worked up and prepared for kidney transplantation.

▶ RENAL REPLACEMENT THERAPIES

When electrolyte abnormalities, acidosis, volume overload, or uremia cannot be managed medically, dialysis should be considered. Dialysis may be short-term to allow time for the kidneys to heal, such as in AKI. For chronic or end-stage renal failure, kidneys may require dialysis permanently or until a kidney transplant. Dialysis can be completed in the home, in a dialysis unit, or in the hospital.

PERITONEAL DIALYSIS

Peritoneal dialysis (PD) involves the placement of a catheter in the peritoneal space. Dialysate fluid is infused into the peritoneal cavity causing electrolytes to diffuse across the semipermeable membrane of the peritoneum. PD may be used acutely to manage hypervolemia, hypertension, hyperkalemia, or uremia, or as a long-term solution until kidney function improves or until kidney transplantation. Advantages and disadvantages of PD are listed in Table 7.2 (Dokas, 2019).

Table 7.2. Advantages and Disadvantages of Peritoneal Dialysis

Advantages	Disadvantages
Use in any size patient, even neonates Does not require anticoagulation Catheter can be placed at bedside for short-term use Therapy available in home setting Less risk for rapid fluid and electrolyte shifts	Less reliable ultrafiltration and slow removal Risk for peritonitis: monitor for cloudy dialysate, abdominal pain, and vomiting Risk for complications: leaking, catheter obstruction Contraindications: abdominal wall defects, abdominal infection, severe inflammatory bowel disease Pain during inflow and outflow Compromised diaphragmatic excursion Hyperglycemia

Source: Dokas, M. A. (2019). Renal system. In M. C. Slota (Ed.), *AACN core curriculum for pediatric high acuity, progressive, and critical care nursing* (3rd ed.). Springer Publishing Company.

CONTINUOUS RENAL REPLACEMENT THERAPY

- removes fluid at a slower pace to maintain hemodynamic stability; useful for patients unable to tolerate large fluid volume shifts
- dialyzes in a more physiological way over 24 hours
- avoids complications associated with hemodialysis
- excessive fluids and wastes are removed as blood is passed through a filter
- therapy can be quickly adjusted and titrated

TYPES OF CONTINUOUS RENAL REPLACEMENT THERAPY

- **CAVH** = continuous arteriovenous hemodialysis
- **CAVH/D** = continuous arteriovenous hemofiltration with dialysis
- **CVVH** = continuous venovenous hemofiltration
- **CVVH/D** = continuous venovenous hemofiltration with dialysis

Continuous Venovenous Hemofiltration

Continuous venovenous hemofiltration (CVVH) removes larger volumes of fluid mainly via convection. *Replacement fluid is added.* No dialysate is used. CVVH is effective method for removal of large molecules

Continuous Arteriovenous or Venovenous Hemofiltration/Hemodialysis

CVVH/D removes fluid and solutes mainly by diffusion using dialysate. *No replacement fluid is used.* CVVH/D is an effective method for removal of small to medium sized molecules. This therapy requires vascular (arterial or venous) access and is only performed in the ICU. It is preferred for critically ill patients with unstable hemodynamics. Advantages and disadvantages of CAVH/D and CVVH/D are listed in Table 7.3.

Table 7.3. Advantages and Disadvantages of Continuous Arteriovenous or Venovenous Hemofiltration/Hemodialysis

Advantages	Disadvantages
Requires ICU admission Continuous fluid and electrolyte correction Controlled fluid balance Tolerated by hemodynamically unstable patients	Risk for anticoagulation, filter clotting Risk for line infection Invasive vascular access Hypovolemia

Source: Dokas, M. A. (2019). Renal system. In M. C. Slota (Ed.), *AACN core curriculum for pediatric high acuity, progressive, and critical care nursing* (3rd ed.). Springer Publishing Company.

INTERMITTENT HEMODIALYSIS

Intermittent hemodialysis requires arterial or venous vascular access, a fistula, which is a surgically anastomosed artery and vein, or a graft, an implanted stent which joins an artery and vein. Hemodialysis is highly effective and capable of rapidly correcting fluid, acid–base, and electrolyte abnormalities. In CKD, hemodialysis is typically initiated when GFR is <30 mL/min per 1.73 m². Advantages and disadvantages of intermittent hemodialysis are outlined in Table 7.4.

Table 7.4. Advantages and Disadvantages of Intermittent Hemodialysis

Advantages	Disadvantages
Highly effective in removing toxins (ammonia, uric acid)	Requires special vascular access
Best for life-threatening electrolyte abnormalities (hyperkalemia)	High cost
	Hypotension and hypovolemia may occur
Effective in removing toxins (ammonia, uric acid)	Requires anticoagulation

Source: Dokas, M. A. (2019). Renal system. In M. C. Slota (Ed.), *AACN core curriculum for pediatric high acuity, progressive, and critical care nursing* (3rd ed.). Springer Publishing Company.

▶ HEMOLYTIC UREMIC SYNDROME

Hemolytic uremic syndrome (HUS) is one of the main causes of AKI in children and is characterized by the presence of a triad of features:

- thrombocytopenia
- anemia
- AKI

Renal injury occurs when inflammatory mechanisms damage endothelial cells, platelets aggregate and fibrin is deposited in capillaries and arterioles, and perfusion to the renal parenchyma is decreased. Infections, commonly the Shinga-toxin producing *E. coli* or *S. pneumoniae*, are the cause of HUS in over 90% of cases and children under 5 years of age are primarily affected (Niaudet & Boyer, 2021b). HUS may also be associated with a hereditary disorder, such as with mutations in the genes involved in the coagulation pathway or cobalamin (vitamin B_{12}) metabolism, or be medication related (Box 7.1; Dokas, 2019; Niaudet & Boyer, 2021b; Sethi, 2019).

Box 7.1 Medication Causes of Hemolytic Uremic Syndrome

Calcineurin inhibitors: cyclosporine, tacrolimus
Cytotoxic drugs: mitomycin, bleomycin, gemcitabine, or cisplatin
Quinine
Oral contraceptives

SIGNS AND SYMPTOMS

Children with HUS will present with:

- anemia
- elevated lactate dehydrogenase or low haptoglobin (a protein made by the liver that attaches to a certain type of hemoglobin)
- schistocytes >1% on peripheral smear
- thrombocytopenia
  Other symptoms include:
- fever
- lethargy
- decreased urine output
- hypertension
- pallor
- petechia
- dehydration
  Electrolyte abnormalities may occur due to AKI such as:
- hyperkalemia
- hyperphosphatemia
- metabolic acidosis

In HUS caused by *S. pneumoniae*, children will present with symptoms of sepsis, pneumonia, or meningitis, and have a positive Coombs test. A 2- to 3-week history of bloody diarrhea is common in

E. coli-associated HUS. Infants with cobalamin deficiency will present with symptoms of feeding difficulties, abnormal tone, visual impairment, and developmental delay (Niaudet & Boyer, 2021a).

NURSING IMPLICATIONS AND TREATMENT

TREATMENT AND MANAGEMENT

Treatment of HUS is generally supportive and will include:
- administering isotonic fluids to maintain intravascular volume and avoiding dehydration
- correcting electrolyte abnormalities
- red blood cell transfusions for hemoglobin <7 g/dL or hematocrit <18%
- platelets for significant bleeding

Nurses caring for children with HUS should ensure nephrotoxic drugs are discontinued and anticipate dialysis for children with severe electrolyte abnormalities, fluid overload, symptomatic uremia, or **azotemia**. Generally, in young children, PD is the preferred method of dialysis for HUS.

Severe central nervous system symptoms such as seizures, stroke, or decreased level of consciousness are managed by plasmapheresis or administration of a monoclonal antibody, Eculizumab. Antibiotics should be given for HUS caused by *S. pneumoniae*. Most children have good renal recovery after HUS but some children will have irreversible injury to the kidneys requiring long-term dialysis or renal transplantation (Niaudet & Boyer, 2021a).

Clinical Pearl

Infection with an encapsulated bacterium such as N. meningitis, S. pneumonia, *or* H. influenzae *is a life-threatening risk of treatment with Eculizumab. Children receiving this monoclonal antibody must receive meningococcal vaccination before the first dose. Antibiotic prophylaxis with penicillin is also recommended.*

▶ KIDNEY TRANSPLANT

A kidney transplant is a surgical procedure whereby a healthy kidney from a living or deceased donor replaces a diseased kidney. End-stage renal disease is an indicator for kidney transplantation as children in end-stage renal disease have better long-term survival with a transplant than long term dialysis (Abramyan & Hanlon, 2022). Children with CKD should be considered for kidney transplantation when GFR is less than 30 mL/min per 1.73 m² (stage 4). Contraindications for kidney transplants include severe comorbidities that may affect transplant success:
- cardiac or pulmonary disease
- malignancy
- active infection
- drug use
- uncontrolled diseases
- history of noncompliance

NURSING IMPLICATIONS AND TREATMENTS

TREATMENT AND MANAGEMENT

Postoperative considerations include management of a postoperative patient and surgical complications. Postoperative management of a kidney transplant often requires strict fluid status monitoring and hydration to ensure adequate blood flow to the new kidney and urine production (Abramyan & Hanlon, 2022).
- pain management
- strict, hourly inputs, and outputs
- care of an indwelling urinary catheter
- Vasopressors may be used to maintain peak blood flow to the kidneys.

COMPLICATIONS

Surgical complications include hemorrhage, thrombosis, infection, arterial stenosis, and urinoma.
- ***Hemorrhage*** is classically identified by tachycardia and hypovolemia; however, postoperative transplant recipients often are on beta-blockers and may not present with tachycardia. Hypertension

(rather than hypotension) may be noted due to parenchymal compression. Nurses caring for patients post-transplant should look for physical signs of hemorrhage: acute flank pain and a bulge near the incision.

- **Thrombosis** is rare and associated with graft loss. Diagnostic renal ultrasounds can identify postoperative blood flow concerns. New-onset hematuria and sudden-onset oliguria are indicators of diminished flow to the kidney.
- **Infections** are common as patients are immunosuppressed immediately following surgery. Patients are commonly placed prophylactically on antivirals and antibiotics especially in the first 3 to 6 months. Common causes of infection are from Epstein-Barr virus (EBV) and cytomegalovirus (CMV), and BK virus (polyomavirus).
- **Arterial stenosis** is a late complication that is often asymptomatic but noted by elevated serum creatinine, an indicator of diminished graft function, and by ultrasound and angiography.
- **Lymphocele** is a complication caused by lymphatic tissue disruption resulting in a painful bulge or bump overlying the kidney. Treatment includes percutaneous draining of the lymph collection.
- **Urinoma** is the collection of urine within the retroperitoneum, as urine leaks from the kidney. Decompression of the bladder is necessary. Treatment involves placing an indwelling urinary catheter or surgical placements of stents and revisions.

Clinical Pearl

Diseased, existing kidneys are often left in place as the newly transplanted kidney is placed in the iliac fossa; the renal artery is connected to the external iliac artery and the renal vein is connected to the external iliac vein (see Figure 7.2). The donor ureter is anastomosed to the bladder. Biopsy of a kidney is typically done from the back, with the patient lying on their stomach. However, to biopsy a transplanted kidney, patients lie on their back and are accessed from the lower abdomen.

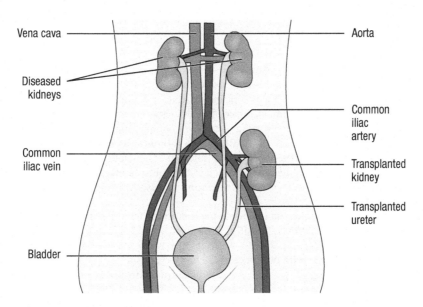

Figure 7.2 Kidney transplantation
Source: **Demchick, W. S. (2017).** *Kidney location after transplantation.*

▶ LIFE-THREATENING ELECTROLYTE IMBALANCES

Alterations in serum sodium, potassium, phosphate, calcium, and magnesium occur in renal failure when GFR is reduced and the kidney is unable to effectively manage electrolyte secretion and reabsorption (Blayney, 2013; Burgunder, 2021; Dokas, 2019; Roberts, 2013).

HYPONATREMIA

- Sodium is the extracellular cation responsible for muscle, nerve, and myocardium action potentials. It maintains acid–base balance, fluid balance, and regulates osmolality.
- **Normal serum sodium is 135 to 145 mEq/L.**
- Hyponatremia may occur from vomiting, diarrhea, gastrointestinal (GI) losses, increased water intake, or decreased sodium intake. In renal disease, hyponatremia is due to increased water intake or dilution from fluid retention.
- Signs and symptoms of hyponatremia include nausea, headache, muscle cramps, weakness, confusion progressing to lethargy, seizure, and coma.
- Treatment of hyponatremia is by restricting fluids and correcting the underlying cause. If a patient is experiencing mental status changes then hypertonic saline is administered. Serum sodium must be corrected slowly to avoid cerebral edema.

HYPERKALEMIA

- Potassium is the intracellular cation responsible for skeletal and cardiac muscle activity and maintains acid–base balance.
- **Normal serum potassium is 3.5 to 5 mEq/L.**
- Hyperkalemia may occur from tumor lysis, hemolysis, metabolic acidosis, from medications including angiotensin blockers, potassium-sparing diuretics, or ACE inhibitors, or hypoaldosteronism. In renal failure, hyperkalemia occurs as excretion by the kidneys is reduced.
- Signs and symptoms of hyperkalemia are skeletal muscle weakness, paresthesia, and EKG changes. EKG changes typically progress from peaked T waves → prolonged and widened QRS → loss of P waves → ST segment depression → bradycardia, AV block, ventricular arrythmias, and cardiac arrest.
- Serum potassium of 6 to 7 mEq/L with a normal EKG can be managed by removing potassium from the diet and intravenous fluids and administration of kayexalate. An abnormal EKG and serum potassium >7 mEq/L will be treated by administering calcium gluconate, sodium bicarbonate, insulin and dextrose, and inhaled albuterol. Dialysis should be considered if there's no improvement.

HYPOCALCEMIA

- Calcium is involved in nerve transmission, bone composition, and muscle contractions. Only about half of the body's calcium is available for use and not bound to protein or anions. This available portion is ionized calcium and essential in clotting, cardiac function, muscle contraction, and nerve impulse transmission. Serum calcium and phosphate levels share an inverse relationship. In renal failure, the kidneys retain phosphate leading to hyperphosphatemia and hypocalcemia.
- **Normal serum calcium is 9 to 11 mg/dL (total), 1.00 to 1.4 mmol/dL (ionized).**
- Causes of hypocalcemia are hypoparathyroidism, vitamin D deficiency, hyperphosphatemia, pancreatitis, and malabsorption. Medications such as calcium channel blockers or anticonvulsants may cause hypocalcemia. Hypocalcemia occurs in tumor lysis syndrome secondary to hyperphosphatemia.
- Signs and symptoms of hypocalcemia include muscle cramps, tetany, paresthesia of the fingertips or hands, fatigue, prolonged QT interval, positive Trousseau's and Chvostek signs, hypotension, and seizures.
- First treat hyperphosphatemia with oral phosphate binders or dialysis in severe hyperphosphatemia. Severe hypocalcemia is managed with intravenous calcium chloride or calcium gluconate.

HYPERPHOSPHATEMIA

- Phosphorus is found in the body's bones and teeth. It provides structure for bones, is involved in energy processes, and maintains acid–base balance.
- Phosphate levels are higher in children because of skeletal growth. **Normal serum phosphate is 4.2 mg/dL in the newborn, 3.5 to 6.5 mg/dL in the young child, 2.5 to 4.5 mg/dL in the older child and adolescent.**
- Causes of hyperphosphatemia include tumor lysis syndrome, rhabdomyolysis, diabetic ketoacidosis, and excessive intake. In renal failure, hyperphosphatemia occurs because the kidney is unable to adequately excrete phosphorus.

■ Signs and symptoms of hyperphosphatemia include tachycardia, hyperreflexia, muscle cramps, nausea and diarrhea, tetany, and hypocalcemia.

■ Hyperphosphatemia in CKD is managed by reducing phosphate in the diet and administering phosphate binders. In the acutely or critically ill child, serum calcium should be monitored closely and corrected. Dialysis may be required.

HYPO- AND HYPERMAGNESEMIA

■ Magnesium is responsible for metabolic and enzyme processes. It's involved in neuromuscular and cardiovascular functions and the metabolism of adenosine triphosphate (ATP).

■ **Normal serum magnesium is 1.5 to 2.5 mEq/L.**

■ Magnesium balance is maintained by the kidneys. In renal failure, reduced GFR decreases reabsorption of magnesium and diuretics given to manage fluid overload cause increased magnesium excretion leading to hypomagnesemia. Hypermagnesemia is common in CKD due to decreased renal excretion of magnesium. Other causes of hypo- and hypermagnesemia are outlined in Table 7.5.

Table 7.5. Electrolyte Imbalances

Electrolyte Imbalance	Etiology	Clinical Manifestations	Management
Hyperkalemia K >5 mEq/L	Renal failure Hypoaldosteronism Tumor lysis syndrome Metabolic acidosis Hemolysis Medications (angiotensin blockers, K sparing diuretics, heparin, ACE inhibitors)	Skeletal muscle weakness Paresthesia EKG changes: peaked T waves → prolonged and widened QRS → loss of P waves → ST segment depression → bradycardia AV block, ventricular arrythmias, cardiac arrest	Correct cause Obtain 12-lead EKG Remove K from diet and fluids Kayexalate Calcium gluconate Sodium bicarbonate Insulin and dextrose Albuterol Dialysis
Hypokalemia K <2.5 mEq/L	Diuretics GI loss (diarrhea, laxatives) Malnutrition Metabolic alkalosis Interstitial nephritis	Skeletal muscle weakness Ascending paralysis Ileus Urinary retention Cardiac arrythmias EKG changes: flat T waves, depressed ST segment, U waves Hyperreflexia	Correct cause Potassium replacement (max 1 mEq/kg/hr)
Hypernatremia Na >135 mEq/L	Diabetes insipidus CKD Diuretics Excess exogenous sodium Deficit of free water Fever Hyperglycemia	Lethargy Weakness Altered mental status Irritability, coma, seizures Muscle cramps Respiratory failure Dry, sticky mucous membranes Intense thirst	Correct cause Slowly correct sodium and free water deficit

(continued)

Table 7.5. Electrolyte Imbalances (*continued*)

Electrolyte Imbalance	Etiology	Clinical Manifestations	Management
Hyponatremia *Na <135 mEq/L*	Vomiting, diarrhea GI losses Burns and wounds Renal diseases Diuretics Increased water intake and decreased sodium intake Malnutrition Fever Excessive diaphoresis DKA	Nausea Headache Muscle cramps Weakness Confusion Apnea Lethargy, seizure, coma Depressed deep tendon reflexes	Correct cause Restrict fluids Sodium replacement with hypertonic saline Correct slowly to avoid cerebral edema
Hypermagnesemia *Mg >4.5mg/dL*	Renal failure Excessive supplementation Status asthmaticus Enemas Phosphate binders Laxatives Lithium ingestion	Hypotonia Hyporeflexia Paralysis Lethargy Confusion Hypotension Prolonged QT, QRS, and PR intervals, AV block Respiratory failure and cardiac arrest >15 mg/dL	Stop any supplements Diuresis Give calcium supplements Dialysis
Hypomagnesemia *Mg <0.7mg/dL*	Diarrhea Short bowel Pancreatitis Genetic: mitochondrial disorders Medications: amphotericin, cyclosporine, loop and thiazide diuretics, mannitol Decreased oral intake Hyperaldosteronism	Tetany Malaise Depression Hyperreflexia EKG changes: flattened T wave and ST segment lengthening, PVC's, Ventricular tachycardia Ventricular fibrillation *Signs are similar to hypocalcemia*	Correct cause IV magnesium sulfate Oral Mg oxide or Mg sulfate Monitor EKG Neuromuscular assessment
Hypercalcemia *Ca >10.5 mg/dL* *iCa >1.34*	Hyperparathyroidism Vitamin D intoxication Excessive calcium administration Prolonged immobilization Thiazide diuretics Hyperthyroidism	Weakness, hypotonicity Irritability Lethargy Seizures Coma Abdominal cramping Anorexia Nausea Vomiting Shortened QT interval	Correct cause Increase urine output by increasing fluids with potassium to 2-3x maintenance rate Diuretics Hemodialysis Steroids Calcitonin or bisphosphonate Correct hyperphosphatemia before hypercalcemia as tissue calcification may form

(*continued*)

Table 7.5. Electrolyte Imbalances (*continued*)

Electrolyte Imbalance	Etiology	Clinical Manifestations	Management
Hypocalcemia *Ca <8 mg/dL* *iCa <1.15*	Hypoparathyroidism Vitamin D deficiency Hyperphosphatemia Pancreatitis Malabsorption Medications: calcium channel blockers or anticonvulsants Tumor lysis syndrome	Tetany Neuromuscular irritability with weakness Paresthesia Fatigue Cramping Altered mental status Seizures Prolonged QT Trousseau's and Chvostek sign Hypotension	Correct cause Treat hyperphosphatemia IV calcium chloride or calcium gluconate Oral supplementation
Metabolic acidosis *Arterial bicarbonate* *<20 mmol/L*	Ketoacidosis: DKA, starvation Lactic acidosis: tissue hypoxia, ingestions Viral gastroenteritis Intoxication (NSAIDs) Acute and chronic renal failure Diarrhea Genetics	Hyperventilation Nausea and vomiting Lethargy Confusion	Correct cause Electrolyte replacements (sodium bicarbonate)
Hyperphosphatemia *PO4 >4 mg/dL*	Tumor lysis syndrome Rhabdomyolysis DKA Renal failure	Tachycardia Muscle cramping Nausea and diarrhea Tetany Hypocalcemia	Correct cause Monitor calcium levels Low phosphorus diet Phosphate binders Dialysis
Hypophosphatemia *PO4 <3 mg/dL*	Decreased intake Decreased GI absorption Excessive antacids Burns Increased renal excretion	Irritability Tremors Confusion, delirium, seizures, coma Decreased myocardial function Respiratory failure	Identify and correct cause IV potassium or sodium phosphate

ACE, angiotensin-converting enzyme; CKD, chronic kidney disease; DKA, diabetic ketoacidosis; GI, gastrointestinal; PVCs, premature ventricular contractions.

Source: Burgunder, L. (2021). Fluids and electrolytes. In K. Kleinman, L. McDaniel, & M. Molloy (Eds.), *Harriet Lane Handbook* (pp. 261–282). Elsevier.

■ Signs and symptoms of hypo- and hypermagnesemia include:
- **Hypomagnesemia:** tetany, confusion, seizures, coma, respiratory depression, and coma. EKG changes such as flattened T wave and ST segment lengthening, premature ventricular contractions (PVCs), and ventricular arrythmias.
- **Hypermagnesemia:** hypotonia, hyporeflexia, paralysis, lethargy, confusion, hypotension. EKG changes including prolonged QT, QRS, and PR intervals, AV block

■ Children at risk for hypo- or hypermagnesemia should be monitored closely due to concerns for life threatening ventricular arrythmias and cardiac arrest. The underlying cause should be identified and treated.
- **Hypomagnesemia:** Monitor EKG, perform neuromuscular assessment, and give intravenous (IV) magnesium sulfate.
- **Hypermagnesemia:** Monitor EKG, give calcium, stop any supplemental magnesium, and prepare for dialysis.

Life-threatening electrolyte imbalances, their causes, signs and symptoms, and management are outlined in Table 7.5.

Clinical Pearl

*Hyperkalemia can be treated most acutely following the acronym CBIG for **C**alcium (calcium chloride or calcium gluconate), sodium **B**icarbonate, **I**nsulin, and **G**lucose. In addition, beta-2 agonists like albuterol can also help to move potassium from cells. Kayexalate exchanges sodium for potassium, allowing the body to excrete potassium from the body.*

▶ RENAL AND GENITOURINARY INFECTIONS

Patients are at higher risk for infection due to the presence of invasive lines for therapy, AKI, structural abnormalities that prevent urine flow, reflux of urine from the bladder to the kidneys, and uncontrolled diabetes. See Figure 7.3 for a diagram of the renal system.

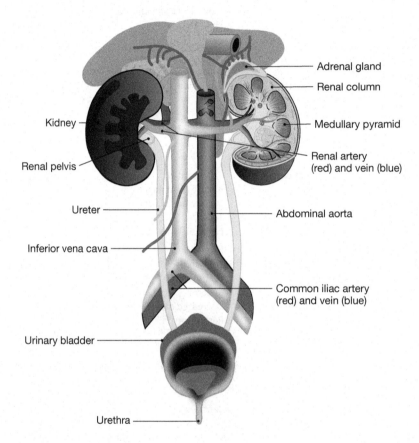

Figure 7.3 The renal system
Source: Gawlik, K. S., Melnyk, B. M., & Teall, A. M. (Eds). (2021). *Evidence-based physical assessment: Best practices for health and well-being assessment.* Springer Publishing Company.

▶ PYELONEPHRITIS

Pyelonephritis is a kidney infection caused by *E. coli* in the urinary tract that begins in the urethra or bladder and eventually moves into the kidneys. If not treated properly, kidney infections can lead to permanent kidney damage, failure, or sepsis.

SIGNS AND SYMPTOMS

Pyelonephritis signs and symptoms include those indicating infection:
- fever and chills
- flank pain

- frequent urination, burning sensation with urination
- nausea and vomiting
- cloudy or potent urine

Patients with any urinary tract blockages are at elevated risk for infection as the bladder is unable to empty completely (Bolick et al., 2021).

NURSING IMPLICATIONS AND TREATMENT

Pyelonephritis is confirmed through a urine sample to measure white and red blood cells, bacteria, and increased protein. Pyelonephritis is treated through antibiotics, pain management, and hydration. In more severe cases, drains may be placed to remove infection.

▶ RENAL AND GENITOURINARY SURGERY

Renal and genitourinary surgeries are often focused on relieving obstructions to proper urine production and flow from the kidneys to the bladder and out the urethra. Diagnostic surgical procedures include renal biopsies, nephrectomies, and cystoscopies and nephrostomies.

Renal biopsies are often done under light sedation. Postoperatively, patients remain flat and complete blood counts (CBCs) are monitored for internal bleeding. Patients may or may not have bloody urine for up to 24 hours postoperatively. Complications include infection, bright red blood or clots in the urine, difficulty urinating, pain at biopsy site, discharge at biopsy site, and bleeding.

Nephrectomy is the removal of a kidney, typically due to kidney cancer. This can be done laparoscopically or via open surgery. Following a nephrectomy, blood pressure and electrolytes are closely monitored. A urine catheter is often in place for a few days for close urine output monitoring. Complications include changes in urination such as frequent urination or changes in urine color, edema in the legs and face, and persistent hypertension. As a single kidney remains, patients should ensure that they do not participate in activities that could injure or put the surviving kidney at risk. Otherwise, patients typically live functional and healthy lives with just one kidney.

Ureteral obstructions are blockages in urine flow in the ureter from the kidney or to the bladder. These are often caused by nephrolithiasis, ureterocele, tumors, or retroperitoneal fibrosis. These blockages cause urinary tract infections that present with fever, pain difficulty urinating, blood in the urine. Untreated, these blockages can result in renal failure. Surgical interventions for these blockages include the placement of indwelling urethral stents to relieve the obstruction and infection. If the stents are inadequate, nephrostomy tubes are percutaneously placed. However, nephrostomy tubes present a high risk for bleeding and infection.

CASE STUDY

A previously healthy 4-year-old female presents to the pediatrician with a 6-day history of abdominal pain, vomiting, and diarrhea. Her mother shares that other children in her preschool program have also been sick with a stomach bug. Her parents describe her as being pale, tired, irritable for the last few days, and have noticed her urine is dark colored. Vital signs are stable other than a mild tachycardia and elevated blood pressure.

1. Which of the following is the most probable cause of renal failure in this patient?
   A. Hepatorenal syndrome
   B. Hemolytic uremic syndrome (HUS)
   C. Acute glomerulonephritis
   D. Hydronephrosis

The pediatrician, suspecting hemolytic uremic syndrome (HUS), refers the family to the pediatric ED where a complete blood count, comprehensive metabolic panel, urinalysis, and arterial blood gas (ABG) are obtained.

2. Expected laboratory results for this patient include:
   A. Thrombocytopenia, anemia, and hyponatremia
   B. Polycythemia, anemia, and schistocytes on peripheral smear
   C. Thrombocytopenia, anemia, and elevated serum creatinine
   D. Hypokalemia, hyperphosphatemia, and hypocalcemia

Laboratory results reveal an elevated serum creatinine, anemia, thrombocytopenia, and electrolyte abnormalities.
- hemoglobin: 6 g/dL
- platelet count: 40,000/uL
- serum creatinine: 5 mg/dL
- sodium: 155 mEq/L
- potassium: 5 mEq/L
- arterial blood gas (ABG): pH 7.24, $PaCO_2$ 30, HCO_3 16

The patient is admitted to the pediatric ICU (PICU) for further management.

3. Which of the following are priority nursing interventions?
   A. Insert an indwelling urinary catheter.
   B. Give kayexalate.
   C. Prepare for intubation for hypocarbia management.
   D. Draw a type and cross in preparation for platelet administration.

Two days postadmission, the patient is noted to have worsening fluid balance. The patient is edematous and daily weights indicate that the patient has become progressively more fluid positive over the course of the PICU admission. Laboratory analyses indicate rising blood urea nitrogen (BUN) and creatinine levels and worrying electrolyte abnormalities including a serum potassium of 6.5 mEq/L. The PICU provider has asked that nursing prepare for peritoneal dialysis (PD).

4. The patient's mother is frightened and asks the nurse why this treatment is necessary. Which of the following is the most appropriate response?
   A. Peritoneal dialysis (PD) will avoid the need for a kidney transplant.
   B. PD is the most effective way to remove fluid and balance electrolytes in the body.
   C. Other methods of dialysis are contraindicated in hemolytic uremic syndrome (HUS) because of the risk for bleeding.
   D. PD will gently remove fluids and correct electrolytes which can be safer than other forms of dialysis.

PD was successful in improving the patient's fluids status and correcting electrolyte abnormalities. After several weeks in the hospital, the patient was discharged home on dialysis where she was followed closely by the pediatric nephrology team as an outpatient.

(See answers next page.)

ANSWERS TO CASE STUDY QUESTIONS

1. B) Hemolytic uremic syndrome (HUS)

HUS is the most common cause of acute kidney injury (AKI) in children. This patient's symptoms are consistent with renal failure from Shinga-toxin producing *E. coli*. Children with HUS have a history of abdominal pain, diarrhea, and vomiting 5 to 10 days prior to HUS. This patient's symptoms are not consistent with hepatorenal syndrome, acute glomerulonephritis, or hydronephrosis.

2. C) Thrombocytopenia, anemia, and elevated serum creatinine

Patients with HUS have anemia, increased schistocytes on peripheral smear, thrombocytopenia, and signs of AKI (elevated serum creatinine, blood urea nitrogen [BUN], and electrolyte abnormalities). Common electrolyte abnormalities in AKI include hyperkalemia, hyperphosphatemia, hypocalcemia, and hypermagnesemia.

3. A) Insert an indwelling urinary catheter.

Close monitoring of urine output is necessary for managing the patient's fluid status. Hyperkalemia is typically not treated until >7 mEq/L. The $PaCO_2$ is acidotic as the patient is compensating for the metabolic acidosis. A type and cross is indicated for a transfusion of packed red blood cells (PRBCs), not platelets unless the patient has active bleeding.

4. D) PD will gently remove fluids and correct electrolytes which can be safer than other forms of dialysis.

Fluid removal is slower with PD and risk for rapid fluid or electrolyte shifts is lessened. PD does not prevent kidney transplantation. Hemodialysis is most effective, compared to PD or continuous venovenous hemofiltration with dialysis (CVVH/D). Bleeding is not a risk factor in hemolytic uremic syndrome (HUS).

KNOWLEDGE CHECK: CHAPTER 7

1. Which of the following are expected laboratory abnormalities in acute kidney injury (AKI)? (Select all that apply.)
   A. Hypercalcemia
   B. Hyperkalemia
   C. Hyperphosphatemia
   D. Hypomagnesemia

2. A nurse is caring for a patient with acute glomerulonephritis in the pediatric ICU (PICU). Over the course of the shift, the patient's urine output has increased to 4 mL/kg/hr. Which of the following interventions is most appropriate?
   A. Restrict fluid intake.
   B. Prepare to assist with continuous renal replacement therapy initiation.
   C. Discontinue all nephrotoxic drugs.
   D. Administer urine replacement fluids as ordered.

3. A nurse recognizes the mother of an 18-month-old patient receiving peritoneal dialysis (PD) understands discharge teaching when she says:
   A. "The outflow bag should be held above the bed to avoid pain."
   B. "It's very important that anyone touching the peritoneal dialysis tubing wash their hands first."
   C. "Antibiotics should be given to prevent infection."
   D. "It's okay if the outflow fluid looks cloudy sometimes."

4. Acute glomerulonephritis is differentiated from other forms of acute kidney injury (AKI) in children in that:
   A. Children do not develop hypertension with glomerulonephritis.
   B. Glomerulonephritis is usually secondary to *E. coli* infection.
   C. Hematuria and proteinuria are common symptoms of glomerulonephritis.
   D. Glomerular filtration rate (GFR) is unaffected.

5. A pediatric ICU (PICU) provider has ordered a red blood cell (RBC) transfusion for your critically ill pediatric patient with hemolytic uremic syndrome (HUS) whose hemoglobin is 6 g/dL. As the nurse prepares to administer the blood transfusion, which of the following do they anticipate?
   A. Transfusing a large volume of 15 to 20 mL/kg RBCs to reduce the number of transfusions the patient receives throughout the hospitalization
   B. The blood bank canceling the order as the patient's hemoglobin is not low enough to transfuse
   C. Receiving RBCs due to expire in the next couple of days to prevent the blood bank from wasting product
   D. Transfusing a small volume of 3 to 5 mL/kg RBCs within 4 hours

6. Laboratory results of a patient recently admitted to the PICU with a 4-day history of vomiting and diarrhea revealed the following:
   - arterial blood gas: pH 7.26, $PaCO_2$ 34, HCO_3 18
   - serum potassium: 5 mEq/L
   - serum sodium: 155 mEq/L
   - serum creatinine: 1.2 mg/dL

   Priority nursing interventions in the care of this patient include: (Select all that apply.)
   A. Placement of an indwelling urinary catheter and measuring urine output hourly
   B. Giving 20 mL/kg of normal saline intravenously
   C. Preparing for bedside hemodialysis catheter placement for continuous venovenous hemodialysis
   D. Administering calcium, sodium bicarb, insulin, and glucose

7. Which of the following symptoms indicates hyponatremia?
   A. Nausea, muscle cramps, and seizures
   B. Muscle weakness, ascending paralysis, and flat T waves
   C. Tetany, fatigue, and cramping
   D. Nausea, weakness, and hyperreflexia

(See answers next page.)

1. B) Hyperkalemia; C) Hyperphosphatemia

Serum potassium and phosphate levels are high in AKI due to decreased renal excretion of potassium and phosphate. Increased urinary retention of phosphate causes low serum calcium. Magnesium is increased due to decreased renal excretion of magnesium.

2. C) Discontinue all nephrotoxic drugs.

Urine output significantly increases in the diuretic phase in acute tubular necrosis as the kidneys are recovering but unable to adequately concentrate the urine. Urine replacement fluids are necessary to avoid hypovolemia and hypervolemia. Restricting fluids will cause hypovolemia and kidney hypoperfusion. There is not enough information to determine if dialysis is necessary. Nephrotoxic drugs are discontinued upon first recognition of kidney injury.

3. B) "It's very important that anyone touching the peritoneal dialysis tubing wash their hands first."

Peritonitis is a frequent complication of PD, especially in diapered infants and young children. Meticulous hand hygiene and good catheter site care is most important in preventing infection. The outflow bag should never be elevated above the bed as it will cause the outflow to flow back into the peritoneal cavity and is a risk factor for infection. Antibiotics are given to treat peritonitis but are not given prophylactically. Cloudy outflow fluid is a symptom of peritonitis.

4. C) Hematuria and proteinuria are common symptoms of glomerulonephritis.

Sudden onset of hematuria with proteinuria are typical symptoms of acute glomerulonephritis. Hypertension is common due to fluid and sodium retention. Streptococcus or staphylococcus are bacterial organisms known to cause acute glomerulonephritis and GFR is reduced (Niaudet, 2021).

5. D) Transfusing a small volume of 3 to 5 mL/kg RBCs within 4 hours

Small volumes of 3 to 5 mL/kg volumes of packed red blood cells (PRBCs) are appropriate in patients with acute kidney injury (AKI) who are experiencing hypertension, hypovolemia, or at risk for hyperkalemia. Patients with HUS may require blood transfusions when hemoglobin is less than 7 g/dL or hematocrit is less than 18%. RBCs should be fresh as older blood has a higher potassium content.

6. A) Placement of an indwelling urinary catheter and measuring urine output hourly; B) Giving 20 mL/kg of normal saline intravenously

Hypovolemia is a common cause of prerenal acute kidney injury (AKI). It is important to correct hypovolemia with fluid boluses of isotonic crystalloid fluid. An indwelling urinary catheter should be placed and urine output measured and documented hourly. There is not enough information to determine if dialysis is necessary at this time. Unless the patient is showing clinical signs and symptoms of hyperkalemia, pharmacologic management is typically not initiated until the serum potassium is greater than 7 mEq/L.

7. A) Nausea, muscle cramps, and seizures

Hyponatremia occurs in acute kidney injury (AKI) from dilution in fluid overload or secondary to diuretic use. Signs and symptoms of hyponatremia include nausea, headaches, muscle cramps, weakness, seizure, and coma. Muscle weakness, ascending paralysis, and flat T waves are signs of hypokalemia. Tetany, fatigue, and cramping are signs of hypocalcemia. Nausea, weakness, and hyperreflexia are signs of hypomagnesemia.

8. A new pediatric ICU (PICU) nurse verbalizes understanding common complications of hemodialysis when they say:
   A. "Metabolic alkalosis, hypokalemia, and hypophosphatemia are complications of hemodialysis."
   B. "A fluid bolus may be needed before starting therapy."
   C. "Hemodialysis requires percutaneous placement of a catheter in the abdomen."
   D. "The circuit is sterile so infection is not a major concern."

9. A patient is considered to have chronic kidney disease when:
   A. The serum creatinine increased from 1 to 2 mg/dL in the last 4 days
   B. Urine output has been 0.5 mL/kg/hr for the last two shifts
   C. The serum creatinine has increased from 0.5 mg/dL to 0.8 mg/dL in 72 hours
   D. Glomerular filtration rate is decreased for 4 months

10. Diseases that cause intrinsic acute kidney injury (AKI) in children include:
    A. Sepsis, burns, and congestive heart failure
    B. Tumor lysis syndrome, bladder dysfunction, and hemolytic uremic syndrome
    C. Glomerulonephritis, tumor lysis syndrome, and renal artery thrombosis
    D. Bladder dysfunction, ureteral obstruction, and hemorrhagic cystitis

(See answers next page.)

8. B) "A fluid bolus may be needed before starting therapy."

Some patients are at risk for hypotension during dialysis. A fluid bolus may be needed to correct blood pressure before starting therapy. Metabolic acidosis, hyperkalemia, and hyperphosphatemia are complications of hemodialysis. Peritoneal dialysis involves the placement of a catheter in the peritoneum through the abdomen. Infection is always a concern for critically ill hospitalized patients and patients with kidney disease are at increased risk.

9. D) Glomerular filtration rate is decreased for 4 months

Chronic kidney disease is abnormal kidney structure or function lasting more than 3 months. According to Kidney Disease: Improving Global Outcomes (KDIGO) guidelines, acute kidney injury (AKI) is defined as an increase in serum creatinine by ≥0.3 mg/dL within 48 hours, or an increase in serum creatinine by ≥1.5 times baseline within the prior 7 days, or urine output ≤0.5 mL/kg/hour for 6 hours.

10. C) Glomerulonephritis, tumor lysis syndrome, and renal artery thrombosis

Glomerulonephritis, tumor lysis syndrome, and renal artery thrombosis all contribute to renal injury through parenchymal damage. Sepsis, burns, and congestive heart failure are causes of prerenal AKI. Postrenal causes include bladder dysfunction, ureteral obstruction, and hemorrhagic cystitis.

REFERENCES

Abramyan, S., & Hanlon, M. (2022). Kidney transplantation. In *StatPearls* [Internet]. StatPearls Publishing. https://www.ncbi.nlm.nih.gov/books/NBK567755/

Blayney, F. (2013). Renal disorders. In M. F. Hazinski (Eds), *Nursing care of the critically ill child* (3rd ed., pp. 703–772). Elsevier.

Bolick, B., Reuter-Rice, K., Madden, M., & Severin, P. (2021). Kidney and genitourinary disorders. In B. Bolick, K. Rueter-Rice, M. Madden, & P. Severin (Eds), *Pediatric acute care: A guide for interdisciplinary practice* (2nd ed.; pp. 732–782). Elsevier.

Burgunder, L. (2021). Fluids and electrolytes. In K. Kleinman, L. McDaniel, & M. Molloy (Eds.), *Harriet Lane handbook* (pp. 261–282). Elsevier.

Demchick, W. S. (2017, February 21). *Kidney location after transplantation.* https://commons.wikimedia.org/wiki/File:Kidtransplant.svg

Dokas, M. A. (2019). Renal system. In M. C. Slota (Ed.), *AACN core curriculum for pediatric high acuity, progressive, and critical care nursing* (3rd ed.). Springer Publishing Company.

Fountain, J. H., & Lappin, S. L. (2022). Physiology, renin angiotensin system. In *StatPearls* [Internet]. StatPearls Publishing. https://www.ncbi.nlm.nih.gov/books/NBK470410/

Gallo, P. M. (2021). Nephrology. In K. Kleinman, L. McDaniel, & M. Molloy (Eds.), *Harriet Lane handbook* (pp. 472–501). Elsevier.

Kidney Disease: Improving Global Outcomes CKD Work Group. (2012). KDIGO 2012 clinical practice guideline for acute kidney injury. *Kidney International Supplement, 1*, 1–138.

Kidney Disease: Improving Global Outcomes CKD Work Group. (2013). KDIGO 2012 clinical practice guideline for the evaluation and management of chronic kidney disease. *Kidney International Supplement, 3*, 1–150.

Niaudet, P. (2021). Overview of the pathogenesis and causes of glomerulonephritis in children. In F. B. Stapleton & L. Wilkie (Eds.), *UptoDate.* https://www.uptodate.com/contents/overview-of-the-pathogenesis-and-causes-of-glomerulonephritis-in-children

Niaudet, P., & Boyer, O. G. (2021a). Overview of hemolytic uremic syndrome in children. In T. K. Mattoo & K. Wilkie (Eds.), *UptoDate.* https://www.uptodate.com/contents/overview-of-hemolytic-uremic-syndrome-in-children

Niaudet, P., & Boyer, O. G. (2021b). Treatment and prognosis of Shiga toxin-producing *Escherichia coli* (STEC) hemolytic uremic syndrome (HUS) in children. In T. K. Mattoo & L. Wilkie (Eds.), *UptoDate.* https://www.uptodate.com/contents/treatment-and-prognosis-of-shiga-toxin-producing-escherichia-coli-stec-hemolytic-uremic-syndrome-hus-in-children

Ogobuiro, I. & Tuma, F. (2022). Physiology, renal. In *StatPearls* [Internet]. StatPearls Publishing. https://www.ncbi.nlm.nih.gov/books/NBK538339/

Patel, M., & Hu, E. W. (2021). Trousseau sign. In *StatPearls* [Internet]. StatPearls Publishing. https://www.ncbi.nlm.nih.gov/books/NBK557832/

Roberts, K. E. (2013). Fluid, electrolyte, and endocrine problems. In M. F. Hazinski (Eds.), *Nursing care of the critically ill child* (3rd ed., pp. 679–701). Elsevier.

Sethi, S. K. (2019). Hemolytic uremic syndrome. In S. Sethi, R. Raina, M. McCulloch, & T. Bunchman (Eds.), *Critical care pediatric nephrology and dialysis: A practical handbook*. Springer. https://doi.org/10.1007/978-981-13-2276-1_15

Srivastava, T., & Warady, B. A. (2021). Chronic kidney disease in children: Overview of management. In T. K. Mattoo & L. Wilkie (Eds.), *UpToDate.* https://www.uptodate.com/contents/chronic-kidney-disease-in-children-overview-of-management

Tobias, A., Ballard, B. D., & Mohiuddin, S. S. (2022). Physiology, water balance. In *StatPearls* [Internet]. StatPearls Publishing. https://www.ncbi.nlm.nih.gov/books/NBK541059/

Warady, B. A., & Weidemann, D. K. (2021). Chronic kidney disease in children: Definition, epidemiology, and course. In T. K. Mattoo & L. Wilkie (Eds.), *UpToDate.* https://www.uptodate.com/contents/chronic-kidney-disease-in-children-definition-epidemiology-etiology-and-course

Young, M. & Leslie, S. W. (2022). Renal biopsy. In: *StatPearls* [Internet]. StatPearls Publishing. https://www.ncbi.nlm.nih.gov/books/NBK470275/

Integumentary System Review

Erin Dwyer and Molly Stetzer

The integumentary system is the largest organ in the body and is the first line of defense against external insults. The integumentary system is often underrated in its importance. In a critically ill child, the assessment of the skin can inform the status of other organs. The skin is a barrier against external forces such as chemicals and microorganisms and assists with fluid, temperature, and electrolyte regulation. A breach in the integumentary system in a critically ill patient can provide the perfect opportunity for a bacterial insult. Pediatric patients in the ICU are at high risk of complications related to skin integrity.

> ## Clinical Pearl
>
> *When choosing an adhesive or type of tape, use one that will cause the least amount of trauma to the skin while effectively securing a medical device. Consider protecting the skin with silicone-based skin protectants. Also, when inserting an IV, make sure the advancing flange is up and not downward pushing into the skin. This may cause skin breakdown.*

▶ INTRAVENOUS INFILTRATION

Peripheral intravenous (PIV) infiltration is an event where fluids and/or medications infuse outside of the blood vessel and into the surrounding tissue. Extravasation is the infiltration of a vesicant solution or medication. The term *infiltration* will be used throughout this text, but the principles discussed apply to both infiltration and extravasation. When fluid or medication is infused into the tissue outside of the blood vessel, the fluid collection may put pressure on the surrounding tissues and structures, leading to a decrease in blood supply and the risk of compartment syndrome. Extravasation may lead to cell death in the local tissue. Vasoactive medications may cause constriction in the capillary beds, resulting in ischemic necrosis of the local tissue.

Pediatric-specific risks of PIV infiltration include:

- ▪ inability to explain to small children in a developmentally appropriate way the importance of the PIV
- ▪ Need for additional securement devices may obscure the insertion site from being thoroughly assessed.
- ▪ Preverbal children are unable to communicate pain specific to the PIV site.
- ▪ smaller or more fragile veins (Garcia et al., 2021; Tofani et al., 2012)

Additional patient-specific factors that increase the risk of infiltration:

- ▪ patients with altered sensation in the area of the PIV
- ▪ patients receiving sedation/who have altered consciousness
- ▪ difficult PIV access related to history of multiple venipunctures
- ▪ PIV dwell time (longer catheters more likely to infiltrate)
- ▪ ultrasound-guided insertion with less than two-thirds of the catheter in the vein (Gorski et al., 2021)

PIV infiltration may cause injury to the surrounding tissues depending on the degree of infiltration and the infusate that infiltrates. Particularly in the ICU environment, there are many high-risk medications that may be administered through a PIV, which increases the risk of infiltrate injury. Characteristics of vesicant medications include pH, osmolarity, vasoconstrictive potential, and cytotoxicity (Table 8.1).

Table 8.1 pH and Osmolarity

pH	Osmolarity
▦ Ideal pH 5–9 ▦ Increased infiltrate risk with acidic and alkaline infusions ▦ Extreme pH reduces vein tolerance, damages cell proteins, and increases risk for rupture or infiltrate	▦ Ideal osmolarity 281–282 mOsm/L ▦ Extravasation of hypertonic solutions → swelling and increased pressure and disrupted cell function ▦ Extravasation of hypotonic solutions → cell swelling and rupture Common examples: Dextrose >10%, IVF w/ high amino acid or electrolyte additives, undiluted electrolytes

IVF, intravenous fluids.

Long-term sequelae of intravenous (IV) infiltration may include skin, muscle, or nerve damage. IV infiltration can lead to long-term scarring that inhibits the child's mobility if over a joint. A variety of grading scales are available to evaluate the severity of infiltration and should be used when infiltrate injury is identified.

SIGNS AND SYMPTOMS

Nurses caring for critically ill pediatric patients with PIVs should routinely assess PIVs in accordance with their organization's standards.
- ▦ Assess PIVs every hour or more frequently if receiving infusions of vesicant medications.
- ▦ Assess PIVs prior to administering medications.
- ▦ Ensure insertion site is easily visualized, PIV is properly stabilized and protected, and tape and dressings are not too tight.
- ▦ Monitor for pain, burning, redness, or swelling with PIV use.

NURSING IMPLICATIONS AND TREATMENT

It is crucial for nurses to select the most appropriate site when inserting a PIV in order to reduce the risk of infiltration or extravasation (Gorski et al., 2021).

LABS AND DIAGNOSTICS

If infection is present after an infiltrated IV, a wound culture may be required. Breaches in skin integrity may require a wound consult, special dressings, and surgical interventions if severe.

TREATMENT AND MANAGEMENT

Nurses should also be familiar with medications that are **vesicants** and/or **irritants** and prepare to offer treatment for an infiltration should one occur during infusion of a high-risk medication. Frequent and thorough assessment of PIV sites may help to identify infiltrations early and avoid extensive tissue damage. Assessment should include comparison with contralateral extremity to identify signs of swelling. Observation should also include assessment for color change, fluid leaking from additional puncture sites, blistering, and patient report of pain (if patient is verbal). When a PIV infiltrate occurs, the nurse should immediately stop all infusions running through the PIV. Emergency medications, such as vasopressors, should be immediately infused through another point of vascular access to avoid patient decompensation. The nurse should not flush the PIV as this will further infuse into the tissue and could cause additional damage (Gorski et al., 2021). The nurse may attempt to withdraw any solution from the tissue by gently aspirating with an empty syringe connected to the PIV. Depending on the specific infusate, it may be appropriate to inject the tissue with an antidote or dispersal enzyme to prevent long-term tissue damage.
- ▦ **Phentolamine** is preferred for extravasation of vasopressors and may help promote prompt reperfusion of the surrounding tissue (Gorski et al., 2021).
- ▦ **Hyaluronidase** is an enzyme that increases the absorption of some vesicants and promotes dispersion of the medication into the tissue (Gorski et al., 2021). Hyaluronidase may be used with cytotoxic medication and is also used for a variety of other vesicants including both acidic and alkalotic drugs, as well as hyperosmolar solutions such as parenteral nutrition (Gorski et al., 2021).
  After discontinuing infusions and finding alternate IV access for life-sustaining infusions, the nurse should:
- ▦ elevate the extremity to promote reabsorption of the infiltrated fluid/medication

- loosen any securement devices and/or adhesive and remove the IV
- consult with the IV specialty nurse and/or the medical care team
- remove the infiltrated catheter
- perform a neurovascular assessment of the extremity and immediately report any compromise in tissue perfusion to the medical team
- apply heat or cold therapy as indicated, based on infusate. Compresses should be dry to avoid causing maceration of the surrounding tissue. Pay particular attention to which medications require heat versus cold therapy based on the goal of medication reabsorption into the tissue.

Cold compresses are indicated for medications such as DNA-binding agents where the goal is vasoconstriction/isolation of the medication to the localized tissue and decreased inflammation.

Heat therapy should be applied when the goal is to increase local blood flow (vasodilation) and disperse the medication through the tissue. One example would be with a vasopressor infiltration (Gorski et al., 2021).

The nurse is responsible for ongoing assessment of the affected area to monitor for swelling, blistering, and perfusion. Serial neurovascular checks *distal* to the point of infiltration should be performed (Gorski et al., 2021). Patients that experience severe PIV infiltrates are at risk of compartment syndrome, which is a medical emergency. Prompt removal of securement devices and adhesive may aid in the prevention of compartment syndrome. Neurovascular checks including: capillary refill time, quality of pulses, and temperature of the tissue distal to the infiltration should be assessed frequently and until resolution of the infiltrate.

Some high-risk medications for tissue damage include:

- acyclovir
- amiodarone
- calcium
- dextrose >12.5%
- mannitol
- potassium >60 mEq
- sodium bicarbonate
- sodium chloride >1%
- total parental nutrition >900 mOsm/L
- vasopressors (dopamine, epinephrine, norepinephrine, etc).

Consider central venous access (either a central venous catheter or a peripherally inserted central catheter line) for administration of high-risk medications.

▶ PRESSURE INJURIES

A pressure injury is an area of localized damage to the skin and underlying soft tissues, which frequently occurs over a bony prominence (National Pressure Injury Advisory Panel [NPIAP], 2016). Pressure injuries may present as intact skin or an open ulceration and may be painful. Often, injuries at advanced stages are not painful once the nerve endings have become so damaged that the patient can no longer feel pain. Pressure injuries result from intense and/or prolonged pressure, or pressure in combination with shear. Predisposing factors to pressure injury include poor nutrition, altered mobility, friction and/or shearing effect, and alteration in the microclimate of the skin during a period of acute illness (NPIAP, 2016). Patients in the ICU are at an increased risk of developing pressure injuries for a number of reasons, including hospital-acquired impaired mobility, presence of medical devices, and alteration in nutritional status (extended nothing by mouth [NPO] times).

Clinical Pearl

*Remember some of the simplest things a nurse can do to prevent skin breakdown in the pediatric ICU (PICU) is to **turn the patient every 2 hours**, keep the head of bed (HOB) at 30° to prevent sliding down in bed of the patient, use pillow of foam wedges to protect boney prominences from coming in contact with each other, use gel pads to protect the occiput and boney surfaces, and keep pillows under the heels to raise the heels up off the bed.*

SIGNS AND SYMPTOMS/PRESSURE INJURY STAGING

Pressure injuries often present as an area of erythema over a bony prominence and result from a period of prolonged pressure that results in a decrease in blood flow to the affected area. Pressure injuries are staged based on the most advanced part of the wound.

Stage 1 pressure injury is **nonblanchable** erythema of intact skin (NPIAP, 2016). Nonblanchable indicates that there is no color change when fingertip pressure is applied to the erythematous area. If the injury does blanch (there is color change with pressure) then the injury is a *pre-stage 1* injury and is not yet classified as a pressure injury. Pressure offloading may prevent this pre-stage 1 injury from advancing to a true pressure injury (Figure 8.1).

In patients with darkly pigmented skin, erythema may be difficult to appreciate so a thorough head-to-toe skin assessment in a well-lit room is essential.

Stage 2 pressure injury involves partial-thickness skin loss with exposed epidermis or may present as a fluid-filled blister (NPIAP, 2016; Figure 8.2).

Stage 3 pressure injuries have advanced to the point of full-thickness skin loss and may have visible adipose tissue (NPIAP, 2016). Depending on the area of the body where the pressure injury develops, a

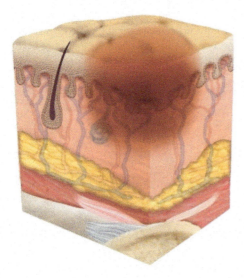

Figure 8.1 Stage 1 A. Lightly pigmented skin

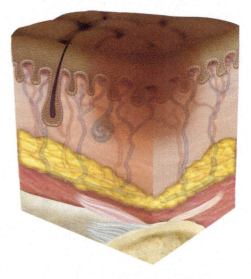

Figure 8.1 Stage 1 B. Darkly pigmented skin
Source: A,B: © 2016, National Pressure Injury Advisory Panel (NPIAP). *NPIAP Pressure Injury Stages.* Reprinted with permission.

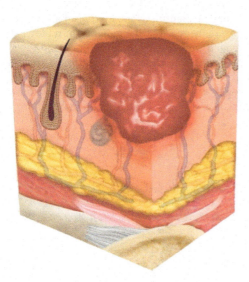

Figure 8.2 Stage 2 A. Lightly pigmented skin

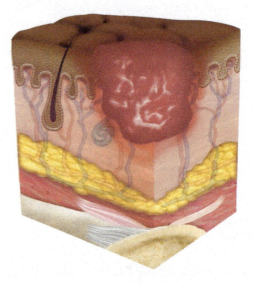

Figure 8.2 Stage 2 B. Darkly pigmented skin
Source: A,B: © 2016, National Pressure Injury Advisory Panel (NPIAP). *NPIAP Pressure Injury Stages.* Reprinted with permission.

stage 3 injury can be very deep or more superficial. Areas of significant adiposity can have deeper injuries that remain stage 3 before they become more advanced (Figure 8.3).

Stage 4 pressure injuries involve full-thickness skin and tissue loss, with exposed bone, tendon, or cartilage (NPIAP, 2016). These injuries will require advanced therapies for healing, directed by a wound care specialist. These injuries may not be painful for the patient as they have often surpassed the level of the nerve endings (Figure 8.4).

Unstageable pressure injuries are full thickness (stage 3 or 4 injuries) where the wound bed is occluded by the presence of eschar (dead tissue; NPIAP, 2016). The wound bed must be debrided before a stage can be determined. Some wounds with stable eschar will remain classified as unstageable if the appropriate healing is taking place and eschar is not fully removed (Figure 8.5).

Deep tissue pressure injuries (DTPIs): DTPIs appear as a dark purple or maroon discoloration, or as a blood-filled blister. These deep injuries represent intense or prolonged pressure, and the skin may stay intact or may open to reveal a full thickness injury (NPIAP, 2016). Clinicians should be careful to not misclassify vascular injuries (bruises, petechiae) as DTPIs (Figure 8.6).

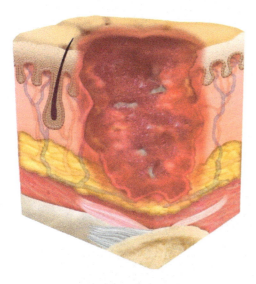

Figure 8.3 Stage 3 A. Lightly pigmented skin

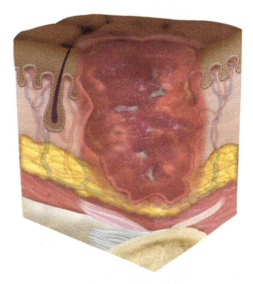

Figure 8.3 Stage 3 B. Darkly pigmented skin
Source: A,B: © 2016, National Pressure Injury Advisory Panel (NPIAP). *NPIAP Pressure Injury Stages*. Reprinted with permission.

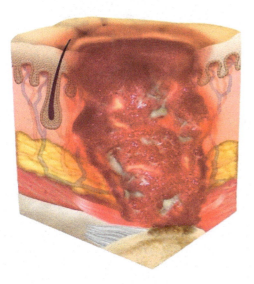

Figure 8.4 Stage 4 A. Lightly pigmented skin

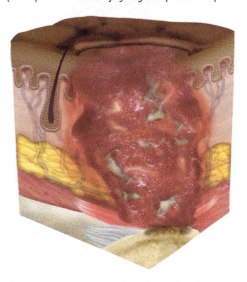

Figure 8.4 Stage 4 B. Darkly pigmented skin
Source: A,B: © 2016, National Pressure Injury Advisory Panel (NPIAP). *NPIAP Pressure Injury Stages*. Reprinted with permission.

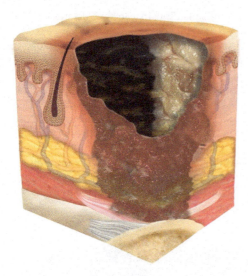

Figure 8.5 Unstageable pressure injuries A. Half slough, lightly pigmented skin

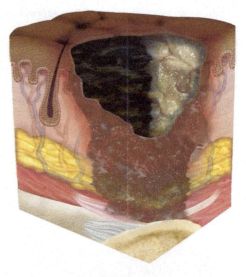

Figure 8.5 Unstageable pressure injuries B. Half slough, darkly pigmented skin
Source: A,B: © 2016, National Pressure Injury Advisory Panel (NPIAP). *NPIAP Pressure Injury Stages*. Reprinted with permission.

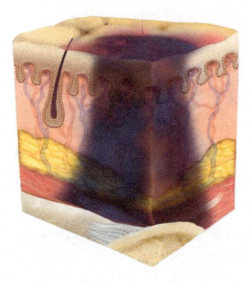

Figure 8.6 Deep tissue pressure injury A. Lightly pigmented skin

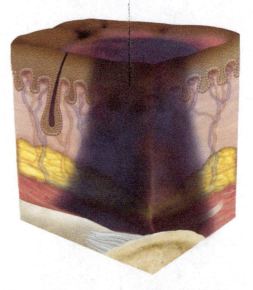

Figure 8.6 Deep tissue pressure injury B. Darkly pigmented skin
Source: A,B: © 2016, National Pressure Injury Advisory Panel (NPIAP). *NPIAP Pressure Injury Stages*. Reprinted with permission.

Helpful illustrations of pressure injury staging and other free resources can be found by visiting the National Pressure Injury Advisory Panel website (NPIAP.com).

NURSING IMPLICATIONS AND TREATMENT

ASSESSMENT

A thorough head-to-toe skin assessment should be performed on all children upon admission to the ICU and at least once per shift thereafter. The nurse should evaluate the patient's skin for any signs of redness/discoloration, bogginess, or indentations from medical devices. A validated pressure injury risk assessment tool should be utilized to identify patients at high risk of developing pressure injuries. In pediatrics, the Braden QD is commonly used to predict immobility and medical device-related pressure injury. Patients should be assessed for risk on admission and daily. Total scores range from 0 (low risk) to 20 (highest risk). Patients who score ≥13 are considered at risk and interventions are needed. The downloadable Braden QD Scale can be found online at http://www.marthaaqcurley.com/uploads/8/9/8/6/8986925/braden_qd_tool.pdf.

TREATMENT AND MANAGEMENT

Interventions should be based on the level of risk and specific areas of risk for a patient. ICU nurses should be cognizant that visible manifestations of pressure injuries may take up to 72 hours to present following an operative procedure and should increase the frequency of skin assessment during this high-risk period (Papantonio et al., 1994). Pediatric patients have different anatomical areas of risk as compared to adult patients, such as the occiput due to the larger size of the pediatric patient's head relative to their body surface area. Other areas of risk include the sacrum, elbows, heels, scapulae, and nasal septum/bridge of nose for patients with respiratory support devices.

Primary prevention of pressure injury is the most effective nursing intervention. Care to pad bony prominences should be taken, and medical devices should be diverted away from the patient's skin whenever possible. All medical devices affixed to the patient should be rotated at regular intervals, when possible (i.e., blood pressure cuff, pulse ox probe). Regular repositioning should be part of nursing care, and patients should be turned at least every 2 hours while in bed. Children who are at in increased risk of pressure injury (as determined by pressure injury risk assessment score or decreased mobility) should be evaluated for placement on a specialty mattress. Specialty surfaces include air- and fluid-immersion mattresses, which redistribute pressure based on the patient's body positioning. Some surfaces offer turn-assistive technology. For patients on specialty surfaces, pay special attention to minimizing linen layers and reduce use of other pressure injury prevention devices to allow for maximum benefit from the pressure reducing surface.

Patients who will undergo lengthy procedures in the operating room that require supine positioning may benefit from side-to-side repositioning on the shift prior to and following their procedure. This will help to decrease the cumulative amount of time spent in the supine position. Patients with hemodynamic instability that inhibits the ability to fully turn the patient will benefit from microturns, as even minor repositioning can help to reestablish blood flow and redistribute pressure. Prophylactic dressings are beneficial in the prevention of pressure injuries, especially for patients with impaired mobility. Silicone-based dressings are often used and should be changed at the frequency defined in the hospital's standard of care. Other methods of pressure offloading include floating heels and elbows off the bed, use of gel pads for bony prominences, and placing the patient on a specialty bed/pressure redistributing mattress. Additional clinical pearls in pressure injury prevention include lifting a patient off of the bed as much as possible during repositioning or "boosting" to avoid a shearing injury, minimizing linen layers, and removing braids/barrettes from the hair of children with decreased mobility to prevent scalp injuries.

If a patient develops a pressure injury, the patient's care team should be notified, and appropriate consultations should be placed for the patient to be evaluated by a healthcare professional with advanced training in the management of pediatric wounds. Immediate interventions should include staging of the pressure injury and implementation of pressure offloading from the affected area of the body. For skin that is intact, a protective dressing (such as a silicone-based dressing) may be applied. For injuries where a fluid-filled blister is present, care should be taken to keep the blister intact. In the event of a stage 3 or stage 4 injury, wound care may include application of ointments, packing the wound, and/or debridement.

Nursing interventions should include regular assessment of the wound and surrounding skin, applying ointments as ordered, and performing dressing changes as ordered. In order to promote healing, a dressing may be left in place for several days during which nursing should monitor the surround skin and evaluate the dressing to be clean, dry, and intact. Nursing is also responsible to divert any contaminating substances (i.e., stool or urine) away from dressings. Implementation of a toileting schedule or increased frequency of diaper changes may be necessary to promote wound healing. General principles of wound management are covered later in this chapter.

Wounds that are advanced or slow to heal may require negative pressure wound therapy (NPWT), hyperbaric therapy, or other advanced wound therapies. ICU nurses are responsible for the nursing assessment of the patient's tolerance to these therapies and support of the patient's condition throughout the duration of therapy.

▶ SKIN FAILURE

Pediatric skin failure has several unique characteristics that set it apart from traditional skin alterations such as pressure injury. Skin failure is typically sudden in onset, full thickness in depth, and occurring in patients with two or more dysfunctional organ systems. Notably, patients with skin failure have a much higher mortality rate (42%) compared to overall PICU mortality rates (1.8%; Cohen et al., 2017).

SIGNS AND SYMPTOMS

The Kennedy terminal ulcer (KTU) was first described in adult literature in 1989 as a dark red and rapidly progressing pear-shaped wound on the sacrum (Figure 8.7). The KTU has a sudden onset; it has been described as not being present for the daily assessment, but then appearing within hours (Reitz & Schindler, 2016).

Apart from the sacrum, deep red to purple localized injuries over nonpressure bearing anatomic locations can appear rapidly, these are called the Trombley-Brennan terminal tissue injury (Figure 8.8), and may assist clinicians in prognosticating patient's death within hours (Jacob et al., 2020).

Patients with significant edema may experience partial thickness wounds related to third spacing, such as striae stretched to splitting and bullae. Patients with multiple organ dysfunction syndrome, sepsis or shock, and use of vasopressors are at increased risk for developing skin failure.

NURSING IMPLICATIONS AND TREATMENT

For the nurse caring for the critically ill child experiencing skin failure, priorities can include patient comfort, providing high-quality skin and wound care, and the promotion of undisrupted family time as able. Offer both pharmacologic and nonpharmacologic pain interventions prior to, during, and following care such as repositioning and hygiene. Time activities that may cause discomfort around scheduled pain medication administration. Weigh pain management with desire for wakeful interactive time with family and incorporate the patient and family's values and preferences.

If there is a single position of comfort, reinforce with the patient and family the need to give that bony prominence a chance to off-load pressure by switching positions, if only briefly or slightly. Continue to provide bathing, moisturization, and moisture barrier in incontinent patients. Cluster care whenever possible to maximize undisrupted family time. Anticipatory guidance can prepare families for the planned interruptions to assess and provide care. Offer acceptable choices to encourage routine care. For example, "I can reposition you at 10 or 10:30. Which works better for you?"

For children at life's end, the facility's pressure injury prevention bundle may be insufficient to keep the child free from pressure injury. Consult wound care specialist to collaborate in enhancing prevention strategies. Understand that skin injury is distressing to patients and families, and clinicians as well, as a visible manifestation of the patient's severe illness.

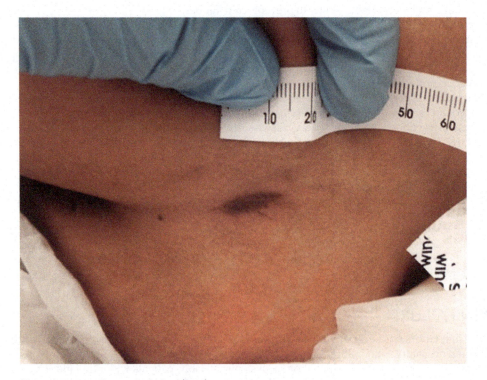

Figure 8.7 Kennedy terminal ulcer (KTU)

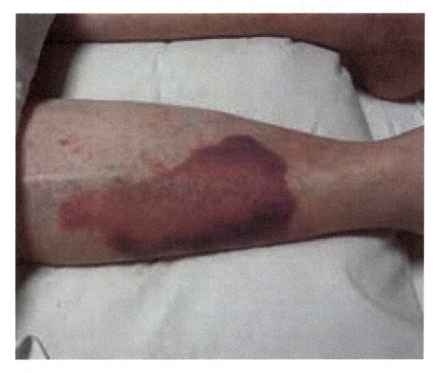

Figure 8.8 Trombley-Brennan terminal tissue injury
Source: Trombley, K., Brennan, M. R., Thomas, L., & Kline, M. (2012). Prelude to death or practice failure? Trombley-Brennan terminal tissue injuries. *American Journal of Hospice and Palliative Medicine®, 29*(7), 541–545. https://doi.org/10.1177/1049909111432449

▶ WOUNDS

Pediatric patients experience wounds of myriad etiologies, ranging from burns, traumatic, surgical, or pressure injuries to congenital anomalies. Regardless of the etiology of the wound, principles of wound healing are largely the same. Goals of care can include mitigating the cause of the wound, maintaining moisture balance, obliterating dead space, removal of devitalized tissue, and palliating patient symptoms.

Clinical Pearl

The types of wounds included in penetrating wounds are puncture wounds, surgical wounds and incision, thermal, chemical, or electric burns, bites or stings, and high velocity projectiles that injury the body (bullets). Blunt force trauma includes abrasions, lacerations, or skin tears.

SIGNS AND SYMPTOMS

Unlike many conditions that present with nonspecific signs and symptoms, wounds are visible and, in many cases, evident to family members and lay people. The etiology or treatment may not be as evident, however, and it is important to recognize when management of the skin alteration requires consultation to a specialist, such as a certified wound, ostomy, and continence nurse, or physician for medical or surgical management.

NURSING IMPLICATIONS AND TREATMENT

Assessment of a pediatric patient with a wound or concern for a wound should include visual inspection and palpation. Especially in darkly pigmented patients, early signs of skin changes can be difficult to visualize, and palpation may reveal tissue that is warmer or cooler, boggier or firmer than surrounding skin. Nonverbal patients may show signs of pain such as increased heart rate, blood pressure, cry, or grimace. Verbal patients may complain of pain from the wound, but if wound pain is overshadowed by other symptoms (e.g., reason for hospitalization), this can be unreliable. Caregivers familiar with the patient are often more insightful about the presence and source of discomfort. See Table 8.2 for characteristics of the wound that must be assessed and supplemental guidance.

Table 8.2 Wound Assessment Guidance

Wound Assessment Component	Supplemental Guidance
Anatomic location	Refer to bony prominence if immobility-related pressure injury. Clarify laterality.
Length	Measure the largest measurement from head to toe.
Width	Measure the largest measurement from side to side (e.g., hip to hip or shoulder to shoulder).
Depth	Measure perpendicular to skin surface at the deepest point of the wound.
Wound edges	Document whether the wound edges are well demarcated or diffuse, attached to the wound bed or unattached, do the wound edges roll under (epibole)?
Undermining	The ability to pass a cotton-tipped applicator under the skin at the wound edge; **undermining** is demonstrated as a significant portion of the wound edge. Document the portion of the wound edge involved as hours on a clock face, e.g., undermining 10–2 o'clock would represent the superior 120° of a wound.
Tunneling	The ability to pass a cotton-tipped applicator under the skin at the wound edge; **tunneling** is unidirectional in its tract. Document the direction of the sinus tract as an hour on a clock face, e.g., tunneling at 12 o'clock would represent a sinus tract tunneling towards the head.
Wound bed description	Describe the color of the tissue in the wound bed, pink, red, yellow, white, brown, grey, brown, black, etc. If there are multiple colors, describe in approximate percentages (e.g., 30% yellow, 70% red).
Exudate description	Describe the color and consistency of the wound exudate.
Exudate volume	Describe the quantity of the exudate, from none for a dry wound, scant for a moist wound with no drainage in dressing, small amount fills 1%–25% of dressing, moderate for drainage that fills 26%–75% to copious when wound drainage fills >76% of dressing.
Wound odor	Describe the odor of the wound following cleansing. Note odor of drainage on the removed dressing.
Peri-wound skin	Describe the skin surrounding the wound. Assess for changes in color, temperature, firmness (e.g., fluctuance or induration).

LABS AND DIAGNOSTICS

While labs can be informative of the patient's conditions that contribute to risk for wounds, the diagnosis and treatment of a wound are based on physical assessment. Poor nutritional status contributes to the risk of wound development, and traditionally measures of **albumin and prealbumin** have been used to assess nutritional status. Anemia should be assessed as low iron can negatively impact wound healing. Anthropometric data can also inform nutritional status. Patients may need protein and calories beyond maintenance to achieve healing. For patients with nutritional deficiencies, vitamin C, iron, and zinc supplements can be considered to promote wound healing.

When concern for infection arises, lab values such as white blood cells, erythrocyte sedimentation rate, and C-reactive protein can inform diagnosis and treatment. Radiographs may show signs of osteomyelitis if concern for bone involvement, MRI is more sensitive and noninvasive, but the gold standard for diagnosis of osteomyelitis is bone biopsy. Fluctuance near a wound can indicate fluid collection and can be assessed with ultrasound. Cultures of the wound should be collected judiciously. Chronic wounds will be colonized with skin flora. If the decision is made to culture the wound, the wound must first be cleansed with normal saline to remove exudate and debris from the wound surface. A swab is rotated on a 1 cm area of the clean wound bed, and pressure adequate to express fluid is applied. Care must be taken to ensure the swab is not contaminated by adjacent skin and that the delivery to lab is timely.

TREATMENT AND MANAGEMENT

Treatment of the wound should address the underlying cause. Pressure should be offloaded from pressure injuries either by turning the patient off of the bony prominence affected or removing, rotating site, or padding underneath medical devices causing pressure injury. Wounds caused by exposure to moisture will benefit from moisture management. Moisture management for wounds in the pelvic region, for example, a sacral pressure injury, may benefit from indwelling or noninvasive urinary and/or fecal management systems to prevent contamination of urine and stool into the wound.

Moist wound healing promotes faster wound healing than allowing the wound bed to dry or scab over. For dry wounds without endogenous moisture, donation of moisture with a wound gel can achieve the desired moisture balance. Wound gels are available with additives such as antimicrobials silver or metronidazole. Highly exudative wounds will require an absorbent dressing that manages the exudate to protect peri-wound skin and promote moist wound healing. Peri-wound skin should be protected from moisture using an alcohol-free skin barrier film. Wounds with undermining, tunneling, or significant depth may require packing to obliterate dead space. Packing should be one continuous piece of material such as roll gauze or hydrofiber ribbon, and a 2 to 3 cm tail should remain outside the wound for easy removal of packing.

Negative pressure wound therapy (NPWT), also known as a vacuum-assisted closure, has successfully been used in pediatric patients, especially those with large and/or slow-healing wounds. Benefits of NPWT include improved exudate management and decreased frequency of dressing changes to every 2 to 3 days rather than daily or more often (McNichol et al., 2022). It is important for the nurse to be aware of proper settings and make sure the device is working properly.

Wound beds obscured by necrotic tissue should be debrided. Methods of debridement include surgical, conservative-sharp, autolytic, mechanical, and enzymatic. Nonselective methods of debridement, such as mechanical debridement in the form of wet to dry dressings, take both nonviable and viable tissue and should be avoided. Refer to facility policy for guidance on how to choose an appropriate wound product and when to refer to a specialist in wound care.

Patients with wounds are often affected by pain, itching, odor, and the stress and discomfort of dressing changes. Pain management principles should be applied including pharmacologic and nonpharmacologic techniques. Itch can be improved with pharmacologic interventions like antihistamines, topical, or systemic steroids and nonpharmacologic interventions such as cool compress and emollient use. Odor can be managed with antimicrobial agents for wound irrigation (e.g., hypochlorous acid) and antimicrobial wound dressings. Collaboration with the patient and their caregiver can help to determine the frequency of dressing changes. Dressings should be changed often enough that the wound is not permitted to dry out nor become over-wet from saturated dressings. If drainage volume changes, the dressing strategy will need to change as well in order to have appropriate moisture balance at an acceptable frequency of dressing change. Child life specialists are valuable partners in promoting coping through wound care procedures.

⬤ CASE STUDY

The nurse is caring for a 10-year-old with a history of static encephalopathy, cerebral palsy, seizure disorder, developmental delay, and G-tube dependence. They are admitted to the pediatric ICU (PICU) in respiratory distress, are found to be rhino/enterovirus positive, and are requiring noninvasive positive pressure ventilation (NIPPV). The patient is nonverbal and nonambulatory at baseline. They have a peripheral intravenous (PIV) in each hand; one is infusing maintenance intravenous fluids (IVF) and the other is currently saline-locked.

Over the course of the last 2 hours, the nurse has observed a 10% increase in the patient's heart rate (HR) and blood pressure (BP). The patient is afebrile and has good urine output in the brief. Oxygen saturation is 93% on 50% FiO_2. The patient is intermittently moaning. The parents have stepped away from the bedside for a few hours. The nurse believes the patient could be in pain and begins a head-to-toe assessment to identify possible sources of pain. The patient's PIV site appears to be swollen, but the nurse is unsure if this is edema or the patient's normal anatomy.

CASE STUDY QUESTIONS

1. The nurse's next steps in assessing the peripheral intravenous (PIV) site should include:
   A. Pause the maintenance intravenous fluids (IVF)
   B. Compare the patient's two hands to identify the presence of swelling
   C. Palpate both hands to evaluate for firmness around the intravenous (IV) site
   D. All of the above

The nurse identifies that the patient's IV has infiltrated. The nurse removes the IV, elevates the hand, switches the maintenance IVF to the other IV, and utilizes an infiltration grading scale to evaluate the infiltrate. The infiltrate is graded as mild, and the patient thankfully does not require any additional therapy at this time.

2. The patient still appears to be in pain, so the nurse continues the assessment. The nurse asks the respiratory therapist (RT) to assist in assessing the skin under the noninvasive positive pressure ventilation (NIPPV) mask. Upon assessment, the nurse identifies that the bridge of the patient's nose has nonblanching erythema. The nurse identifies that the patient:
   A. Has a stage 2 pressure injury
   B. Has a stage 1 pressure injury
   C. Has a pre-stage 1 pressure injury
   D. Does not have a pressure injury

The nurse works with the RT to identify an alternate NIPPV interface that will allow for pressure offloading of the patient's nose. The nurse develops a plan with the RT and the medical team to rotate interfaces every 4 hours to decrease the risk of additional pressure injuries and obtain a foam-based dressing to provide padding under the NIPPV interface.

3. Due to the patient's increased risk of pressure injury, what other prophylactic measures might the nurse consider?
   A. Prophylactic silicone or foam-based dressings
   B. Floating heels
   C. Frequent turning
   D. Rotating medical devices
   E. All of the above

(See answers next page.)

ANSWERS TO CASE STUDY QUESTIONS

1. D) All of the above

Pausing the maintenance IVF, comparing the patient's hands, and palpating both hands are all appropriate next steps in assessment for this patient.

2. B) A stage 1 pressure injury

The nonblanching erythema on the patient's nose is indicative of a stage 1 pressure injury. Partial-thickness skin loss would indicate a stage 2 injury, which is not present here.

3. E) All of the above

All of these listed are prophylactic measures the nurse would utilize for her patient.

KNOWLEDGE CHECK: CHAPTER 8

1. A serous fluid-filled blister is staged as what type of pressure injury?
   A. Stage 1 pressure injury
   B. Stage 2 pressure injury
   C. Deep tissue pressure injury
   D. A blister is not a pressure injury

2. What should be the nurse's priority when an intravenous (IV) infiltrate is discovered?
   A. Notifying the physician
   B. Placing a new IV
   C. Removing any adhesive dressings from the site
   D. Elevating the extremity

3. Which anatomic location for pressure injury is more prevalent in children than adults?
   A. Sacrum
   B. Heels
   C. Occiput
   D. Elbows

4. A novice nurse is assisting a patient's primary care nurse who is caring for the terminally ill patient in performing a brief/diaper change. At the conclusion of care, the assisting nurse reaches for the turning wedges and suggest repositioning the patient to a side-lying position. The patient's primary nurse states, "He is comfort care only; we aren't turning him anymore." What is the most appropriate response by the assisting nurse?
   A. Agree with the nurse and leave the patient in the supine position.
   B. Encourage the nurse to continue with routine repositioning.
   C. Suggest that the nurse discontinue all intravenous fluids (IVF) and medications as part of comfort care.
   D. Remove the wedges from the room to avoid further efforts to reposition.

5. The nurse is performing wound care on a patient with a deep wound. What action demonstrates understanding of safe wound packing practices?
   A. Utilize one continuous piece of packing material.
   B. Ensure all packing is tightly packed into the wound.
   C. Avoid packing material into the wound, placing the dressing over the outside of the wound.
   D. Ensure the previous dressing is fully dry before removing it from the wound.

6. The nurse is caring for a patient who was just placed on extracorporeal membrane oxygenation (ECMO) for respiratory failure and severe acute respiratory distress syndrome (ARDS). The most appropriate intervention for the patient would be:
   A. Waiting until the patient is hemodynamically stable to turn them
   B. Placing a foam donut under the patient's head
   C. Performing micro turns at least every 2 hours
   D. Full side-to-side turning every 4 hours

7. A patient's severe edema has led to their striae weeping serous fluid. Because of the patient's fragile skin, the nurse is worried about placing an adhesive dressing at the site. Which action is most appropriate?
   A. Place an absorbent underpad beneath patient to catch drainage.
   B. Apply an adhesive dressing and plan to remove with an adhesive removing wipe.
   C. Place dry gauze over striae and change as needed.
   D. Consult the wound care nurse to determine plan of action.

(See answers next page.)

1. B) Stage 2 pressure injury
A stage 2 pressure injury can either be seen as partial-thickness loss of skin OR a serous fluid-filled blister. A blood-filled blister would be a deep tissue pressure injury.

2. C) Remove any adhesive dressings from the site
Adhesive may be tightly applied and cause strangulation of tissue in the presence of swelling. Adhesive dressings should be removed, along with the IV, to decrease the risk of compartment syndrome. The nurse would notify the physician but not immediately. The nurse would want to assess the site first. A new IV may need to be placed later. Elevating the extremity would also be done later to decrease edema.

3. C) Occiput
Children have much larger heads relative to their body size than adults, especially during infancy and early childhood. Children are more prone to occipital pressure injuries than adults and should have occipital offloading measures implemented when critically ill.

4. B) Encourage the nurse to continue with routine repositioning.
Repositioning at the end of life can promote comfort for patients. Development of pressure injuries at the end of life can cause pain and distress for patients and their families.

5. A) Utilize one continuous piece of packing material.
This is important to prevent retained wound packing. If all of the packing is tight into the wound without a 2 to 3 cm tail, it may be difficult to remove packing from the wound, and wound should not be packed tightly so the wound has space to contract as it heals. Deep wounds require packing to obliterate dead space, so dressings should not just be placed on the outside of the wound. Finally, wet-to-dry dressings are not recommended as they will remove both dead and healthy tissue from the wound bed.

6. C) Performing micro turns at least every 2 hours
Waiting until the patient is hemodynamically stable could be hours to days before the patient can be fully turned. The patient is a low-flow state during this time and especially vulnerable to pressure injury development. Using donut-like devices places the skin in the middle of the donut at risk of strangulation of blood flow and should be avoided. Completing full side-to-side turning should be done when the patient's hemodynamic status will tolerate it and should be done with the assistance of an ECMO specialist every 2 hours. Micro turns will help redistribute blood flow and prevent pressure injuries, as even small shifts in position are helpful. This should be done as frequently as the patient will tolerate, at least every 2 hours.

7. D) Consult the wound care nurse to determine plan of action.
An underpad would not protect skin from moisture weeping. An adhesive dressing, even when removed with adhesive remover, may still cause skin injury on fragile skin. Dry gauze can become adhered to open skin and cause nonselective debridement. An expert should help to create a care plan that promotes skin health.

8. A patient develops blistering following a peripheral intravenous (PIV) infiltration. Which of the following interventions is most appropriate?
   A. Use a 24-gauge sterile needle to aspirate the fluid from the blister.
   B. Cover with a transparent adhesive dressing.
   C. Assist the physician to unroof the blister using a scalpel.
   D. Promote maintenance of blister integrity by protecting the site with a nonadhesive dressing.

9. Which laboratory values should the nurse monitor to assess for development a pressure injury?
   A. High sodium
   B. Increased white blood cells (WBCs)
   C. Decreased platelet count
   D. None of the above

10. A patient experienced a severe intravenous (IV) infiltrate in the previous shift. What findings in assessing the affected limb are most concerning?
    A. Deep purple discoloration
    B. Fluid-filled blisters
    C. Delayed capillary refill
    D. Edema

(See answers next page.)

8. **D) Promote maintenance of blister integrity by protecting the site with a nonadhesive dressing.**

Fluid-filled blisters provide protection to the underlying dermis. Drainage is not recommended unless the blister compromises the surrounding anatomy. Use of an adhesive dressing is contraindicated.

9. **D) None of the above**

Physical assessment is the key in monitoring for development of a pressure injury. Monitoring lab values is important for overall patient status, but nothing replaces the importance of a thorough head-to-toe skin assessment at least once per shift, on admission, and with a change in patient status.

10. **C) Delayed capillary refill**

The other findings could be present following an infiltration, but delayed capillary refill would be the most concerning, as it could indicate compromised perfusion and be a symptom of compartment syndrome. This is a medical emergency, and the physician should be notified immediately.

REFERENCES

Cohen, K. E., Scanlon, M. C., Bemanian, A., & Schindler, C. A. (2017). Pediatric skin failure. *American Journal of Critical Care, 26*(4), 320–328. https://doi.org/10.4037/ajcc2017806

Garcia, M. G., Dutton, H., Samual, K. & Marusich, J. (2021). Purposeful hourly rounding to decrease peripheral intravenous infiltrations and extravasations in pediatrics. *Journal of Pediatric Nursing, 61*, 59–66. https://doi.org.ezp1.villanova.edu/10.1016/j.pedn.2021.03.009

Gorski, L. A., Hadaway, L., Hagle, M. E., Broadhurst, D., Clare, S., Kleidon, T., Meyer, B. M., Nickel, B., Rowley, S., Sharpe, E., & Alexander, M. (2021). Infusion therapy standards of practice, 8th edition. *Journal of Infusion Nursing, 44*(1S Suppl 1), S1–S224. https://doi.org/10.1097/NAN.0000000000000396

Jacob, A., Grabher, D., & Newberry, D. M. (2020). The phenomenon of Trombley-Brennan terminal tissue injury in a neonate: A case study. *Advances in Neonatal Care, 20*(2), 171–175. https://doi.org/10.1097/ANC.0000000000000688

McNichol, L. L., Ratliff, C. R., & Yates, S. S. (2022). *Wound management core curriculum* (2nd ed.) Wolters Kluwer.

National Pressure Injury Advisory Panel (NPIAP). (2016). *NPIAP Pressure Injury Stages*. https://cdn.ymaws.com/npiap.com/resource/resmgr/online_store/npiap_pressure_injury_stages.pdf

Papantonio, C. T., Wallop, J. M., Kolodner, K. B. (1994). Sacral ulcers following cardiac surgery: Incidence and risks. *Advances in Wound Care, 7*(2), 24–36.

Reitz, M., & Schindler, C. A. (2016). Pediatric Kennedy terminal ulcer. *Journal of Pediatric Healthcare, 30*(3), 274–278. https://doi.org/10.1016/j.pedhc.2015.12.001

Tofani, B. F., Rineair, S. A., Gosdin, C. H., Pilcher, P. M., McGee, S., Varadarajan, K. R., & Schoettker, P. J. (2012). Quality improvement project to reduce infiltration and extravasation events in a pediatric hospital. *Journal of Pediatric Nursing, 27*(6), 682–689. https://doi-org.ezp1.villanova.edu/10.1016/j.pedn.2012.01.005

Musculoskeletal Disorders

Maryann Godshall

Musculoskeletal injuries affect the bone, muscles, ligaments, nerves, or tendons that cause pain. In children, this can vary from a strain, sprain, or fracture to a complex injury that impairs circulation. Fractures can require initial immobilization, traction, casting, and surgical repair. The complexities of musculoskeletal injuries can result in damage to soft tissue, ligaments, and tendons. Complications to these injuries, such as impaired circulation, can cause permanent serious conditions that the nurse needs to continually monitor for.

▶ MUSCULOSKELETAL SURGERY

Musculoskeletal surgery is a wide variety of surgical procedures aimed at restoring, improving, or optimizing disorders, conditions, injuries, or congenital conditions to ensure stability and support to the musculoskeletal system. The goal is to restore or optimize function. The nurse's responsibility is to explain, support, and monitor for complications after surgery. Much of the nursing assessment will assess perfusion, monitor for complications, and prevent infection.

▶ FRACTURES

Most fractures are simple and nondisplaced, which require the application of a cast. Fractures can also be closed (do not break the skin) or open (break the skin). Risk for infection increases with open fractures. Doing neurovascular (NV) checks to monitor edema, skin color and temperature, and perfusion is a critical assessment. Excessive swelling can lead to compartment syndrome (CS; Hockenberry et al., 2019).

Bladder rupture can occur very commonly with pelvic fractures. There can also be damage to the femoral artery or vein. This can be life threatening as damage can occur to any surrounding organ.

Clinical Pearl

In any situation when a cervical injury/fracture is suspected with a possible spinal cord injury, the child should be calmed and told not to move until c-spine immobilization is achieved with an appropriately sized cervical collar. At an accident scene, one person should be in charge of holding the cervical spine in a neutral position and maintaining alignment. For infants and small children in car seats, they should not be removed from their car seats unless medically necessary. This care should be continued in the hospital setting.

▶ COMPARTMENT SYNDROME

CS occurs when pressure within the myofascial compartment exceeds capillary perfusion pressure, so blood flow is compromised to the distal tissues. This is usually because of edema but can also be a result of bleeding into the muscle compartment, intravenous infiltration, burn or crush injuries, or external forces. CS is most often seen in the lower extremities compared to the upper extremities. It can also occur in the abdominal compartment (see Chapter 6). If this condition is left untreated it can lead to muscle necrosis, contraction, infections, or permanent nerve damage. Acute CS is a surgical emergency. Pressure is released by performing a fasciotomy, which will restore blood flow to the distal extremity.

SIGNS AND SYMPTOMS

Signs and symptoms of CS can be subtle and should be picked up by the nurse when doing NV checks. Swelling, tenderness, tingling or paresthesia, lack of feeling, pain, decrease or absent pulse (late sign), prolonged capillary refill, temperature change, or color change of the extremity are commonly seen. Pain particularly not relieved by analgesia or if increase analgesia is needed is another sign of possible CS.

NURSING IMPLICATIONS AND TREATMENT

Nursing implications and treatment include keeping the affected extremity level with the heart, removing all dressing and splints that may be causing external pressure, performing frequent NV checks, anticipating a fasciotomy, and monitoring for the development of rhabdomyolysis. The use of a noninvasive regional saturations (NIRS) monitor can be helpful in measuring oxygen saturation to the affected area to help measure for CS. Pressures of 10 to 25 mmHg with signs and symptoms present or and intracompartmental pressure of 30 mmHg indicate the need for a fasciotomy. Early fasciotomy can save an extremity and should be performed ideally within 4 hours of symptoms. A sterile occlusive dressing or wet to dry dressing wrapped in a gauze bandage is or negative pressure wound therapy (NPWT) is usually applied after fasciotomy. The skin may be closed after the swelling has subsided and perfusion is restored to the extremity. It is important to watch for signs of infection during this time. A severe complication of compartment syndrome is amputation if circulation is not restored to the extremity in a timely fashion.

> ### Clinical Pearl
>
> *Assessing for CS includes monitoring for the 5 Ps of ischemia (pain, pallor, pulselessness, paresthesia, and paralysis).*

▶ FAT EMBOLI SYNDROME

Fat emboli is the presence of fat particles in the blood. Fat emboli syndrome (FES) is the systemic manifestation of fat emboli within microcirculation. FES is a common complication of orthopedic trauma. It is often associated with long bone fractures such as the femur and pelvic fractures. Signs and symptoms may be nonspecific. They can occur 12 to 72 hours after injury. FES develops as a result of fat droplets that leak from fractured bone marrow and are transferred to the lung or brain. Most commonly the lungs. The fat droplets are broken down into free fatty acids that are toxic to the pulmonary vasculature. Fat emboli alter pulmonary hemodynamics and pulmonary vascular permeability. The lungs become very edematous and hemorrhagic. This can lead to the development of acute respiratory distress syndrome (ARDS). Adolescents are usually those affected in the pediatric age groups (Rothburg & Makarevitch, 2019).

SIGNS AND SYMPTOMS

The triad of most common symptoms includes pulmonary distress, neurological symptoms, and petechial rash (Maitre, 2006).

NURSING IMPLICATIONS AND TREATMENT

ASSESSMENT
Assessment is made through major and minor criteria (see Table 9.1).

Table 9.1 Fat Emboli Syndrome Criteria

Major Criteria	Minor Criteria
Hypoxia (<60 mmHg O_2), dyspnea, tachypnea Confusion, altered level of consciousness, or seizures Petechial rash	Fever (>39 °C) Tachycardia (>120 bpm) Retinal changes (petechiae) Anuria or oliguria Anemia (Hgb ↓ 20%) Thrombocytopenia (platelets ↓ 50%) Elevated ESR (>71 mm/hr) Fat microglobulinemia

ESR, erythrocyte sedimentation rate.
Source: Slota, M. C. (Ed.). (2019). *AACN core curriculum for pediatric high acuity, progressive, and critical care nursing* (3rd ed.). Springer Publishing Company.

TREATMENT AND MANAGEMENT

Nursing implications are primarily vigilant monitoring for the previously stated signs and symptoms. There is no specific treatment for FES and treatment is supportive. Patients with pulmonary involvement tend to have resolution within 2 weeks while those with cerebral FES gradually resolve within a few weeks to months. It is important to know that when caring for a patient with FES, the extremity should be moved as little as possible before surgical fixation/repair. With supportive hospital care, most people recover.

▶ RHABDOMYOLYSIS

Rhabdomyolysis is a breakdown of skeletal muscle that releases a damaging protein (myoglobin) into the blood. Myoglobin can damage the kidneys. When the myocytes are injured, they cause a massive influx of calcium ions, sodium ions, and fluid into the cytoplasm. Myoglobin, potassium, phosphate, and lactate are released into the intracellular fluid space. This can result in electrolyte disturbances: hypocalcemia, hyperkalemia, hyperphosphatemia, and metabolic acidosis. Uric acid levels may also be elevated. This condition may be fatal or cause permanent disability.

Some predisposing conditions that are cause rhabdomyolysis are (Torres et al., 2015):
- crush injuries
- electrical shock
- severe burns
- extended immobility
- snake venom
- substance abuse (drug and alcohol)
- toxins
- infections
- prolonged seizures
- muscle ischemia
- electrolyte and metabolic disorders
- temperature induced states like neuroleptic malignant syndrome (NMS)

SIGNS AND SYMPTOMS

Clinical signs of rhabdomyolysis include:
- dark reddish-brown "tea-colored" urine
- serum creatinine kinase (CK) equals or exceeds a level five times normal
- Myoglobin is present in the urine (reason for the dark reddish-brown color).
- Urine dipstick is (+) for blood but no red blood cells (RBCs) are present.
- elevated blood urea nitrogen (BUN) and creatinine (indicate acute renal insufficiency)
- electrolyte imbalances

Symptoms include muscle pain (myalgia), weakness, decreased urine output, and cramping. Tachycardia, nausea and vomiting, and fever are present. Neurological symptoms like confusion and agitation may be present. Renal manifestations include decreased urine output, possible renal failure, and electrolyte abnormalities. Disseminated intravascular coagulation (DIC) may also occur (Torres et al., 2015).

NURSING IMPLICATIONS AND TREATMENT

Nursing implications and treatment include first recognizing the disorder and preventing further damage. Then replace electrolyte abnormalities and administer intravenous (IV) crystalloids. Prevention of subsequent kidney dysfunction is paramount through aggressive administration of IV fluids. IV fluids increase renal blood flow and decrease the concentration of nephrotoxic pigments. Monitor lab values, and if hyperkalemia is present, treat with sodium bicarbonate, insulin, and glucose. Administering phosphate binding antacids, antacids, and diuretics has been studied, but their roles have not firmly established (Mondor, 2021). Strict intake and output (I&O) is required, and urine output should be at least 1 mL/kg/hr to ensure adequate flushing of the kidneys (Torres et al., 2015).

CASE STUDY

A 4-year-old was hit by a car. He suffered a large subdural hematoma that was evacuated. He has a ventriculostomy in place. He also had a left tibia/fibula fracture that is loosely splinted with an elastic bandage (ACE™ wrap). It has not yet been repaired. He has multiple abrasions to his face, arms, and lower extremities. He was intubated and sedated. He is in the pediatric ICU (PICU) with q1h neurologic and neurovascular (NV) checks. The nurse gets a report, and the off-going nurse said his NV checks were fine all night. Upon the nurse's first assessment, she notes the patient's left foot is cold and pale. The nurse cannot obtain a pedal pulse. His capillary refill is 3 to 4 seconds.

1. In regard to the neurovascular (NV) checks, if the nurse cannot feel a pedal pulse, what should the next course of action be?
   A. Document unable to obtain a pulse.
   B. Check for a pulse using a Doppler.
   C. Put a sock on the foot to warm it.
   D. Prepare to go to the operating room (OR).

The nurse is unable to get a pulse utilizing that course of action.

2. What would the next course of action be?
   A. Notify the attending physician.
   B. Document the findings and continue to observe.
   C. Prepare for a bedside fasciotomy.
   D. Call for a lower extremity scan.

The physician shares that they are busy with another trauma patient. The physician will be up to the unit as soon as they can. The pediatric ICU (PICU) intensivist is aware and starts rounds. Hourly neurovascular (NV) checks remain unchanged. No pulse to the left foot. Two hours later the trauma attending has not yet arrived in the unit. The nurse grows increasingly concerned. The intensivist then calls the trauma attending and gets the same response. They are busy and will come to the PICU later. Two hours later, the trauma attending arrives in the unit. They assess the foot and note indeed there is no pulse. Compartment syndrome (CS) or a deep vein thrombosis (DVT) is suspected. An order is received to go to interventional radiology (IR) for an angiography. No clot is detected.

3. What would be the expected treatment for this child now?
   A. Q1h neurovascular (NV) checks
   B. Medicinal leeches
   C. Fasciotomy
   D. An MRI

(See answers next page.)

ANSWERS TO CASE STUDY QUESTIONS

1. B) Check for a pulse using a Doppler.

If a pulse cannot be manually palpated, the nurse should try to obtain a Doppler pulse. Documenting the inability to obtain a pulse is insufficient. Warming the foot is not appropriate in this instance, and preparing for the OR is not indicated.

2. A) Notify the attending physician.

If the nurse cannot get a Doppler pulse, the physician needs to be notified. Simply documenting and observing are not sufficient. Bedside fasciotomy or lower extremity scans are not indicated at this time.

3. C) Fasciotomy

An angiogram may be performed to rule out a DVT. Once that is ruled out, it is most likely CS. The treatment for CS is a fasciotomy either at bedside or in the OR. Continued observation or an MRI without intervention is not adequate. Medicinal leeches are not indicated.

KNOWLEDGE CHECK: CHAPTER 9

1. A 12-year-old patient is admitted to the pediatric ICU (PICU) after a motor vehicle crash (MVC) where the patient was ejected from the car is diagnosed with compartment syndrome (CS). What would the expected treatment be?
   A. Intravenous (IV) steroids
   B. Immediately apply ice and elevate
   C. Fasciotomy
   D. Frequent neurovascular checks

2. Which is the priority action to reduce the risk of a fat emboli in a patient with a closed humerus fracture?
   A. Administer low dose heparin.
   B. Regular use of compression socks.
   C. Limiting fractured limb movement.
   D. Apply a sequential compression device.

3. When caring for a child with rib fractures, what should the nurse include in their care?
   A. Reinforce that they must refrain from contact sports until medically cleared.
   B. Inform the child to wrap a binder around the chest to decrease pain.
   C. Teach the child to cough and deep breath once a shift.
   D. Tell the child to notify the doctor if pain occurs when taking a deep breath.

4. Following x-rays for an injured wrist, the adolescent is informed his wrist is badly sprained. What statement made by the adolescent indicates that teaching was effective?
   A. "I will use a compression bandage continuously."
   B. "I will apply a heat pad to decrease muscle spasms."
   C. "I will use a pillow to keep my arm above my heart."
   D. "I will exercise every day to keep my joint mobile."

5. A 10-year-old child arrives in the ED with ankle swelling and pain after twisting their ankle playing soccer. Which order should the nurse implement first?
   A. Administer naproxen sodium (Naprosyn) 300 mg PO.
   B. Wrap the ankle and apply an ice pack.
   C. Give acetaminophen with codeine (Tylenol #3).
   D. Take the patient to the radiology department for an x-ray.

6. The nurse is caring for a patient with bilateral femur fractures. Twelve hours after admission the patient becomes confused, tachypneic, and tachycardic. The nurse should assess the patient for:
   A. Compartment syndrome (CS)
   B. Fat emboli syndrome (FES)
   C. Deep vein thrombosis (DVT)
   D. Cardiogenic shock

7. After being admitted and treated for compartment syndrome (CS), the patient reports feeling paresthesia. Which of the following symptoms would describe paresthesia?
   A. Numbness and tingling
   B. Pain and discomfort
   C. Change in range of motion
   D. Fever and chills

(See answers next page.)

1. C) Fasciotomy

A fasciotomy is recommended to relieve the pressure. This pressure is usually caused by edema. Applying ice, elevating, and administering IV steroids would not be beneficial treatment for this condition at this time. Neurovascular (NV) checks are important and part of care, but once the child is diagnosed with CS, more frequent checks would not change this diagnosis. An emergent surgical intervention like a fasciotomy must be performed.

2. C) Limiting fractured limb movement

To reduce the risk of dislodging fat emboli, the nurse should limit the movement of the fractured extremity until surgery can be performed. This may require splinting. Heparin would not have any effect on the formation of a fat embolism. Compression socks or a sequential compression device is useful in preventing a venous embolus but not fat emboli. Aggressive fluid resuscitation and maintenance of an adequate circulatory volume have also shown to be protective. Monitoring of pulse oximetry would be beneficial to determine if there is respiratory insufficiency.

3. A) Reinforce that they must refrain from contact sports until medically cleared.

The child cannot participate in any contact sports until the ribs have healed and medically cleared by the doctor. Wrapping a binder around the chest needs to be done with caution as it might restrict respirations. The child should cough and deep breath more frequently than once a shift. The doctor doesn't need to be notified if pain occurs as pain will be expected with rib fractures. Pain medication should be taken to help relieve discomfort.

4. C) "I will use a pillow to keep my arm above my heart."

For comfort and to decrease edema, the injured wrist should be kept elevated above the heart. A compression bandage should not be used as this might increase pain and decrease perfusion to the hand. Heat should not be used initially; an ice pack would better decrease edema. To promote healing the joint should not be moved every day. It needs adequate time to heal and recover.

5. B) Wrap the ankle and apply an ice pack.

The first thing that should be done is to wrap the ankle to support the joint, elevate it, and apply an ice pack to decrease edema formation. The child will likely get an x-ray, but that would not be the first thing to be done. A nurse could provide comfort with ice an immobilization while they wait for the x-ray. Pain medication would need to be ordered by the physician. A mild analgesia like acetaminophen or ibuprofen would be offered first. If pain relief does not occur a medication with an opioid like codeine might be ordered. Naproxen sodium, a nonsteroidal anti-inflammatory, would not be a first choice of pain reliever.

6. B) Fat emboli syndrome (FES)

Even though FES is rare, it most often presents as a pulmonary complication. Cerebral manifestations of FES include confusion to encephalopathy. The patient may also have headaches, seizures, or become comatose. An MRI would be the imaging of choice to determine this. CS and a DVT do not present with neurological changes. A thrombus could travel to the brain and cause a stroke. Cardiogenic shock would present with tachypnea and tachycardia and may experience a loss of consciousness. Given the mechanism of injury and no mention of heart trauma, this would not be a likely manifestation.

7. A) Numbness and tingling

Paresthesia would be exhibited by numbness and tingling of the extremity involved. This is a result of edema formation and decreased blood flow to the extremity. Pain and discomfort might be exhibited but are not a sign of paresthesia. A change in the range of motion might also be noted but as a result of edema verses paresthesia. Fever and chills would be a sign of infection.

8. Compartment syndrome (CS) can develop from which of the following situations?
   A. Immobilization of the extremity
   B. A surgical intervention
   C. Internal or external pressure
   D. Increased blood flow to the extremity

9. Which of the following is an indication of early compartment syndrome (CS)?
   A. Skin pallor
   B. Heat
   C. Edema
   D. Paresthesia

10. When a patient has rhabdomyolysis, a large amount of _____ is released into the bloodstream, which causes a discoloration of urine.
    A. Myoglobin
    B. Albumin
    C. Calcium
    D. Dopamine

(See answers next page.)

8. C) Internal and external pressure

CS can occur from internal pressure (bleeding or edema) or external pressure (cast, brace, or dressing too tight). Immobilization would not cause CS. A surgical intervention like a fasciotomy might be required to treat CS. A surgical procedure to repair the fracture is the cause of CS. With CS there is decreased blood flow to the extremity not increased blood flow.

9. D) Paresthesia

Paresthesia is the first indication of CS. Pain, heat, or edema are also signs but usually occur later. Skin pallor is not an indication of CS but could be an indication of decreased perfusion to the extremity.

10. A) Myoglobin

With rhabdomyolysis, muscle tissue breakdown occurs and a protein (myoglobin) is released into the blood stream. It is eliminated by the kidneys and is why the urine appears reddish-brown, like tea, in color. Myoglobin can damage the kidneys. Albumin is a protein made by the liver but not released when a muscle is damaged or with rhabdomyolysis. Calcium is an electrolyte and is not released into the bloodstream with rhabdomyolysis. Initially hypocalcemia might be present. Dopamine is a neurotransmitter and is not released in large quantities into the blood stream with rhabdomyolysis.

REFERENCES

Hockenberry, M., Wilson, D., & Rodgers, C. (2019). *Wong's nursing care of infants and children* (11th ed.). Elsevier.

Maitre, S. (2006). Causes, clinical manifestations, and treatment of fat embolism. *Virtual Mentor, 8*(9), 590–592. https://doi.org/10.1001/virtualmentor.2006.8.9.cprl1-0609

Mondor, E. (2021). Trauma. In L. D. Urden, K. M. Stacy, & M. E. Lough (Eds.), *Priorities in critical care nursing* (8th ed., p. 453). Elsevier.

Rothburg, D. L., & Makarevitch, C. A. (2019). Fat embolism and fat emboli syndrome. *Journal of the American Academy of Orthopaedic Surgeons, 27*(8), e346–e355. https://doi.org/10.5435/JAAOS-D-17-00571

Torres, P. A., Helmstetter, J. A., Kaye, A. M., & Kaye, A. D. (2015). Rhabdomyolysis: Pathogenesis, diagnosis, and treatment. *The Oshner Journal, 15*(1), 58–69.

Neurological Systems Review

Megan Snyder, Kenya Agarwal, and Kristen Lourie

The brain is divided into the cerebrum, diencephalon, brainstem, reticular formation, and the cerebellum. There are four lobes that make up the cerebral hemispheres:

- fontal lobe (thinking, memory, behavior, and movement)
- parietal lobe (comprehension of language, spatial relations, and touch)
- temporal lobe (reception and interpretation of auditory information, emotions, and visceral responses, and retention of recent memory)
- occipital lobe (reception and interpretation of visual information; Vernon-Levett, 2019)

The corpus callosum transfers information between the cerebral hemispheres. The brainstem helps regulate breathing, heart rate, temperature, and swallowing. The cerebellum helps with balance and coordination.

The spinal cord is an extension of the medulla oblongata, and the spinal column contain 33 vertebrae (7 cervical, 12 thoracic, 5 lumbar, 5 fused sacral, and 4 fused coccygeal segments; Vernon-Levett, 2019). The subarachnoid space surrounds the spinal cord and contains cerebrospinal fluid (CSF) and blood vessels. The inner core of the spinal cord is comprised of both gray and white matter. The gray matter consists of the anterior horn (motor neurons to skeletal muscles), posterior horn (sensory input to the spinal cord), and gray commissure (preganglionic fibers of the autonomic nervous system; Vernon-Levett, 2019). White matter surrounds the gray matter and is subdivided into pathways that serve different functions.

- The ascending tract is more sensory related and transmits pain, temperature, touch, and pressure.
- The descending tract is the motor pathway and plays a major role in voluntary motor movement (Vernon-Levett, 2019).

It takes several years for the nervous system to fully mature and develop after birth. Therefore, neurologic assessments of pediatric patients must be tailored to reflect the patient's development. Assessing level of consciousness requires that the clinician assess content (mental function) and arousal (e.g., wakefulness; Vernon-Levett, 2019).

The Glasgow Coma Scale (GCS) is the most widely used scoring system to assess neurologic status using verbal response, eye opening, and motor response (Table 10.1). Total scores range from 3 (least responsive) to 15 (normal). The scale can be applied without modification to children >5 years old but as younger children and infants are unable to verbalize orientation or follow commands, must be modified in these groups. A GCS is used to determine the severity of a traumatic brain injury (TBI).

It is classified as:

- mild TBI (GCS 13–15)
- moderate (GCS 9–12)
- severe (GCS 3–8; Denke et al., 2020)

Table 10.1 Glasgow Coma Scale

Behavior	Score	Infant Response	Score	Child/Adolescent/Adult
Eye opening	4	Spontaneously	4	Spontaneously
	3	To speech	3	To speech
	2	To pain	2	To pain
	1	None	1	None
Verbal	5	Coos and babbles	5	Oriented
	4	Irritable cry	4	Confused
	3	Cries to pain	3	Inappropriate words
	2	Moans to pain	2	Incomprehensible sounds
	1	None	1	None

(continued)

Table 10.1 Glasgow Coma Scale (*continued*)

Behavior	Score	Infant Response	Score	Child/Adolescent/Adult
Motor	6 5 4 3 2 1	Normal spontaneous movement Withdraws to touch Withdraws to pain Abnormal flexion (decorticate posturing) Abnormal extension (decerebrate posturing) None	6 5 4 3 2 1	Obeys commands Localizes pain Withdraws to pain Abnormal flexion (decorticate posturing) Abnormal extension (decerebrate posturing) None

Source: Vernon-Levett, P. (2019). Neurologic system. In M. C. Slota (Ed.), *AACN core curriculum for pediatric high acuity, progressive, and critical care nursing* (3rd ed., pp. 349–444). Springer Publishing Company.

▶ CONGENITAL NEUROLOGICAL ABNORMALITIES

Neural tube defects (NTD) are among the most common of the congenital anomalies and affect the brain and spinal cord (Centers for Disease Control and Prevention [CDC], 2020a). The most common NTDs are spina bifida, encephalocele, and anencephaly (CDC, 2020a). NTDs occur in approximately 3,000 births per year in the United States.

SIGNS AND SYMPTOMS

- **Spina bifida cystica:** An incomplete fusion of one or more vertebral laminae, which results in external protrusion of spinal tissue, is present.
- **Myelomeningocele:** A sac outside of the back area, containing meninges, CSF, and neural tissue, is present.
- **Meningocele:** A sac outside the back area, containing only meninges and CSF, is present.
- **Encephalocele:** A sac-like protrusion of the brain and membranes is visible through an opening in the skull (CDC, 2020a).
- **Anencephaly:** Serious NTD in which parts of the brain and skull never develop. Almost all newborns with this condition die shortly after birth. Although the etiology is not completely understood, a deficiency in maternal folic acid is highly associated with NTDs (Vernon-Levett, 2019).

PATHOPHYSIOLOGY

NTD abnormalities occur in early embryonic development, by the 17th to 30th day. In spina bifida, the most common part of the spine affected is the lower thoracic lumbar and sacral areas. In some cases, patients with NTDs develop tethered cord syndrome where the spinal cord becomes fastened to a fixed structure, such as bone (Vernon-Levett, 2019).

NURSING IMPLICATIONS AND TREATMENT

ASSESSMENT

- history
  - Open NTDs are immediately apparent at birth.
  - Closed NTDs have more varied presentation. For example, spina bifida occulta can go undetected since there is no protrusion of neural structures. Newborns may have a history of asymmetry of legs or foot or hammering of the toes. Other symptoms may include weakness or sensory loss in one leg, and bowel and/or bladder dysfunction.
- **Physical exam:** A full neurological exam of the newborn is needed to identify and document structural and functional abnormalities.

LABS AND DIAGNOSTICS

- neuroimaging
  - **spinal radiographs:** help identify the exact location of the deformity
  - **CT scan:** provides direct visualization of the defect and anatomy
  - **MRI:** most desired study for NTDs as it shows intracranial and intraspinal defects

- **ultrasound:** used during pregnancy to help identify a NTD
- Clinical course depends on the type of NTD. Infants with open NTDs have varied clinical courses depending on the location of the defect, and mild closed NTDs may go undetected or have subtle neurological findings (Vernon-Levett, 2019). Infants with anencephaly usually die shortly after birth.

TREATMENT AND MANAGEMENT

- Screen patient for latex allergies.
- **Preventative care:** The American Academy of Pediatrics (AAP) supports the U.S. Public Health Service recommendation that all women of childbearing age consume 400 mcg of folic acid to prevent NTDs (1999). Several studies, including two randomized controlled trials, have shown that 50% or more of NTDs are prevented if women consume folic acid supplementation before and during the early weeks of pregnancy (Czeizel & Dudás, 1992; MRC, 1991).
- **Direct care:** There is no cure for NTDs. The priority is prevention of infection, and it is now recommended to immediately close the sac with a goal to preserve neural tissue (Vernon-Levett, 2019).
- Supportive care includes:
  - Management depends on the type of NTD and severity of the neurologic impairment.
  - Newborns with myelomeningocele present challenges during vaginal delivery related to protecting the sac from trauma and during neonatal resuscitation if positive pressure ventilation is needed.
  - For open NTDs, the sac is protected with a sterile saline moist dressing prior to surgical repair. Keep the patient in a prone or side-lying position before and immediately postoperatively to promote wound healing.
  - Routine postoperative care includes keeping the wound free from bodily fluids (such as urine and feces).
  - Provide a latex free environment for children with NTDs to help decrease risk of developing latex allergy.
  - Bowel and bladder elimination may be altered for many patients so intermittent catheterization and bowel regimens may be needed (Vernon-Levett, 2019).
- Outcomes depend on the etiology, severity of defect, and associated environmental factors. In general, children with spina bifida lead active lives but may require assistive devices for ambulation or activities of daily living (Vernon-Levett, 2019).

▶ HYDROCEPHALUS

Hydrocephalus is a disorder of CSF physiology that results in abnormal expansion of the cerebral ventricles due to inadequate passage of CSF from its point of production within the ventricular system to its point of absorption into the systemic circulation (Rekate, 2009). Hydrocephalus is a pathological condition, and not a disease (Vernon-Levett, 2019). Prevalence of hydrocephalus diagnosed at birth occurs in about 78 out of 100,000 births in developed countries and 106 out of 100,000 births in low- and middle-income countries (Viscidi et al., 2021).

SIGNS AND SYMPTOMS

Hydrocephalus can begin in utero or develop later in life (Rekate & Blitz, 2016). An infant and toddler's brain is unique from that of the older child or adult in several important ways: the brain continues to grow during the third trimester and for the first few years of life, the blood vessels in this region do not yet have a blood-brain barrier and remain very fragile, and the skull is expandable since the sutures have not fused (Rekate & Blitz, 2016).

PATHOPHYSIOLOGY

- **Based on the CSF theory:** CSF is actively produced, passively reabsorbed, and flow is unidirectional from the secretion site to the reabsorption site. Based on this theory, any obstruction that blocks flow or reabsorption leads to hydrocephalus (Vernon-Levett, 2019).
- The cause of hydrocephalus varies, but it is commonly described as *communicating* or *noncommunicating*. There are several congenital abnormalities that affect drainage of CSF including Arnold-Chiari type II, aqueductal stenosis, and congenital arachnoid cyst. A patient can also acquire

a disorder/disease process (e.g., neoplasm, hemorrhage, infection, trauma) that can impact CSF production or absorption. Overproduction of CSF can also be a cause of hydrocephalus such as CSF-producing tumors, but this is rare (Wright et al., 2016).

▦ **Communicating hydrocephalus:** normal anatomic flow of CSF in the ventricular system, but improper CSF absorption

▦ **Noncommunicating hydrocephalus, also known as obstructive hydrocephalus:** impeded flow of CSF within the ventricular system (Wright et al., 2016)

NURSING IMPLICATIONS AND TREATMENT

ASSESSMENT

▦ history
  ● can be diagnosed in utero
  ● Clinical presentation depends on age of the patient, cause of hydrocephalus, location of the obstruction, duration of the condition, and speed of onset (Vernon-Levett, 2019).
▦ **Physical exam:** Complete a physical exam and assess for presenting symptoms in Table 10.2.

Table 10.2 Presenting Symptoms of Hydrocephaly

Infant	Older Child
Increased head circumference	Headaches
Tense or bulging fontanelle	Unsteady gait with history of falling
Apnea and bradycardia	Declining school performance
Splaying of the cranial sutures	Visual complaints (blurred or spotty)
Irritability	Papilledema
High pitched cry	Decreasing level of consciousness
Lethargy	Behavioral changes (irritable, lethargic)
Vomiting and weight loss/poor feeding	Nausea and vomiting
Seizures*	Seizures
Sunset sign*	
Macewen's sign	

*Indicate late-stage signs of hydrocephalus
Source: Wright, Z., Larrew, T. W., & Eskandari, R. (2016). Pediatric hydrocephalus: Current state of diagnosis and treatment. *Pediatrics in Review, 37*(11), 478–490. https://doi.org/10.1542/pir.2015-0134

LABS AND DIAGNOSTICS

▦ While imaging is needed to diagnose hydrocephalus, the practice of serial head circumference in long-term management of hydrocephalus is very useful (Wright et al., 2016).
▦ No lab test is diagnostic of hydrocephalus.
▦ diagnostic tests
  ● neuroimaging
    ❑ **Ultrasound** is most useful up to 12 to 18 months of age while the anterior fontanelle is open to help evaluate progression of hydrocephalus as well as intraventricular hemorrhages. However, ultrasound images may not be sufficient for diagnosis (Wright et al., 2016).
    ❑ **MRI and CT** are both used to diagnose hydrocephalus. MRI produces greater anatomic detail and is more helpful in identifying the underlying cause of hydrocephalus (Wright et al., 2016).
  ● Clinical course depends on the cause of hydrocephalus. Acute presentation of hydrocephalus is a clinical emergency, especially after the cranial sutures have closed. Neurosurgical consultation is required for this patient population (Wright et al., 2016).

TREATMENT AND MANAGEMENT

▦ **Preventative care:** If the condition that caused the hydrocephalus is treatable, temporary CSF diversion may control or stop CSF accumulation. The risk of acquired hydrocephalus can be minimized by keeping vaccines current to help prevent meningitis, and by preventing TBI by wearing appropriate safety equipment (i.e., seatbelts, helmets; Vernon-Levett, 2019).

- **Direct care:** Rapid onset hydrocephalus requires emergent procedures to relieve pressure and potentially divert CSF. A lumbar puncture can be used in cases of hydrocephalus that are anticipated to resolve spontaneously, such as an intraventricular hemorrhage, and imaging may be warranted prior to the procedure. Many patients will require a **ventricular shunt** to divert CSF from the intraventricular space into an alternate space for reabsorption. The peritoneal space of the abdomen is the most common distal location for the shunt and is called a ventriculoperitoneal (VP) shunt. A ventriculoatrial (VA) shunt is when the distal end of the shunt is placed in the right atrium of the heart.
- **Supportive care:** Includes performance of serial neurologic assessments, monitoring for signs of increased intracranial pressure, and monitoring fluid and electrolyte status. Provide routine postoperative care by providing pain control, incisional care, and monitoring for signs and symptoms of an infection.
  - Outcomes vary depending on the cause of the hydrocephalus, and children with well controlled hydrocephalus have demonstrated better outcomes (Vernon-Levett, 2019).
- Postsurgical intervention risks include:
  - strokes
  - hemorrhage
  - catheter misplacement resulting in a nonfunctioning shunt and need for further surgical interventions (Wright et al., 2016)
  - Shunts can malfunction in a few different ways, including mechanical hardware failure, infection, or overdrainage. A patient with a shunt malfunction will have a similar presentation to that of a patient with initial hydrocephalus, but the onset may be more rapid (Wright et al., 2016).

▶ STROKE

A stroke occurs when blood flow to the brain is disrupted or when blood vessels rupture (National Institute of Neurological Disorders and Stroke, 2021). Although information on strokes in the adult population is readily available, pediatric acute ischemic stroke is "less understood" (Sutherly & Malloy, 2020, p. 58).

Both symptoms and risk factors are variable. Pediatric strokes affect 1,000 pediatric patients per year in the United States with higher occurrences in neonates and premature infants (McKinney et al., 2018). Due to the prolonged timing of presentation following symptom development, most patients are not eligible for tissue plasminogen activator (tPA) administration (McKinney et al., 2018; Table 10.3).

Table 10.3 Stroke Types, Symptoms, Causes, and Treatment

Type	Symptoms	Cause	Treatment
Ischemic	Focal manifestations (such as weakness), speech or language changes, visual changes, headache, altered mental status Younger children more commonly present with altered mental status and seizures	Arteriopathies, cardiac disorders, thrombophilia, infection, trauma, and migraines Cerebral sinovenous thrombosis Sickle cell disease Moyamoya syndrome Medications (cocaine, amphetamines) Thrombus Embolus	Dissolve or remove blood clot, possible anticoagulation
Hemorrhagic	Refer to ischemic symptoms	Vascular malformations AVM Aneurysm Cavernous malformation Spontaneous hemorrhage into tumor Trauma	Supportive care Stop the bleeding if known bleeding disorder or abnormal labs Consider holding or reversing current anticoagulation therapy

(continued)

Table 10.3 Stroke Types, Symptoms, Causes, and Treatment (*continued*)

Type	Symptoms	Cause	Treatment
Neonatal	Differentiate between neonatal stroke and diffuse hypoxic-ischemic injury via neuroimaging	Majority are ischemic versus hemorrhagic; Combination of factors from the mother, fetus, and placenta	Maintain homeostasis and prevent seizures

AVM, arteriovenous malformations.

Sources: Bernson-Leung, M. E., & Rivkin, M. J. (2016). Stroke in neonates and children. *Pediatrics in Review, 37*(11), 463–477. https://doi.org/10.1542/pir.2016-0002; Ferriero, D. M., Fullerton, H. J., Bernard, T. J., Billinghurst, L., Daniels, S. R., DeBaun, M. R., deVeber, G., Ichord, R. N., Jordan, L. C., Massicotte, P., Meldau, J., Roach, E. S., Smith, E. R., & American Heart Association Stroke Council and Council on Cardiovascular and Stroke Nursing. (2019). Management of stroke in neonates and children: A scientific statement from the American Heart Association/American Stroke Association. *Stroke, 50*(3), e51–e96. https://doi.org/10.1161/STR.0000000000000183; Sutherly, L. J., & Malloy, R. (2020). Risk factors of pediatric stroke. *The Journal of Neuroscience Nursing: Journal of the American Association of Neuroscience Nurses, 52*(2), 58–60. https://doi.org/10.1097/JNN.0000000000000489

SIGNS AND SYMPTOMS

▨ Symptoms to assess for include mental status, symmetry of motor strength or weakness, facial symmetry, seizures, and headaches, aphasia, or visual disturbances (as developmentally able to convey).

▨ Pediatric symptoms may mirror other conditions such as seizure, failure to thrive, hemiparesis, or dysphagia (Ghofrani et al., 2018) as well as migraines, conversion disorder, and syncope (McKinney et al., 2018).

NURSING IMPLICATIONS AND TREATMENT

ASSESSMENT

▨ Regardless of stroke etiology, basic nursing assessment fundamentals include assessing and monitoring the patient's airway status, vital signs, and frequent neurologic exams. Symptoms may progress or change over time and early identification of these changes can lead to timely patient intervention and prevention of subsequent sequelae.

LABS AND DIAGNOSTICS

▨ **Diagnostic imaging:** Brain MRI is more sensitive than a CT scan (McKinney et al., 2018). However, in the immediate presentation, a CT scan may be obtained to assess for immediate causes.
  ● Additionally, a magnetic resonance angiography (MRA) of the head and neck should be obtained in any suspected stroke patient (McKinney et al., 2018).

▨ Labs to anticipate include serum chemistry, electrolytes, coagulation, and complete blood count (CBC; McKinney et al., 2018).

TREATMENT AND MANAGEMENT

▨ Treating risk factors is a primary focus. These may include hypertension, atrial fibrillation, and diabetes (National Institute of Neurological Disorders and Stroke, 2021) as well as sickle cell disease, trauma, sepsis, encephalitis, cardiac disorders, and other major infections (McKinney et al., 2018).

▨ Care is focused on prevention of further effects. Measures should include providing supplemental oxygenation, maintaining euvolemia, addressing hyperthermia, possible antithrombotic therapy, preventing hyperglycemia, and maintaining normal blood pressures (BP; McKinney et al., 2018). The head of the bed (HOB) is traditionally flat unless there are concerns for increased intracranial pressure (in which case the HOB would be elevated to >30°).

COMPLICATIONS

Complications of stroke include hemiplegia, paralysis, speech difficulties, and difficulty controlling emotions (National Institute of Neurological Disorders and Stroke, 2021).

▶ INTRACRANIAL HEMORRHAGE

Nontraumatic intracranial hemorrhage (ICH) is uncommon in pediatrics but is an important cause of death or lifelong injury (Lo et al., 2008).

SIGNS AND SYMPTOMS

▦ ICH refers to bleeding within the intracranial vault, inclusive of the brain parenchyma and surrounding meningeal spaces (Caceres & Goldstein, 2012). Several causes of hemorrhagic stroke in pediatrics include ICH and subarachnoid hemorrhage (Vernon-Levett, 2019). The primary etiology for hemorrhagic stroke is from intracranial vascular anomalies (e.g., aneurysm or arteriovenous malformations [AVMs]), although underlying disease or trauma can also cause an ICH (Vernon-Levett, 2019). Hematologic disorders, hypertension, and genetic vasculopathies are additional causes of ICH (Vernon-Levett, 2019).

PATHOPHYSIOLOGY

▦ **Arteriovenus malformations** can occur early in fetal development when the capillaries fail to develop. Blood supply to adjacent brain tissue is diminished or absent because arterial flow without capillaries doesn't allow diffusion of oxygen and glucose. Because of the malformation, increased blood flow through this vascular malformation is increased and the malformation continues to grow. Without capillaries and inherent resistance to blood flow, arterial blood empties directly into thin walled veins. The veins are at high risk to rupture leading to a hemorrhage.

▦ An **aneurysm** is a bulge in a blood vessel caused by a weakness in the blood vessel wall, and this usually occurs near a branch. A ruptured aneurysm is a critical event requiring emergent interventions. Patients develop acute symptoms with bleeding into the subarachnoid space. There is a risk of rebleeding after a post aneurysm clot dissolves, which occurs 7 to 10 days after rupture (Vernon-Levett, 2019).

NURSING IMPLICATIONS AND TREATMENT

ASSESSMENT

▦ Clinical presentation varies and depends on the child's age, cause, size, and location of the hemorrhage (Lanni et al., 2011; Table 10.4).

Table 10.4 Clinical Presentation of Intracranial Hemorrhage by Age

Newborn	Infants	Older Children
Focal seizures	Focal seizures	Seizures
Apnea	Apnea	Headache
Lethargy	Lethargy	Altered level of consciousness
	Poor feeding	Vomiting
	Respiratory distress	Focal signs based on location of hemorrhage

Source: Lanni, G., Catalucci, A., Conti, L., Di Sibio, A., Paonessa, A., & Gallucci, M. (2011). Pediatric stroke: Clinical findings and radiological approach. *Stroke Research and Treatment, 2011*. https://doi.org/10.4061/2011/172168

▦ **Physical exam:** All body systems are examined with a focus on neurologic function (Vernon-Levett, 2019).

▦ **Clinical course:** AVMs are present at birth, but the patient may not be symptomatic for years. In a multicenter review, Hofmeister et al. (2000) reported mean age at diagnosis was 31.2 years. Overall risk of hemorrhage from an untreated AVM in any age group is 2% to 4% annually (El-Ghanem et al., 2016). Aneurysms can be congenital or acquired, and the progression of the disease is dependent on many variables (Vernon-Levett, 2019).

LABS AND DIAGNOSTICS

Neuroimaging and lab testing is similar to acute ischemic stroke.

TREATMENT AND MANAGEMENT

▦ **Preventative care:** There is no known way to prevent the formation of an aneurysm or AVM. Treatment for a hemorrhagic stroke is supportive while also attempting to reduce risk of a rebleed (Vernon-Levett, 2019). If a vascular malformation has been identified prior to rupture, then the goal is to prevent a hemorrhage. Other preventive care instructions are focused on controlling BP, avoiding smoking, and avoiding stimulant drugs (Vernon-Levett, 2019).

▦ direct care
  ● **Hemorrhagic stroke:** Depending on size and location, surgery is controversial and individualized for the patient (Vernon-Levett, 2019).
  ● **Arteriovenous malformations:** Treatment depends on the size and location of the AVM, age of the patient, cerebral dominance, condition of patient, and characteristics of the feeder vessels. Total surgical resection is ideal, but certain vascular malformations are inoperable (Vernon-Levett, 2019). Gamma Knife radiosurgery and embolization are other options of treatment available in designated pediatric centers.
  ● **Aneurysm:** The most common surgical treatment option is occluding the aneurysm at its neck with clips. If the aneurysm ruptures, the goal is to prevent rebleeding and control cerebral vasospasm (Vernon-Levett, 2019). Other options include cardiovascular coiling and instilling a glue-like liquid delivered through a microcatheter.

▦ Supportive care is focused on optimizing respiratory function, controlling systemic hypertension, controlling increased intracranial pressure (ICP), and controlling seizures (Vernon-Levett, 2019).

Clinical Pearl

Normal ICP is 9 to 21 mmHg. Sustained ICP >20 mmHg for longer than 5 minutes is abnormal and requires immediate intervention.

▦ Outcomes for an intracranial hemorrhage depend on numerous factors including location of the hemorrhage, extent of bleeding, time between rupture and treatment, and baseline health of the patient (Vernon-Levett, 2019). Most patients will experience long-term neurologic, motor, and cognitive impairments (Greenham et al., 2016). Mortality from hemorrhagic strokes range from 6% to 54%, but mortality rates have been declining possibly related to improvements in clinical management (Greenham et al., 2016). Outcomes are best for vascular malformations when the risk of hemorrhage is minimized or if the malformation can be removed (Vernon-Levett, 2019).

▶ SPACE OCCUPYING LESIONS

Space occupying lesions include conditions that can occur in the brain and therefore impact the distribution of brain contents as relevant in the Monro-Kellie doctrine. These can include tumors (benign or malignant), cysts, bleeds, and AVMs.

The Monro-Kellie doctrine provides an overview of the components and distribution of brain contents within the fixed space of the skull. These include CSF (10%), blood (10%), and brain matter (80%). If one category is increased, another must decrease. As ICP increases, the brain is initially able to compensate by decreasing CSF production and minimizing or shunting blood flow. After this primary compensation, the brain is unable to regulate further.

Primary malignant central nervous system (CNS) tumors are the most common pediatric solid organ tumor and the second most common childhood cancer (Lau & Teo, 2020). They surpass the pediatric mortality rate of acute lymphoblastic leukemia (Lau & Teo, 2020). Oncologic complications are discussed in Chapter 5.

SIGNS AND SYMPTOMS

▦ "Cushing's triad" is a common phrase used to describe symptoms of increased ICP; however, this often occurs late.
▦ The triad includes an **irregular breathing pattern**, **hypertension**, and **bradycardia**.
▦ In the critical care environment, these symptoms may be masked by care interventions (such as intubation and ventilation) and should not be relied on as earlier indicators of increased ICP.

- The location of the tumor can influence presenting symptoms. Tumor locations include posterior fossa, brainstem, spinal cord, and supratentorial and central tumors (Lau & Teo, 2020). The most common location is the posterior fossa (Children's Hospital of Philadelphia [CHOP], 2022).
- The most common presenting symptom for CNS tumors is headache. These headaches are often worse in the morning, relived by vomiting, and not responsive to analgesics (such as acetaminophen). Other symptoms include nausea and vomiting particularly due to posterior fossa tumors (Lau & Teo, 2020), ataxia and gait disturbances, seizures, cranial nerve palsies, impaired vision, torticollis, papilledema, macrocephaly, endocrinopathies, developmental delay, and behavioral changes.

PATHOPHYSIOLOGY

- Varies depending on the primary agent
- CNS tumors may include gliomas, medulloblastomas, craniopharyngiomas, ependymoma, germ cell tumors, never sheath tumors, spinal cord tumors, tuberous sclerosis, meningiomas and others (Lau & Teo, 2020; Table 10.5).

Table 10.5 Common Pediatric Brain Tumors

Type of Brain Tumor	Presentation	Treatment
Gliomas	Most common type regardless of age	
Astrocytomas Malignant gliomas Ependymomas	Most common of gliomas	Surgery
	More aggressive than astrocytomas	Require surgery, radiation and chemotherapy
	Arises from cells lining the ventricles; slow growing	May reoccur
Mixed neuronal-glial tumors		
Ganglioglioma Subependymal glial cell tumor Pleomorphic xanthoastrocytoma	Childhood/early teens	Majority benign, treatment with surgery
	Common in tuberous sclerosis	Majority benign
	Teens/young adults	Majority benign
Embryonal tumors		
Atypical teratoid/rhabdoid tumor PNET	More common in ≤2 years old; often involve chromosome 22, typically in cerebellum or kidneys	At diagnosis, 1/3 have spread
	Most commonly in cerebellum (termed *medulloblastoma*)	Newer effective treatment

PNET, primitive neuroectodermal tumor.
Source: Children's Hospital of Philadelphia. (2022). *Pediatric brain tumors*. https://www.chop.edu/conditions-diseases/pediatric-brain-tumors

NURSING IMPLICATIONS AND TREATMENT

ASSESSMENT

- The patient's neurologic status should be monitored closely for signs of increased ICP. This presentation can vary depending on patient's age and location of the space occupying lesion.

LABS AND DIAGNOSTICS

- Diagnosis of a CNS tumor is performed via neuroimaging (CT or MRI) and histology studies (often via biopsy by a neurosurgeon). Based on these results, treatment may include surgical resection, chemotherapy, and/or radiation.

TREATMENT AND MANAGEMENT

- Treatment is determined based on the type of the space occupying lesion and may include surgery, radiation, chemotherapy, or targeted therapy medications.
- Cysts have many variations in care depending on location and internal contents.
- See previous section on ICHs for further details on management of bleeds and AVMs.

COMPLICATIONS

Complications of space occupying lesions include the risks discussed in other sections pertaining to ICH as well as specific risks depending on the primary causative agent.

▶ ACUTE SPINAL CORD INJURY

Spinal cord injurty (SCI) in pediatrics is rare compared to adults. Pediatric patients have anatomical differences from adults. Children's heads are often larger than their bodies, creating a higher center of gravity and therefore risk of injury. There are also more varied mechanisms of injury in pediatrics. These include motor vehicle crash (MVC), falls, and sports related injuries. Pediatric cervical SCI are rare and affect <1% of patients (Mandadi et al., 2022). Understanding SCI patterns and how they relate to mechanism, treatment, and outcome is especially important in pediatrics (Leonard et al., 2014).

There are two defined types of SCI: complete cord injury and incomplete cord injury.

- **Complete cord injury** is the complete loss of motor and sensory function as a result of nerve interruption below the level of injury (Vernon-Levett, 2019).
  - **Quadriplegia:** complete loss of leg function and complete loss or limited use of arms
  - **Paraplegia:** loss of leg function only
- **Incomplete cord injury** causes some loss of motor and sensory function, but there is usually some level of function spared below injury (Vernon-Levett, 2019). Incomplete cord injury can result in many different syndromes that are largely dependent on the location of injury.
- Younger children suffer more upper cervical spine injuries than adolescents and adults and are more often associated with higher morbidity and mortality rates (Leonard et al., 2014). Children also have a higher incidence of SCI without radiographic abnormality (SCIWORA; Vernon-Levett, 2019). Younger children with an immature spinal column have more elastic ligaments, where the spinal cord itself cannot sustain the same amount of stretch, resulting in injury. SCIWORA is as a result of a hyperextension injury.
  - Blunt trauma is by far the most common mechanism of injury, accounting for 95% of SCI, largely a result of MVCs (Copley et al., 2019). Falls are more commonly the cause of SCIs in those <8 years of age, and sports related injuries are more prevalent in those >8 years of age and adolescents (Copley et al., 2019). Nontraumatic causes of SCI, including tumors and herniated discs, occur across all age groups.

PATHOPHYSIOLOGY

- SCI involves a primary injury from direct impact and often results in secondary injury. Primary SCI includes the following cord injuries: concussion, contusion, transection, or hemorrhage. Laceration or damage to blood vessels surrounding the cord can also occur. Secondary injuries include edema and ischemia. The mechanism of secondary injury is often complex and not widely understood (Vernon-Levett, 2019).
- Spinal shock occurs in the autonomic nervous system (ANS), which produces venous pooling, sinus bradycardia, and hypotension. Spinal shock can last up to 7 days (Vernon-Levett, 2019).
- **Autonomic dysreflexia** is a rare but *life-threatening complication*. Patients with a high thoracic SCI or cervical spine injury are more susceptible to the disorder, and account for up to 90% of autonomic dysreflexia occurrences (Allen & Leslie, 2022). It is caused by stimulation of sensory nerves below level of injury usually T6 or above, usually bowel or bladder distention, or pressure to the skin. Profound sinus bradycardia and vasodilation occurs due to overstimulation of the vagus nerve. The peripheral nervous system (PNS) cannot receive signals due to cord injury. Common symptoms include:
  - severe headache
  - bradycardia
  - hypertension
  - facial flushing
  - pallor, clammy skin, and sweating can occur in lower extremities
  - anxiety or feeling of apprehension
  - sometimes blurry vision (Allen & Leslie, 2022)
- Temperature regulation is impaired with injury above T1 vertebrae (Vernon-Levett, 2019).

NURSING IMPLICATIONS AND TREATMENT

ASSESSMENT

- Patient history should focus on symptoms surrounding the injury to the vertebral column. Details surrounding any motor or sensory deficits are important. The physical exam often includes the following:
  - Depressed GCS <14 in children <3 years, altered mental status, focal neurologic deficits, neck and back pain, sensory and motor dysfunction/deficits
  - Pain is a common complaint.
  - The patient's clinical course depends on the type and location of injury.
  - Neurologic deficits often increase in immediate hours and plateau at 3 to 6 months post injury.
- **Assessments (Table 10.6):** Physical findings on clinical exam are predictive of SCI after suffering blunt trauma. These include altered mental status, neck pain, injury to torso, and focal neurologic deficits (Leonard et al., 2014). Cervical tenderness is the most common physical exam finding in pediatric patients with SCI (Baker et al., 1999). The degree of sensory and motor dysfunction is dependent on location of injury.

Table 10.6 Clinical Exams to Assess Motor Dysfunction

Exam	Location of Assessment	What to Assess	Scoring Tool
Sensory exam	Completed in all 28 dermatomes (right and left)	Light touch and pinprick sensation scored	Scale: 0 = absent 1 = altered 2 = normal
Motor exam	Muscle functions in 10 paired myotomes (C5–T1 and L2–S1)	Strength of each muscle function scored	Scale: 0 = total paralysis 1 = palpable or visible contraction 2 = full ROM without gravity 3 = full ROM against gravity 4 = full ROM against gravity and moderate resistance 5 = normal full ROM, full resistance

ROM, range of motion.
Source: Adapted from Slota, M. (Ed.). (2019). *AACN core curriculum for pediatric high acuity, progressive, and critical care nursing* (3rd ed.). Springer Publishing Company.

Clinical Pearl: Respiratory Assessment

Be alert for anxiety and hypoxia without signs of increased work of breathing. The patient may not be able to use accessory muscles to increase ventilation (Sweeney, 2020).

LABS AND DIAGNOSTICS

- Lab tests for patients suffering from SCI include routine blood work. This usually includes CBC with differential, basic metabolic panel, coagulation studies (prothrombin time/partial thromboplastin time [PTT]/fibrinogen), and serial glucose monitoring.
- Neuroimaging includes standard radiographic films, CT scans, and MRI. MRI is most helpful in evaluating soft tissue injuries (Vernon-Levett, 2019).

TREATMENT AND MANAGEMENT

- Nursing care includes protection and prevention of progression. Immobilization such as cervical collar/backboard or backboard is recommended as soon as possible.
- Direct care includes mostly surgical interventions. These include decompression (laminectomy or debridement), traction, fixation with spinal fusion, bone grafts, metal rods, or halo.
- The role of the critical care nurse during hospitalization should include the following:
  - serial neurologic exams

- prevention of bowel/bladder distension (which can result in life-threatening autonomic dysreflexia)
- oxygenation/ventilation support as needed
- maintaining adequate circulation (vasopressors, fluids)
- monitor for sinus bradycardia
- deep vein thrombosis (DVT) prophylaxis
- serial skin assessments
- thermoregulation
- Most current guidelines do not recommend high dose steroids as treatment for SCI (Leonard et al., 2014).

COMPLICATIONS

Prompt recognition and treatment of SCI is critical due to rarity and morbidity in children (Leonard et al., 2014). The level and extent of injury often predict recovery. High cervical injuries may cause immediate death (Vernon-Levett, 2019). Infants often have a higher rate of mortality.

Clinical Pearl

Autonomic dysreflexia is a life-threatening, sudden increase in BP that is the result of a stimulus below the level of a SCI, often in SCIs at T6 or above. Immediate intervention is needed.

It is usually triggered by constipated bowel, distended bladder (over-retention secondary to kinked or clogged Foley catheter or need for urinary catheterization), or painful stimulus to the skin (tight braces or clothing). Intervention to relieve these symptoms must be done at once. First, sit upright with legs dependent (lowered) and remove any restrictive clothing or bracing devices. Address constipation and bladder distention, if appropriate. If hypertension is not resolved after these interventions, an antihypertensive should be given to prevent severe hypertensive crisis. There is a significantly increased risk of stroke by 300% to 400%. The higher SCI, the more likely this can occur.

▶ NEUROGENIC SHOCK

- Neurogenic shock occurs when there is sudden loss of autonomic tone due to a SCI above T6 (Mack, 2013). Disruption of the sympathetic pathway allows the parasympathetic pathway to go unchecked. This causes decreased systemic vascular resistance and uncontrolled vasodilation. The resulting hypotension from neurogenic shock makes the patient more susceptible to secondary spinal cord ischemia. Neurogenic shock is a type of distributive shock. There is no single diagnostic test (Mack, 2013).
- **Etiology:** Patients with SCIs above T6 are more likely to develop neurogenic shock.

NURSING IMPLICATIONS AND TREATMENT

ASSESSMENT

Patients classically exhibit:
- hypotension as a result of vasodilation and relative hypovolemia
- wide pulse pressure
- relative bradycardia
- warm skin, normal pink in color in the periphery
- unstable core temperature and inability to sweat below the level of injury

Initially, the skin is often warm and flushed from the uncontrolled vasodilation. The patient may develop hypothermia due to the profound vasodilation and heat loss (Mack, 2013).

NURSING IMPLICATIONS AND TREATMENT

Initial management is focused on **hemodynamic stability**, with the first line of treatment being intravenous (IV) fluid resuscitation to treat the hypotension. If the patient is in fluid refractory shock, then the second line treatment is to start vasopressors. **Phenylephrine** is a commonly used agent as it is a pure alpha-1 agonist that causes peripheral vasoconstriction to help offset the loss of the sympathetic tone. **Atropine and glycopyrrolate** can be used to treat bradycardia (Mack, 2013). Immobilization of the cervical spinal cord is also important to prevent further SCI. Surgical interventions may be warranted. Overall prognosis depends on the extent of the SCI and response to treatment (Allen & Leslie, 2022).

▶ HEAD TRAUMA AND TRAUMATIC BRAIN INJURY

TBI is an alteration in brain function that is caused by external force (Silverberg et al., 2020). Depending on the mechanism of injury and timeliness of treatment this injury can be temporary or cause permanent neurologic damage. Falls, MVC, and sports related traumas are some of the most common causes of TBI in infants and young children. Protective devices such as helmets and car seats can minimize extent of injury.

SIGNS AND SYMPTOMS

- TBI consists of a primary injury, often resulting in secondary injuries.
- **Primary injury** occurs at the time of the impact or force. These include skull fractures, epidural and subdural hematomas, subarachnoid and intraventricular hemorrhage, and diffuse axonal injury (DAI; Kannon et al., 2014).
- **Secondary injuries** develop after the event and can include extradural hematoma, brain herniation, infarct, or diffuse cerebral swelling (Vernon-Levett, 2019). Secondary impact syndrome (referred to as diffuse cerebral swelling) occurs when a child suffers a second TBI before the first TBI has been completely resolved. Injury to the brain impairs the brain's ability to autoregulate cerebral blood flow and cerebral perfusion pressure. This can lead to massive brain edema, herniation, and death within minutes (Denke et al., 2022). This can also be as a result of a hypoxic brain injury. Secondary brain swelling occurs usually 48 to 72 hours after the initial traumatic insult.
- Exam findings are dependent on the classification based on the severity of injury (Tables 10.7 and 10.8).

Table 10.7 Common Primary Traumatic Brain Injuries and Presentation

Primary TBI	Presentation
Simple linear fracture	Symptomatic
Basilar fracture	Battle sign: postauricular hematoma and swelling Raccoon sign: periorbital blood collection Rhinorrhea: CSF leakage into middle ear cavity Hemotympanum: blood collection behind tympanic membrane Vertigo
Cerebral contusion	Depends on location of injury. Monitor for signs and symptoms of swelling and increased ICP
Concussion	Loss of consciousness. Variety of symptoms including headache, nausea, retrograde amnesia
Epidural hematoma	Symptoms vary. Infants may have bulging fontanelle and significant bleeding. Older children may have hemiparesis, hemiplegia, or unequal pupils
Subdural hematoma	Nonspecific, may include drowsiness, irritability, and lethargy. Infants should be assessed for retinal hemorrhage
DAI	Loss of consciousness, increased ICP, shock, hypoxia, and apnea usually resulting in a poor outcome

CSF, cerebrospinal fluid; DAI, diffuse axonal injury; ICP, intracranial pressure.
Source: Vernon-Levett, P. (2019). Neurologic system. In M. C. Slota (Ed.), *AACN core curriculum for pediatric high acuity, progressive, and critical care nursing* (3rd ed., pp. 349–444). Springer Publishing Company.

Table 10.8 Traumatic Brain Injury Severity Classifications

Criteria	Mild	Moderate	Severe
Imaging	Normal	Normal or abnormal	Normal or abnormal
Loss of consciousness	0–30 minutes	>30 minutes and <24 hours	>24 hours
Alteration in consciousness	Up to 24 hours	>24 hour (severity based on other criteria)	>24 hour (severity based on other criteria)

(continued)

Table 10.8 Traumatic Brain Injury Severity Classifications (*continued*)

Criteria	Mild	Moderate	Severe
Posttraumatic amnesia	0–1 day	>1 day and <7 days	>7 days
GCS (best score in last 24 hours)	13–15	9–12	<9

GCS, Glasgow Coma Score.

Source: O'Neil, M. E., Carlson, K., Storzbach, D., Brenner, L., Freeman, M., Quiñones, A., Motu'apuaka, M., Ensley, M., & Kansagara, D. (2013, January). *Complications of mild traumatic brain injury in veterans and military personnel: A systematic review.* Department of Veterans Affairs (U.S.). https://www.ncbi.nlm.nih.gov/books/NBK189784/

- Most head traumas are considered "mild" TBIs (mTBI) and are managed largely outside the hospital (Silverberg et al., 2020). An mTBI involves loss of consciousness for <30 minutes and has a <24hr period of posttraumatic amnesia (Mild Traumatic Brain Injury Committee, 1993). A concussion is a type of mTBI with an absence of intracranial abnormalities (Silverberg et al., 2020).

PATHOPHYSIOLOGY

- The pathophysiology of TBI is largely dependent on the mechanism, location, and severity of injury. Care is directed at monitoring and addressing changes in ICP.
- Intensive monitoring of intracranial compliance and cerebral autoregulation should be considered (Laws et al., 2022)

NURSING IMPLICATIONS AND TREATMENT

ASSESSMENT

It is important to note if a change in mental status occurred directly following the trauma. This can present as observed unresponsiveness, memory gaps or inability to follow commands (Silverberg et al., 2020). The critical care nurse should complete thorough and frequent neurologic assessments (minimum every hour). These should include GCS, pupillary assessments, motor strength, cough, and gag. More specific physical exams can be helpful depending on the type and severity of the injury.

Clinical Pearl

Consider any alteration in mental status to be a result of decreased cerebral perfusion until proven otherwise.

Postconcussive symptoms include:
- headache
- nausea
- dizziness
- fatigue
- irritability
- sensitivity to light
- forgetfulness

LABS AND DIAGNOSTICS

- Routine bloodwork, including basic metabolic profile (BMP) and CBC, should be completed.
- skull and cervical spine x-rays
- **CT is the gold standard** to rule out intracranial hemorrhage within 72 hours of injury.
- **MRI** can be useful for follow up or when CT is not consistent with clinical presentation.

TREATMENT AND MANAGEMENT

- Early clinical management is prudent.
- Immediate C-spine immobilization should be considered with either C-collar or spinal board.
- Management targets neuroprotective strategies to address the causes of secondary injuries such as cerebral edema and ischemia (Laws et al., 2022). The overall goal is to maintain adequate cerebral

perfusion pressure (CPP) by managing ICP levels and perfusion, specifically mean arterial pressure (MAP). Current pediatric guidelines recommend:

- **maintaining ICPs <20**
- Pediatric patients post-TBI should maintain a minimum CPP of 40, with a threshold of between 40 and 50 mmHg (children 0–11 years old) while adolescents (>12 years old) should be 50 to 60 mmHg (Woods et al., 2022).
  - ❏ Vasopressors may be needed to achieve appropriate CPP depending on severity of ICP values. Risk must be evaluated regarding hypertension and stroke if administered vasopressors for CPP considerations.

Clinical Pearl

CPP is the difference between MAP and ICP. It is calculated by the MAP minus the ICP (CPP = MAP – ICP).

- Critical care nursing interventions should aim at maintaining low ICPs. These strategies include:
  - keeping the head of the bed at 30°
  - keeping the patient's head midline to promote CSF drainage
  - minimizing noxious stimulation (cluster care, reduce noise levels, and dim lights)
  - administering sedation medications as needed (such as prior to noxious stimuli which could raise ICPs)
- Some medical interventions that the nurse should anticipate include:
  - temperature management
  - pain/sedation medications
  - 3% hypertonic saline
  - Mannitol may also be considered to reduce ICP levels; however, it has some adverse side effects that should be considered. These include acute renal failure, pulmonary edema, rebound cerebral edema, and arterial hypotension which can cause a decrease in CPP due to its diuretic action (Schwimmbeck et al., 2021).
  - Both 3% hypertonic saline and mannitol are effective medications at reducing ICP levels in TBI patients; however, 3% has a more sustained effect as it can be given as a continuous infusion so it can effectively increase CPP (Shi et al., 2020).
  - Brain tissue partial pressure of oxygen ($P_{bt}O_2$) is measured by a fiberoptic sensor surgically placed in the brain parenchyma. $P_{bt}O_2$ is a measurement of oxygenation of brain tissue. Treatment should be aimed at addressing oxygen delivery to the brain and increasing CPP when $P_{bt}O_2$ is low (Laws et al., 2022). $P_{bt}O_2$ <5 mmHg for prolonged period is associated with poor outcomes in pediatric TBI (Laws et al., 2022).
    - ❏ Other neuromonitoring modalities include pupillometry, near-infrared spectroscopy (NIRS) and transcranial Doppler (TCD).
    - ❏ Some surgical considerations include externalized ventricular drainage system and complete or hemi craniectomy.

COMPLICATIONS

- Increased ICP is a common complication after TBI (Lovett et al., 2019).
- Additional complications may include cerebral salt wasting, diabetes insipidus, or syndrome of inappropriate anti-diuretic hormone. Refer to Chapter 4 for more details on these complications.
- Neurologic exams are often confounded and limited due to acuity and use of pharmacologic agents aimed at maintaining ICP levels.

Clinical Pearl

In a patient with a TBI as the brain swells, pressure can only move downward. The patient may herniate their brain contents into the brain stem. The signs of Cushing's Triad are:

1. *Increased systolic BP or widening pulse pressure*
2. *Bradycardia*
3. *Decreased respirations or apnea*

▶ CESSATION OF NEUROLOGIC FUNCTION (BRAIN DEATH)

There are many elements of care to consider for patients who may be experiencing cessation of neurologic function (also known as brain death and death by neurologic criteria; Mathur & Ashwal, 2015). Most states have adopted guidelines to clarify brain death for infants, children, and adults but there are variations in implementation of the pediatric death by neurologic criteria guidelines (Francoeur et al., 2021).

The Uniform Determination of Death Act (UDDA) states that for death to occur, one of two conditions must exist:

- irreversible cessation of breathing or circulation
- irreversible cessation of the whole-brain function (i.e., cortical and brainstem; Vernon-Levitt, 2019)

Cessation of neurologic function is defined as irreversible cessation of all functions of the entire brain, including the brainstem (National Conference of Commissioners on Uniform State Laws, 1981). As of 2022, the UDDA is being revised (Lewis, 2022). Not all states have universally agreed on one test or the other or both. This is an ongoing discussion in 2023.

PATHOPHYSIOLOGY

- Cessation of neurologic function may occur because of infections, TBI, intracranial lesions, hypoxic-ischemic brain injury, vascular events, poisoning, and metabolic disorders (Mathur & Ashwal, 2015).
- The patient's age and presenting condition are primary factors in determining evolution of steps and possibility of recovery. Additionally, there must be absence of confounding factors. Care should target:
  - normothermia
  - BP within normal age ranges
  - lack of metabolic disturbances
  - toxicology screening (including doses of prescribed sedatives)
  - allowing adequate liver and kidney clearance of medications
  - ensuring lack of neuromuscular blockage
  - neuroimaging to rule out other causes (Mathur & Ashwal, 2015)
- Following exclusion of confounding factors and other causes, an examination can occur.

NURSING IMPLICATION AND TREATMENT

Note that the physical examination has many components to capture cessation of neurologic function.

ASSESSMENT

- Examinations to determine cessation of neurologic function include the following elements:
  - lack of function of the entire brain
  - loss of all brainstem reflexes (nonreactive pupils, absence of oculocephalic reflex [dolls eyes], and oculovestibular (cold calorics) reflex; absence of a cough and gag reflex
  - Apnea test
  - flaccid tone and absence of spontaneous or included movements or response to painful stimuli (Mathur & Ashwal, 2015)
  - Two exams, including apnea testing, separated by an observational period, must be performed to determine cessation of neurologic function (Vernon-Levitt, 2019). The first exam demonstrates the patient meets criteria and the second exam confirms it (Mathur & Ashwal, 2015). The time frame for patient observation between exams varies by age: the exams are completed 24 hours apart for patients 37 weeks to 30 days and 12 hours apart for patients >30 days to 18 years of age (Mathur & Ashwal, 2015). Recommendations include having two different attendings physicians perform the examinations and that the attendings not be involved in the patient's clinical care (Mathur & Ashwal, 2015). Please note that all states do not require two separate tests. Some states only require one.

LABS AND DIAGNOSTICS

Ancillary studies (EEG and radionuclide cerebral blood flow) may be performed but can yield results that indicate the presence of cerebral blood flow that may not be evident in clinical exams. Providers and families should be educated on this risk. Flow studies do not replace the neurologic examination but may shorten duration between the two examinations (Mathur & Ashwal, 2015). Therefore, these exams are not required to declare cessation of neurological function.

TREATMENT AND MANAGEMENT

Following confirmation of cessation of neurologic function, the family should be informed of the patient's death in clear and definitive language. Clinicians should refer to the patient in past tense. This will help the caregivers to understand that the patient is no longer alive. Institutions that participate in organ procurement partnerships should follow institutional guidelines.

COMPLICATIONS

- As the critical care nurse, the support of caregivers throughout the process of evaluating for cessation of neurologic function is important to consider. This can be a challenging concept for families to understand and consistency across all team members is vital. It is important to reassess the caregivers' understanding of information and have discussions around support needs as appropriate. Engagement of social work, spiritual support, and child life therapists is recommended.

▶ DELIRIUM

Delirium is a common and often unrecognized complication of critical illness. Delirium is a relatively new concept in pediatric critical care (Kalvas & Harrison, 2020), and therefore, best practices for detection and treatment are still being established.

PATHOPHYSIOLOGY

Pathophysiology for delirium is multifactorial and is dependent on the etiology. Assistive mnemonics such as "I WATCH DEATH" (Ozga et al., 2020) may be used to identify causes of delirium:
- I: Infection
- W: Withdrawal: HIV, sepsis, pneumonia
- A: Acute metabolic: alcohol, barbiturate, sedative-hypnotic
- T: Trauma: acidosis, alkalosis, electrolyte disturbances, hepatic failure, renal failure
- C: CNS pathology: closed-head injury, heat stroke, postoperative, severe burns
- H: Hypoxia: abscess, hemorrhage, hydrocephalus, subdural hematoma, infection, seizures, stroke, tumors, metastases, vasculitis, encephalitis, meningitis, syphilis
- D: Deficiencies: anemia, carbon monoxide poisoning, hypotension, pulmonary or cardiac failure
- E: Endocrinopathies: vitamin B_{12}, folate, niacin, thiamine
- A: Acute vascular: hyper/hypoadrenocorticism, hyper/hypoglycemia, myxedema, hyperparathyroidism
- T: Toxins or drugs: hypertensive encephalopathy, stroke, arrhythmia, shock
- H: Heavy metals: prescription drugs, illicit drugs, pesticides, solvents

NURSING IMPLICATIONS AND TREATMENT

ASSESSMENT

- includes clinical manifestations
- Delirium presents "as a disturbance in attention and awareness accompanied by a change in cognition (e.g., disorientation, perceptual disturbance) [that] develops over a short period of time with symptoms fluctuating throughout the day" (American Psychiatric Association, 2013).

LABS AND DIAGNOSTICS

- Delirium can exist in hypoactive, hyperactive, or a mixed presentation and therefore assessment of delirium in pediatric patients can be challenging. A validated delirium tool should be used to assist in assessment. These include the Pediatric and Preschool Confusion Assessment Method for the ICU (pCAM-ICU and psCAM-ICU), the Sophia Observational withdrawal Symptom Scale—Pediatric Delirium (SOS-PD), and the Cornell Assessment of Pediatric Delirium (CAPD; Kalvas & Harrison, 2020).

TREATMENT AND MANAGEMENT

▨ Treatment of delirium in pediatric patients is aimed at a reduction of benzodiazepines and environmental modification although further studies are needed (Kalvas & Harrison, 2020).
- ● Environmental modifications may include:
    - ❑ keeping lights turned on and window blinds open during daytime hours
    - ❑ dimming the lights to incorporate nap times (as age appropriate)
    - ❑ maintaining the lights off as much as possible during nighttime hours
    - ❑ verbalizing care to patients even if they are unable to participate
    - ❑ reorientating patient as often as/when possible
    - ❑ clustering care to minimize disruptions in rest periods

COMPLICATIONS

▨ Delirium is associated with "increased ICU and hospital length of stay, ICU costs, and mortality" (Kalvas & Harrison, 2020, p. 13).
▨ Mechanical ventilation is associated with delirium, but more research is needed to identify the relationship (Kalvas & Harrison, 2020). Pharmacological management of delirium is lacking evidence for efficacy and safety (Kalvas & Harrison, 2020).

◗ NEUROLOGIC INFECTIOUS DISEASE

Neurologic infectious diseases in pediatrics can result in alterations in brain function and include encephalitis and meningitis.

▶ MENINGITIS

PATHOPHYSIOLOGY

▨ **Meningitis** "is an infection of the meninges, the membranes that surround the brain and spinal cord" (National Institute of Neurological Disorders and Stroke, 2022a).
▨ Causes can be bacterial, viral, or noninfectious (such as medications, autoimmune or auto-inflammatory diseases, and neoplasms; Swanson, 2015).
▨ The incidence of meningitis varies based on cause (including bacterial, viral, and others).
▨ **Acute bacterial meningitis**
- ● For children >1 month of age, *Streptococcus pneumoniae* is the most common cause (Swanson, 2015), as well as *Neisseria meningitidis* (Weinberg, 2022). Prior to the utilization of vaccines, *Haemophilus influenzae type b* was the most common cause of meningitis (Weinberg, 2022).
- ● Children <2 months of age have the highest incidence of bacterial meningitis predominantly caused by *Group B Streptococcus* and *Escherichia coli* (Swanson, 2015).
▨ **Viral (aseptic) meningitis**
- ● Meningitis with a negative bacterial culture (without pre-administration of antibiotics) is referred to as aseptic meningitis. Viral causes are most common and therefore the phrase viral meningitis and aseptic meningitis are at times used interchangeably (Di Pentima, 2021).
    - ❑ Symptoms of viral meningitis are often less severe than in bacterial meningitis.
    - ❑ The patient should be treated for bacterial meningitis and care should not be delayed while awaiting test results.

NURSING IMPLICATIONS AND TREATMENT

ASSESSMENT

Meningitis and encephalitis have similar symptoms such as:
▨ fever
▨ seizure
▨ headache
▨ weakness
▨ pyramidal signs
▨ agitation
▨ decreased consciousness (Fraley et al., 2021)

Meningitis may also present with:
- photophobia
- stiff neck
- nausea
- vomiting
- back pain (Swanson, 2015)

In addition to assessing for the symptoms, thorough neurological assessments should be performed. This includes assessment of fontanelles as appropriate. Close cardiopulmonary monitoring should also be implemented. The critical care nurse should anticipate escalation of care needs based on the patient's clinical presentation and progression of symptoms. Meningitis can progress quickly. Fever can last up to 6 days after the start of appropriate therapy (Swanson, 2015).

LABS AND DIAGNOSTICS

The critical care nurse should anticipate the following CSF studies:
- lumbar puncture (following radiographic imaging if warranted)
- opening pressure
- cell count (white blood cell with differential, red blood cell count)
- protein
- glucose
- gram stain and bacterial cultures
- herpes simplex virus polymerase chain reaction (HSV-PCR)
- enterovirus PCR
- complete metabolic panel
- blood cultures (Fraley et al., 2021)
- Video EEG may be warranted if there is concern for/or actual seizure activity
- When the patient is stable, other radiographic imaging can be considered such as a brain MRI

Clinical Pearl

	Bacterial Meningitis	Viral Meningitis
WBCs	Increased—neutrophils	Slightly increased—lymphocytes
Protein (10–30)	Increased	Normal to slightly increased
Glucose (40–80)	Decreased	Normal
Gram stain/culture	Positive	Negative
Color	Cloudy	Clear

Note: Remember bacteria need "food" to eat so they chew up glucose (count will be low) and spit out protein (count will be high). WBCs, white blood cells.

TREATMENT AND MANAGEMENT

- While ruling out causes (such as viruses, fungi, and parasites; Swanson, 2015), treatment with an antibacterial agent has also shown improved outcomes (Fraley et al., 2021).
- Respiratory isolation (Droplet) precautions should be maintained until the patient has received 24 hours of intravenous (IV) antibiotic therapy.
- The use of dexamethasone to reduce hearing loss in non-*Haemophilus influenzae* type B (Hib) meningitis is controversial (Swanson, 2015). The literature is inconclusive, and concerns exist around potentially decreasing efficacy of antibiotics (Swanson, 2015). As such, if dexamethasone is given, recommendations are to administer dexamethasone before or concurrently with first dose of antibiotic (Swanson, 2015).
- Supportive care is important including volume status, BP management, electrolytes, and cerebral perfusion.
- Supporting and encouraging families to vaccinate their children is an important element of care.
- Most children with viral meningitis recover fully.

COMPLICATIONS

In children with bacterial meningitis, 20% of cases lead to long-term effects of "nervous system problems, deafness, seizures, paralysis of the arms or legs, and learning difficulties" (AAP, 2021).

▶ ENCEPHALITIS

PATHOPHYSIOLOGY

- **Encephalitis** is inflammation of the brain itself (National Institute of Neurological Disorders and Stroke, 2022a). It is neurologic dysfunction accompanied by inflammation of the brain parenchyma (Tunkel, et al., 2008) without an identifying cause that also includes two or more findings:
  - fever
  - seizures or other focal neurologic disorders
  - cerebrospinal fluid pleocytosis
  - abnormal neuroimaging and electroencephalographic findings (Venkatesan et al., 2013)
- Infectious encephalitis is believed to be due to the spread of a systemic infection via the blood into the CSF (Bale, 2015).
- The incidence of encephalitis is unclear due to various causes and variable definitions (Fraley et al., 2021).
  - Prior to the widespread use of vaccines, the following were the top etiologies of infectious encephalitis: measles, mumps, varicella, and polio (Fraley et al., 2021). Additional causes include enteroviruses, West Nile Virus, La Crosse Virus, Zika Virus, and autoimmune encephalitis (Fraley et al., 2021).

Clinical Pearl

West Nile and Zika Viruses spread by mosquitos. This can range from asymptomatic to severe. Signs and symptoms include fever, malaise, lymphadenopathy, and difficulty concentration, which could develop into encephalitis and meningitis.

- **Encephalopathy** is a diagnosis determined when other causes are not able to be identified. Encephalopathy entails brain dysfunction of an unknown cause without inflammation of brain parenchyma (Fraley et al., 2021). It can occur in metabolic disturbances, hypoxia, ischemia, intoxication, medications, organ dysfunction, or even systemic infection (Tunkel et al., 2008). Long-term treatment for encephalopathy is aimed at supportive care.

NURSING IMPLICATIONS AND TREATMENT

ASSESSMENT

Meningitis and encephalitis have similar symptoms such as:
- fever
- seizure
- headache
- weakness or pyramidal signs
- agitation
- decreased consciousness (Fraley et al., 2021)

LABS AND DIAGNOSTICS

See labs and diagnostics for meningitis (the same).

TREATMENT AND MANAGEMENT

- While ruling out causes (such as viruses, fungi, and parasites; Swanson, 2015), treatment with an antibacterial agent has also shown improved outcomes (Fraley et al., 2021).
- The most severe form of encephalitis is caused by herpes simplex virus (HSV); treating early with acyclovir can improve the patient's prognosis (Fraley et al., 2021).
- Respiratory isolation (Droplet) precautions should be maintained until the patient has received 24 hours of IV antibiotic therapy.
- Supportive care is important including volume status, BP management, electrolytes, and cerebral perfusion.
- Supporting and encouraging families to vaccinate their children is an important element of care.
- Encephalitis outcomes vary widely, but more than 40% of patients do not return to their previous level of neurologic function (Khandaker et al., 2016).

▶ SEIZURE DISORDERS

Seizures in pediatrics can present with a variety of symptoms and frequency. They can originate from the brain focally, generally, or unknown.

SIGNS AND SYMPTOMS

The motor component of a seizure disorder can include the following movements:
- epileptic spasms
- **atonic:** slumping to ground, loss of motor tone
- **clonic:** rhythmic jerking
- **tonic:** clonic
- **myoclonic:** brief motor movements
- **tonic:** sustained extension/flexion
- hyperkinetic
- myoclonic-atonic
- myoclonic-tonic-clonic (Fine & Wirrell, 2020)

Nonmotor presentations can include absence onset, behavior or cognitive changes, and others.

PATHOPHYSIOLOGY

- Seizures are caused by abnormal electrical discharge from cortical neurons.
- Risk factors include: "positive family history, high temperature, mental disability, delayed discharge from NICU or premature birth, mother's alcohol abuse, and smoking in pregnancy" (Minardi et al., 2019, p. 3).
- Causes of recurrent seizures (formerly called epilepsy), defined as "two or more unprovoked seizures" (World Health Organization, 2022) are grouped as "genetic, structural, metabolic, immune, infectious and unknown" (Fine & Wirrell, 2020, p. 326).
  - Of note, most patients who present with febrile seizures do not develop recurrent seizures (Annegers et al., 1979).
    - ❏ Febrile seizure criteria: age 6 months through 5 years, temp ≥38 °C, and absence of CNS infection (AAP Subcommittee on Febrile Seizures, 2011).
    - ❏ A simple febrile seizure is "a primary generalized seizure that lasts for <15 minutes and did not recur within 24 hours" (AAP Subcommittee on Febrile Seizures, 2011, p. 390).
    - ❏ Patients should be evaluated for fever source with considerations for meningitis risk and considering patient's immunization status.
- **Status epilepticus** is defined as a *seizure lasting >5 minutes in duration* or *resumption of seizure activity without complete resolution to neurologic baseline after a previous seizure*. The most common causes for status epilepticus in the pediatric population are: "fever, infection of the CNS, hyponatremia, accidental ingestion of toxic agents, abnormalities of the CNS, genetic and metabolic disorders (phenylketonuria, hypocalcemia, hypoglycemia, and hypomagnesemia)" (Minardi et al., 2019, p. 3).

NURSING IMPLICATIONS AND TREATMENT

ASSESSMENT

- It is important to ensure the patient's safety during these events including airway assessment, vital sign monitoring, and treatment of any identifiable causes. Do not place any objects in the mouth to prevent biting of tongue, as this can lead to harm for the patient and increases risk of aspiration. Seizure pads can help prevent injury within the bed due to uncontrolled body movements.
- During the seizure, it is important to note the start of the seizure for duration, vital signs and any changes, movement of the patient (including symmetry vs. asymmetry), and any other features (such as audible noises).
- Movement that cannot be stopped by placing a hand over the extremity is likely to be seizure activity. Clonus can be stopped when the provider applies pressure to the extremity.
- A postictal phase may follow a seizure. During this time, the patient may present as confused, tired, and have difficulties with language and focal weakness (Fine & Wirrell, 2020).

LABS AND DIAGNOSTICS

▣ It is important to rule out potential causes of seizures. These may include electrolyte disturbances (Fine & Wirrell, 2020), meningitis, encephalitis, cerebral abscess (Haspolat et al., 2002), hypoglycemia, neoformations, head injury, hemorrhages, and/or cerebral infarcts (Minardi et al., 2019).

▣ If concern for other causes, a head CT should be obtained.

▣ Video EEG can be helpful for seizure identification, monitoring, and treatment determination.

TREATMENT AND MANAGEMENT

▣ There is increased risk of patient harm the longer a seizure lasts due to potential to irreversibly damage neural cells (Minardi et al., 2019).

▣ Nursing management of seizures should focus on maintaining the airway, providing ventilatory support as needed, ensuring circulation, and checking serum glucose.

▣ Prompt administration of seizure medication is a high nursing priority. Seizures are managed in a stepwise progression.

● The initial medication recommendation is benzodiazepines (Glauser et al., 2016; Minardi et al., 2019). Consider IV benzodiazepines as the first-line choice. Monitor for sleepiness, respiratory compromise, and hypotension (Table 10.9). If seizure persists, treat with additional anti-seizure medications.

Table 10.9 Common Initial Seizure Medications for Status Epilepticus

Medication	Dosage	Considerations
Lorazepam (Ativan)	IV or IM: 0.1 mg/kg (max 4 mg/dose)	Dilute prior to IV administration with equal volume of D5W, NSS, or sterile water for injection. Give via slow IV push. May also be administered IM
Diazepam (Valium)	IV (preferred): 0.15–0.2 mg/kg (max 10 mg/dose) Rectal gel: 2–5 years: 0.5 mg/kg 6–11 years: 0.3 g/kg 12 years: 0.2 mg/kg	Administer undiluted IV or IM
Midazolam (Versed)	IV or IM: 0.2 mg/kg (max 10 mg/dose) Intranasal: 0.2 mg/kg (max 10 mg/dose)	May be administered as a continuous infusion (0.05–2 mg/kg/hr) for refractory seizures. Administer intranasal with mucosal atomizer or needleless syringe. Give half the dose in each nostril, max 1 mL per nostril
Additional Seizure Medications		
Phenobarbital (Luminal)	IV: 15–20 mg/kg (max 1,000 mg/dose)	First-line treatment in neonates. May be administered as a continuous infusion for refractory seizures. Monitor for hypotension, bradycardia, sleepiness, and respiratory depression. Be prepared to provide respiratory support
Phenytoin (Dilantin)	IV: 20 mg/kg loading dose (max 1,000 mg/dose)	Administer slowly. Vesicant, follow with NSS flush. Consider Fosphenytoin for patients with hypotension and bradycardia
Fosphenytoin (Cerebyx)	IV: 20 mg PE/kg/dose (max 1,500 PE/dose) May follow with additional load if seizures continue	Prescribed in mg of PE to avoid dosing errors. Administer slowly. Monitor for hypotension and arrhythmias
Levetiracetam (Keppra)	IV: 20–60 mg/kg loading dose	Well tolerated with minimal side effects

D5W, 5% dextrose in water; IM, intramuscular; IV, intravenous; NSS, normal saline solution; PE, phenytoin sodium equivalents.
Sources: Marks, J., & Eschbach, K. (2021). Seizures. In B. N. Bolick, K. Reuter-Rice, M. A. Madden, & P. M. Severin (Eds.), *Pediatric acute care. A guide for interprofessional practice* (2nd ed., pp. 860–867). Elsevier; Lexicomp. (2022). *Pediatric and neonatal dosage handbook* (29th ed). Wolters Kluwer.

- Second-line medications include a loading dose of phenytoin or fosphenytoin.
- Third-line medications may be considered in consultation with neurology and include phenobarbital (Luminal), valproic acid (Valproic), and levetiracetam (Keppra; see Table 10.9).

Clinical Pearl

Diazepam (Diastat) is available as a rectal gel and can be administered at home or in the hospital. Keep it refrigerated. It comes in a variety of dosages.

- A seizure action plan may be developed and seizure precautions should be implemented.

COMPLICATIONS

- When administering antiseizure medications, it is important to closely monitor cardiac and respiratory status as some patients may no longer be able to protect their airway given the dosages needed to control the seizure activity.
- Depending on patient presentation during the seizure, there may be increased risk for physical harm due to seizure activity. In the hospital environment, seizure pads may be recommended on certain sleep surfaces. Ensuring emergency equipment is available (such as suction and oxygen) is a nursing priority. The patient's bed should be kept in the lowest and locked position; side rails for cribs and beds should be raised appropriately based on the patient's physical abilities.

▶ NEUROMUSCULAR DISORDERS

Neuromuscular disorders in pediatric patients can include muscular dystrophy, Guillain-Barré, myasthenia gravis, and spinal muscular atrophy (SMA). This list is not all inclusive. We will discuss a few of the most common. There are varying characteristics of these disorders that can help to classify and identify treatment. Please see Table 10.10 for guidance.

Table 10.10 Common Neuromuscular Disorders in Pediatrics

Disorder	Cause	Progression	Distinctive Symptoms	Treatment	Prognosis
Duchenne muscular dystrophy	Rare, x-linked neurogenetic disease	Peripheral to central vs. central to peripheral	Male children present with abnormal muscle function Gower's sign (Requires using a hand-and-knees position and then climbs to a standing position by "walking" the hands up the leg due to the weakness in the proximal muscles) Increased serum creatinine kinase Increased AST and ALT	Early identification and assessment of motor development Glucocorticoids	All patients are predisposed to respiratory failure and will require noninvasive mechanical ventilation by teenage years

(continued)

Table 10.10 Common Neuromuscular Disorders in Pediatrics (*continued*)

Disorder	Cause	Progression	Distinctive Symptoms	Treatment	Prognosis
Guillain–Barré	Autoimmune disorder that can be triggered by diarrhea or respiratory illness and rarely post vaccines	Ascending muscle weakness and possibly paralysis secondary to damaged myelin sheath is not contagious	Symptoms often start in bilateral lower extremities and progress to bilateral arms and upper body	Plasma exchange, IVIG	Recovery can take a few weeks up to years
Myasthenia gravis	Chronic, autoimmune destruction of the acetylcholine receptor	Can be sudden	Weakness worse after periods of activity; improves after rest	Thymectomy, monoclonal antibodies, anticholinesterase medications, immunosuppressive drugs, plasmapheresis and IVIG	Chronic, supportive care with therapies; remission is possible
SMA	Genetic, some variants are autosomal recessive, pan-ethnic	Atrophy and progressive symmetrical muscle weakness	Categorized as non-sitters, sitters, and walkers	Supportive, ethical, and palliative care issues	Respiratory failure is primary cause of death

ALT, alanine aminotransferase; AST, aspartate aminotransferase; IVIG, intravenous immunoglobulin; SMA, spinal muscular atrophy.
Sources: Centers for Disease Control and Prevention. (2022, April 18). *Guillain–Barre syndrome*. https://www.cdc.gov/campylobacter
/guillain-barre.html#:~:text=Guillain%2DBarr%C3%A9%20(Ghee%2DYAN,some%20have%20permanent%20nerve%20damage;
Finkel, R. S., Mercuri, E., Meyer, O. H., Simonds, A. K., Schroth, M. K., Graham, R. J., Kirschner, J., Iannaccone, S. T., Crawford, T. O., Woods,
S., Muntoni, F., Wirth, B., Montes, J., Main, M., Mazzone, E. S., Vitale, M., Snyder, B., Quijano-Roy, S., Bertini, E., . . . SMA Care group.
(2018). Diagnosis and management of spinal muscular atrophy: Part 2: Pulmonary and acute care; medications, supplements and immunizations; other organ systems; and ethics. *Neuromuscular Disorders: NMD, 28*(3), 197–207. https://doi.org/10.1016/j.nmd.2017.11.00
4; National Institute of Neurological Disorders and Stroke. (2022, April 25). *Myasthenia gravis fact sheet*. https://www.ninds.nih.gov/
health-information/patient-caregiver-education/fact-sheets/myasthenia-gravis-fact-sheet#:~:text=Myasthenia%20gravis%20is%20
a%20chronic,including%20the%20arms%20and%20legs; Parsons, J. A. (2021). Current updates and advances in diagnosis and treatment
of spinal muscular atrophy. *Journal of Managed Care Medicine, 24*(2), 20–25. https://doi.org/10.www.namcp.org

PATHOPHYSIOLOGY

Refer to Table 10.10.

NURSING IMPLICATIONS AND TREATMENT

ASSESSMENT

Refer to Table 10.10.

LABS AND DIAGNOSTICS

- genetic screening
- **muscular dystrophy:** muscle biopsy or DNA test (CDC, 2020b)
- **myasthenia gravis:** physical exam, assessing acetylcholine receptors, diagnostic imaging (for thymoma; National Institute of Neurological Disorders and Stroke, 2022b)

TREATMENT AND MANAGEMENT

Differential diagnosis should include botulism and acute flaccid paralysis.

▶ SPINAL FUSION

Scoliosis "in early childhood is defined as abnormal curvature of the spine of any etiology that arises before the age of 10" (Ridderbusch et al., 2018, p. 371). It usually requires a lateral curvature of >10°. Table 10.11 indicates major types of scoliosis.

Table 10.11 Classification of Scoliosis and Descriptions

Type of Scoliosis	Causes	Description	Disease Progression	Complications
Syndromic scoliosis	Systemic disease	For example, Down syndrome, Marfan syndrome, neurofibromatosis, Rett syndrome, Prader-Willi, and osteogenesis imperfecta	Unpredictable due to varied causal syndromes	Higher incidence of surgical complications
Congenital scoliosis	Embryonic malformation (5th and 8th weeks of embryo development)	▦ Mostly spontaneous ▦ Maternal diabetes, alcohol, some medications ▦ Associated with anomalies such as genitourinary, respiratory, and cardiac ▦ Failure of formation or segmentation (or both) of the spine	May progress	Some patients require treatment
Neuromuscular scoliosis	Secondary to neuropathic or myopathic diseases. Nerves and muscles do not maintain a balance and alignment in the spine	▦ Central motor neuron (cerebral palsy) ▦ Peripheral motor neuron (infantile spinal amyotrophy, motor neuropathy) ▦ Neuromuscular junction (myasthenia) ▦ Muscular (Duchenne myopathy, arthrogryposis)	Likely to progress to spinal curve	Can continue into adulthood, TIS may develop
Idiopathic scoliosis	Most common, can occur at any age, based on age of appearance/recognition	▦ Infantile: occurs in first 3 years of life, no known cause, effects males/females equally ▦ Juvenile: between 4 and 10 years, lateral curve usually to the right of thoracic region, cause unknown ▦ AIS: older than 10 years, most common (represents 90% of all cases), most cases have family history, multifactorial etiology	▦ Infantile: Resolves without treatment in >90% of cases ▦ Juvenile: 30° curves often progress ▦ Adolescent: <30° curve at maturity usually do not progress, thoracic curves 50°–75° usually progress; Lumbar curves >30° usually progress	▦ Juvenile: 70% of cases require surgery

AIS, adolescent idiopathic scoliosis; TIS, thoracic insufficiency syndrome.
Source: Vernon-Levett, P. (2019). Neurologic system. In M. C. Slota (Ed.), *AACN core curriculum for pediatric high acuity, progressive, and critical care nursing* (3rd ed., pp. 349–444). Springer Publishing Company.

PATHOPHYSIOLOGY

Scoliosis is the result of a variety of causes and can often be multifactorial. It usually progresses gradually and becomes much worse during growth spurts and adolescence. It begins in the soft tissues of the spine, through a shortening that occurs on the concave side of the curve. The deformity is a direct result of unequal forces applied to the growth plates (Vernon-Levett, 2019). The larger the curve the more physically disabling the deformity becomes, often causing compromise to the respiratory and cardiovascular systems. It can eventually progress to thoracic insufficiency syndrome (TIS). In TIS, the thorax is unable to support adequate breathing and lung growth, due to inadequate lung volumes and compromised ventilation (Vernon-Levett, 2019). This is a result of the extreme curvature compromising the lungs' ability to fully expand due to flattening of the chest. As this limits the rib cage's ability to expand, ventilation becomes dependent solely on the diaphragm.

NURSING IMPLICATIONS AND TREATMENT

ASSESSMENT

- A diagnosis of scoliosis is dependent upon a thorough history, physical exam, and diagnostic testing. History should include any birth defects, previous spinal/skeletal trauma, genetic syndromes, familial history of scoliosis, related genetic syndromes, and back pain. Determining the age of onset is extremely important in identifying the type of scoliosis. Female adolescents should include a menstrual history.
- Physical exams should include a thorough assessment as they can be highly variable based on age, underlying syndrome, and the degree of curvature. Gait assessment is important as it can be abnormal in all forms of scoliosis (Vernon-Levett, 2019). Balance and coordination of trunk, neck, and head should be observed. Pelvic unevenness is often the first sign and should be assessed for a tilt or one side sitting higher than the other on exam. In idiopathic scoliosis there may also be an unevenness in the shoulders. The Adam's forward bend test the child is asked to bend over and touch their toes. In visualizing from behind a "torso" lean may be observed, which the body leaning more towards the left or the right (Kuznia et al., 2020).
- Most types of scoliosis (see Table 10.11) are pain free. Neurologic disorders and other possible etiologies should be considered if severe pain is associated. Left thoracic curves are more frequently associated with other processes such as spinal tumors, Arnold-Chiari malformation, and neurologic disorders (Horne et al., 2014).

LABS AND DIAGNOSTICS

- Primary care physicians are critical in early identification of patients with high risk of progression. These screenings are more beneficial than previous mandatory school screening as they help prevent over testing and unnecessary radiographs (Horne et al., 2014).
- Diagnostic tests for scoliosis include radiographs and MRI. The Cobb angle measurement is taken using a standard posterior-anterior film and is needed to diagnosis scoliosis (Horne et al., 2014). Serial radiographs are used to assess and monitor the progression of curvature.
- An inclinometer can be used to quantify any asymmetry or curvature of the spine.
- Pulmonary function tests and echocardiograms may be needed to trend lung capacities and cardiac function in more extreme cases.

TREATMENT AND MANAGEMENT

- The clinical course for scoliosis is dependent on type and degree of curvature.
- There is no preventative care for scoliosis. Treatment is aimed at preventing progression of curvature. In majority of cases no active treatment is required, and the patient's curve is monitored for progression. Treatment is based on risk of curve progression, etiology, pattern of curve, and the patient's age (Vernon-Levett, 2019).
- The three treatment options for scoliosis are observation, casting or bracing, and surgery.
  - **Observation** is the typical approach for mild or moderate curves, especially in patients who have fully developed spines. They are evaluated frequently, particularly during growth spurts, as this is when curves typically progress.
  - **Serial casting** can be used to "achieve derotation and straightening of the curve" (Ridderbusch et al., 2018) in early onset scoliosis (EOS).

❏ This treatment can be used for children up to 5 years of age. A cast is applied to patient's trunk utilizing a special casting table called a Risser table (Ridderbusch et al., 2018). A new cast application is usually required every 8 weeks.

● **Rigid bracing** is the most common nonoperative treatment for scoliosis. It is a conservative treatment usually for idiopathic EOS and includes an individually fitted brace worn on the trunk. The goal of bracing is to reduce the primary curve by 50% (Ridderbush et al., 2018). Success of treatment depends on compliance with wearing the brace and ongoing follow up with treating physicians, likely primary care intensivists or orthopedic specialists. Those that wore a correctly fitted brace for >12.9 hours/day had a 90% to 93% success rate with curvature improvements (Ridderbush et al., 2018).

❏ Bracing relies on compliance of wear and needs both emotional support and education.

● **Surgery** is typically indicated for EOS curves >40 to 50 who have not reached skeletal maturity or those who have reached skeletal maturity with curves >50° (Vernon-Levett, 2019; Table 10.12).

Table 10.12 Surgical Approaches to Scoliosis Treatment

Surgical Approach	Typical Indications	Advantages/Disadvantages
Posterior approach	Idiopathic scoliosis	**Advantage:** Surgeon able to exert more force to correct deformity due to use of malleable rods
Anterior approach	Used for significant lumbar curves, lordosis, hypokyphosis	**Advantage:** Restore thoracic kyphosis
		Disadvantages: Associated with longer length of hospitalization and more complications
Anterior approach with VATS	Newer option for AIS	**Advantage:** Restore thoracic kyphosis; fewer blood transfusions, smaller incisions, less operative loss
		Disadvantages: Single lung ventilation, risk for bleeding
MAGEC	Severe or rapidly progressing curves	**Advantage:** Avoids multiple surgeries utilizing noninvasive magnets and external remote control
		Disadvantage: Lengthening procedure every 3–4 months (but without surgery)
VEPTR	Usually for patients with TIS	**Advantage:** Newer procedure where prothesis is used to expand the ribs
		Disadvantage: Subsequent expansion procedures every 2–3 months until spinal maturity

MAGEC, Magnetic expansion control; TIS, thoracic insufficiency syndrome; VATS, video-assisted thorascopic surgery; VEPTR, vertical expandable prosthetic titanium rib.
Source: Vernon-Levett, P. (2019). Neurologic system. In M. C. Slota (Ed.), *AACN core curriculum for pediatric high acuity, progressive, and critical care nursing* (3rd ed., pp. 349–444). Springer Publishing Company.

❏ Spinal fusion surgery is the standard of care for major adolescent scoliosis (Ridderbush et al., 2018). Goals include limiting the invasiveness of surgery and correcting the imbalance/curvature.

Clinical Pearl

Nursing care of a patient postoperative posterior spinal fusion includes monitoring for blood loss, changes in respiratory status, and performing frequent neurovascular checks.

▪ Outcomes vary and are dependent on etiology, age of onset, severity, and comorbidities.

COMPLICATIONS

▪ Possible complications include surgical site infections (SSI) and skin injury or tearing if rods become displaced.

▪ If infantile progressive scoliosis is left untreated the outcomes are usually unfavorable, leading to high morbidity and mortality due to cardiopulmonary complications (Ridderbush et al., 2018).

▶ PAIN: ACUTE AND CHRONIC

▪ Pain is not optimally assessed, treated, or evaluated in pediatrics (Manworren & Stinson, 2016). Inadequate pain management can impact recovery time as well as increase a patient's length of stay. Pain can be acute, recurrent, chronic, or a combination of the prior. Pain is very subjective to an individual. Ongoing assessment of pain and response to interventions is essential in effectively treating pain (Manworren & Stinson, 2016). Use of valid and reliable pain assessment tools and scales is recommended to provide consistency among providers (Vernon-Levett, 2019). There are numerous types of pain scales used. FLACC (Face, Legs, Activity, Cry, Consolability), FACES, and Numeric (0–10) are the most common scales used. It is vital that nurses educate the patient and family regarding pain management strategies to increase their understanding of pain interventions (pharmacologic and nonpharmacologic) being utilized. Assessing pain in a sedated patient requires close examination of vital sign trends as well as garnering information from the family on the patient's normal response to pain. Assessing pain and agitation in patients with an altered level of consciousness is challenging and requires close analysis of the physiologic status, as well as response to pharmacologic and nonpharmacologic interventions. In patients with a neurologic disease or disorder, the goal is maximum comfort without diminishing patient responsiveness (Vernon-Levett, 2019; Table 10.13).

Table 10.13 Types of Pain: Physiologic and Behavioral Cues

Type of Pain	Physiologic Cues	Behavioral Cues
Acute pain	▪ Increased or decreased HR. Infants may be bradycardic ▪ Increased RR ▪ Increased BP ▪ Decreased oxygen saturation ▪ Diaphoresis ▪ Dilated pupils ▪ Palmar sweating ▪ Change in appetite, sleep pattern	▪ Crying, moaning, groaning, screaming, whimpering, gasping ▪ Facial expression of pain: brow bulging, nasolabial furrowing, eye squeezing, open mouth, chin quiver ▪ Reluctance to move or be moved ▪ Anxiety, restlessness, desperation, highly motivated to get help/relief from pain ▪ Frequent request for analgesia/use of PCA ▪ Disorganized suck in infants ▪ Hypertonicity
Chronic pain	▪ May exhibit very few or no physiologic signs of pain	▪ Decreased spontaneous movement ▪ Irritability/depression/apathy ▪ Learned helplessness behaviors seems passive in decision-making regarding pain management ▪ Flat affect ▪ Poor feeding ▪ Failure to thrive ▪ Absent or weak cry ▪ Utilizes distractive behavior: eating, talking on the phone, playing, and sleeping
Patients who cannot display behavioral signs of pain: ▪ Unconscious ▪ Sedated ▪ Paralyzed	▪ Increased or decreased HR. Infants may be bradycardic ▪ Increased BP ▪ Decreased oxygen saturation ▪ Diaphoresis ▪ Dilated pupils ▪ Palmar sweating	▪ May be unable to display behavioral signs of pain

BP, blood pressure; HR, heart rate; PCA, patient controlled analgesia; RR, respiration rate.

▪ Pharmacologic agents are often a component of the plan to manage a patient's pain. Specific interventions may differ from these guidelines based on a patient's individual needs as determined by the clinical judgment of the interdisciplinary team providing care. Relevant factors in managing the patient's pain include but are not limited to pain type and intensity, duration of pain, age, past exposure, prior response to analgesics (both pain relief and side effects), comorbidities, end organ function, and concomitant administration of other drugs and pharmacokinetics of the analgesics ordered. Optimal pain management will sometimes require using more than one analgesic at the same time. Nonopioids can be given with opioids for moderate or severe pain because different classes of medications have different mechanisms of action and consequently provide better pain relief together than alone.

- IV opioids (e.g., morphine, hydromorphone, fentanyl) are indicated for patients who:
  - ❑ are not tolerating liquids
  - ❑ exhibit or report severe pain of sudden onset
- Oral opioids (e.g., oxycodone) are indicated for patients who:
  - ❑ are tolerating liquids
  - ❑ exhibit or report moderate to severe pain
- Nonopioid analgesics (e.g., acetaminophen, ketorolac, ibuprofen for infants >6 months old) are indicated for patients who:
  - ❑ are taking an opioid and have moderate to severe pain
  - ❑ are having mild, moderate, or severe pain
- Neuropathic pain may be managed with the use of an antidepressant or anticonvulsant medication (gabapentin).
- Nonpharmacologic interventions are also an important part of the pain management plan. Nonpharmacologic interventions include but are not limited to positioning/repositioning, cold or warm compresses, decreasing environmental light/noise, caregiver support, relaxation techniques (e.g., deep breathing, guided imagery, Therapeutic Breathwork), massage, and distraction.
- Patient controlled analgesia (PCA) has limited use in pediatrics related to the child's age and ability to use. PCAs are very helpful with some pediatric disorders requiring frequent pain medication administration.

▶ AGITATION

- Agitation can be challenging in pediatrics. In a neurologically injured patient who is agitated, it is important to identify potential causes. These may include toxins, medication reactions, traumatic brain injury, delirium, and other causes. Care should be tailored to address primary cause when possible.
- Patients with a head injury can become agitated and it is important to manage pain to not increase their ICP.
- Most pediatric ICU (PICU) patients who are intubated and ventilated require medications to make them comfortable. The patient may be on continuous medication infusions of a benzodiazepine and opioid. If the patient is demonstrating physiologic or behavioral cues of discomfort (Table 10.13) then a PRN medication should be administered. Selection of the PRN agent should be based on the patient's pain score. If pain is present, the opioid PRN should be administered. If no pain is present, then the benzodiazepine PRN should be administered to treat agitation.
- Common medications used are benzodiazepines (e.g., midazolam). It is also important for the critical care nurse to assess and monitor for delirium. If delirium is suspected, the nurse would collaborate with the interdisciplinary team and could anticipate that the team would want to wean the benzodiazepine continuous infusion and may consider adding another agent such as dexmedetomidine.

CASE STUDY

M is a previously healthy child whose mother took him to a local ED for several days of gastrointestinal symptoms (including vomiting and decreased energy). There, they drew labs and upon receiving the results, immediately arranged for transport to a children's hospital for an oncologic workup. M was intubated for placement of a central line and started plasmapheresis immediately. The plan was to keep M intubated until a bone marrow aspiration and possibly lumbar puncture could be performed the following day. The plan for your shift after morning rounds is to give M platelets, cryoprecipitate then fresh frozen plasma and reassess his coagulation status. As soon as the nurse starts the platelet transfusion, he perform M's pupillary check as part of his hourly neurological assessments. The nurse notes a change from his previous assessment of bilaterally 4 and briskly reactive to light. M's left pupil is now a 5/sluggishly reactive and his right pupil is now 2/nonreactive.

CASE STUDY QUESTIONS

1. In the scenario, what should the critical care nurse do next?
   A. Notify the critical care provider team.
   B. Wait 30 minutes and then recheck pupils to confirm findings.
   C. Stop the platelet infusion.
   D. Draw coagulation labs.

2. What does the critical care nurse anticipate needing available at the bedside?
   A. Pastoral care to support the family
   B. Extra nursing assistance and ordered emergency medications
   C. The provider to give verbal orders
   D. Neurosurgical team for specialty consultation

3. The critical care nurse knows to administer the following medication first:
   A. Mannitol
   B. Epinephrine
   C. 3% hypertonic saline
   D. Normal saline bolus

4. Where does the critical care nurse anticipate going immediately with this patient?
   A. STAT MRI
   B. STAT head CT
   C. Operating room (OR)
   D. Nowhere, remain in the pediatric ICU (PICU)

(See answers next page.)

ANSWERS TO CASE STUDY QUESTIONS

1. A) Notify the critical care provider team.

This patient has had a critical change in status and requires immediate intervention and new orders from the provider team. Waiting 30 minutes would delay the patient necessary care. Stopping the platelet infusion and drawing labs do not address his neurological status.

2. B) Extra nursing assistance and ordered emergency medications

The provider is needed but the nurse anticipates needing extra nursing hands to administer emergency medications. The neurosurgical team may be consulted but is not the immediate best choice.

3. C) 3% hypertonic saline

3% hypertonic saline is the recommended first line medication for treatment of elevated intracranial pressure (ICP; Schwimmbeck et al., 2021). Mannitol may be given if 3% hypertonic saline is not available; however, it has a potent diuretic effect and can subsequently decrease the cerebral perfusion pressure (CPP). A normal saline bolus and epinephrine may raise the CPP through raising of the blood pressure; however, it will not fix the immediate problem of elevated ICPs.

4. B) STAT head CT

STAT heat CT provides the quickest diagnostic read of what is happening for this patient. An MRI would take too long to obtain. The OR may be warranted but a head CT is needed first.

● KNOWLEDGE CHECK: CHAPTER 10

1. The nurse is admitting a 3-year-old following a motor vehicle accident. The patient's blood pressure (BP) is 70/40. The nurse anticipates the initial management to include:
   A. Administration of packed red blood cells (PRBCs).
   B. Initiation of a vasopressor
   C. Administration of 20 mL/kg of isotonic saline solution
   D. Administration of 5 mL/kg of isotonic saline solution

2. A nursing student is listing the places where the distal catheter of a cerebrospinal fluid (CSF) shunt can be placed. Which response indicates a need for further teaching?
   A. Pleural space
   B. Right atrium
   C. Peritoneal space
   D. Pericardial space

3. A 10-year-old patient with a ventriculoperitoneal (VP) shunt presents to the ED with headache, temperature (39°C/102.2°F), abdominal pain, and nausea/vomiting. On exam, they are sleepy and difficult to arouse. What intervention do you anticipate the provider asking for first?
   A. Provide acetaminophen for the patient's fever.
   B. Obtain a chest x-ray (CXR).
   C. Consult neurosurgery.
   D. Obtain a head CT.

4. A nurse admits a newborn with an unrepaired myelomeningocele to the pediatric ICU (PICU). What is the best nursing intervention to protect the myelomeningocele sac prior to surgery?
   A. Apply petrolatum gauze using sterile technique.
   B. Apply moist saline gauze using sterile technique.
   C. Leave the sac open to air.
   D. Cover with dry sterile gauze.

5. What is the **best** position for a neonate with an unrepaired myelomeningocele?
   A. Prone
   B. Supine
   C. Right side-lying
   D. Left side-lying

6. A 16-year-old patient is being treated in the pediatric ICU (PICU) after suffering from a spinal cord injury (SCI) as a result of a diving accident a month ago. The nurse caring for him notices the following vital signs (VS) on the monitor: heart rate (HR) 42, respiratory rate (RR) 12, blood pressure (BP) 184/100. The patient is cool to touch. This patient is suffering from the following complication:
   A. Laceration
   B. Spinal shock
   C. Autonomic dysreflexia
   D. Battle sign

7. A 16-year-old patient is being treated in the pediatric ICU (PICU) after suffering from a spinal cord injury (SCI) as a result of a diving accident a month ago. The nurse caring for him notices the following vital signs (VS) on the monitor: heart rate (HR) 42, respiratory rate (RR) 12, blood pressure (BP) 184/100. The patient is cool to touch. Based on this scenario, the nurse should assess the following as a likely cause:
   A. Temperature
   B. Bleeding
   C. Headache
   D. Distended bladder

(See answers next page.)

1. C) Administration of 20 mL/kg of isotonic saline solution

Initial treatment for this patient is intravenous (IV) fluids. PRBCs and initiation of a vasopressor are not appropriate initial treatments. The team would not start with 5 mL/kg since no history of cardiac or renal disorder was provided.

2. D) Pericardial space

The pericardial space is not a location for the distal end of the shunt. The peritoneal space of the abdomen is the most common distal location for the shunt and is called a VP shunt. The shunt can also terminate in the right atrium and is called a ventriculoatrial (VA) shunt. Shunts can also terminate in the pleural space, but this is not as common.

3. D) Obtain head CT.

The patient is exhibiting signs of increased intracranial pressure (ICP), so obtaining a head CT is important to rule out shunt malfunction. Providing the patient with acetaminophen will treat the fever, but this is not the top priority given their symptoms of increased ICP. Consulting neurosurgery is important, but the neurosurgeons will need to review the head CT to develop a plan of care. Obtaining a CXR is not correct as the head CT will provide more information for the providers.

4. B) Apply moist saline gauze using sterile technique.

The sac should be kept moist. If left open to air the sac may dry out and use of ointment or dry gauze may be irritating to the skin.

5. A) Prone

A prone position minimizes the tension/pressure on the sac. Side-lying is acceptable but not the best position as it could place tension on the sac with potential to cause a leak. Supine positioning would cause trauma to the sac and potentially could cause it to leak or break.

6. C) Autonomic dysreflexia

Autonomic dysreflexia is a life-threatening complication of spinal cord injury (SCI) that causes severe hypertension. Laceration is a type of spinal cord injury. Spinal shock is a secondary injury that usually resolves in the first few weeks. Battle's sign is a hematoma associated with traumatic brain injury.

7. D) Distended bladder

This patient is suffering from autonomic dysreflexia which occurs from stimulation of sensory receptors below the level of spinal cord injury (SCI). Bladder and bowel distension are the most common causes. Temperature can be impaired with SCI but does not cause autonomic dysreflexia. Bleeding would cause hypotension, not hypertension.

8. Which of the following is considered the "gold standard" diagnostic to rule out intracranial hemorrhage (ICH) within the first 48 hours after suspected traumatic brain injury (TBI)?
   A. CT scan
   B. MRI
   C. X-ray
   D. Obtain complete blood count (CBC)

9. What is the most common form of idiopathic scoliosis?
   A. Infantile scoliosis
   B. Juvenile scoliosis
   C. Adolescent idiopathic scoliosis (AIS)
   D. Congenital scoliosis

10. In preparation for the second clinical exam to evaluate cessation of neurologic function the bedside nurse should:
    A. Administer pain medication so that the patient is not uncomfortable.
    B. Educate the patient's family that if this exam is consistent with cessation of neurological function that the patient is still alive.
    C. Check patient's temperature to ensure they are normothermic.
    D. Move the patient's cervical collar so that the physician can move the patient's head properly.

11. The bedside RN knows that interventions to help prevent delirium include:
    A. Administering ordered sedative medications as soon as the patient awakens
    B. Always keeping the lights on to facilitate patient care
    C. Maintaining a normal sleep/wake cycle
    D. Administering ordered medications for sleep aid (such as melatonin)

12. Treatment of encephalopathy is directed toward:
    A. Treating the bacterial cause
    B. Treating the viral cause
    C. Administering appropriate medications
    D. Supportive management

13. A top priority nursing intervention for a patient having a seizure is to:
    A. Administer ordered first-line anti-seizure medications
    B. Ensure airway management
    C. Monitor vital signs
    D. Educate the family

14. A patient is observed attempting to stand by first getting into a crawling position, straightening their elbows, and then placing their hands on their thighs and slowly coming to a stand. This presentation is most associated with:
    A. Guillain-Barré
    B. Muscular dystrophy
    C. Myasthenia gravis
    D. None of the above

15. A child presents to the hospital with a seizure. The patient is 4 months old, has no history of previous seizures, a core temperature of 37.4°C (99.3°F) and no apparent intracranial infection. The critical care nurse knows that this patient:
    A. Has had a febrile seizure
    B. Cannot be ruled out from having had a febrile seizure
    C. Did not have a febrile seizure due to the patient's age
    D. Did not have a febrile seizure due to the patient's temperature

(See answers next page.)

8. A) CT scan

CT is a faster and more cost effective neurodiagnostic than MRI. X-rays could identify a skull fracture but would not rule out a bleed. CBC levels would identify if red blood cells (RBCs) were low but would not identify a direct source of blood loss.

9. C) Adolescent idiopathic scoliosis (AIS)

AIS represents 90% of all idiopathic scoliosis cases. Congenital scoliosis is an embryonic malformation. Juvenile scoliosis only represents 10% to 15% of idiopathic scoliosis cases.

10. C) Check patient's temperature to ensure they are normothermic.

Confounding variables (such as hypothermia) must be eliminated prior to evaluating for cessation of neurologic function. Administering pain medication is incorrect because pain medication is a confounder for the exam. Since this is the second exam, the patient would be pronounced dead if they meet criteria for cessation of neurologic function. The RN should not remove the cervical collar as this could cause harm to the patient.

11. C) Maintaining a normal sleep/wake cycle

Maintaining a normal sleep/wake cycle can help to prevent delirium. Administering sedative medications is incorrect because benzodiazepines are linked to higher rates of delirium. Keeping the lights on continuously is incorrect because lights disrupt normal sleep/wake cycle and can lead to higher delirium. There is little evidence regarding the safety of pharmacologic management for delirium; therefore, melatonin is not the best choice.

12. D) Supportive management

Encephalopathy is a diagnosis based on exclusion of other causes. It entails brain dysfunction without "inflammation of brain parenchyma that lacks the additional criteria outlined by the International Encephalitis Consortium" (Fraley et al., 2021, p. 72). Its treatment is supportive care.

13. B) Ensure airway management

Airway management is the priority for basic life support needs, although administering medications, monitoring vital signs, and educating the family are correct, they are not the top priority.

14. B) Muscular dystrophy

The movement described is the Gowers' sign. This is a classic finding in muscular dystrophy. It indicates proximal muscle weakness and is most often associated with muscular dystrophy. Guillain-Barré and myasthenia gravis are not applicable.

15. D) Did not have a febrile seizure due to the patient's temperature

The general age range for febrile seizures is 1 month to 6 years, temperature >38°C (99.3°F), no evidence of intracranial infection, no history of epilepsy. This patient's temperature excludes them from having a febrile seizure.

16. A 3-year-old child is admitted directly to the pediatric ICU (PICU) from the trauma bay after a fall on the playground with a witnessed trauma to the head. Vital signs on arrival are the following: heart rate (HR) 145, respiratory rate (RR) 22, SpO$_2$ 98%, and blood pressure (BP) 131/72. His neurologic exam on arrival included a Glasgow Coma Scale (GCS) of 15, pupil, equal, round, reactive to light, and accommodation (PERRLA), and crying inconsolably in the mother's arms. On assessment 2 hours post admission, the RN found the patient unarousable to painful stimulation, the right pupil 4 mm and nonreactive, and left pupil 3 mm and sluggish to light. Using this head trauma scenario, what are some nursing interventions to consider?
    A. Suction the patient
    B. Bag mask ventilate the patient
    C. Elevate head of bed (HOB) to >30°
    D. Administer 3% hypertonic saline

17. Regarding neuroimaging, the critical care nurse knows the following:
    A. MRI is superior to CT scan and should therefore always be performed first.
    B. CT scan is more widely available and is quicker to perform so is often the preferred imaging.
    C. MRI and CT scan are equal in imaging quality and provider preference can drive the decision.
    D. MRI usually does not require the patient to be sedated so should be chosen.

(See answers next page.)

16. C) Elevate head of bed (HOB) to >30°

Increasing the HOB can improve cerebral blood flow by improving venous drainage but no higher or lower than 30° as it will increase intracranial pressure (ICP). Suctioning is a noxious stimulus that can increase ICP. 3% hypertonic saline would need to be ordered by a provider.

17. B) CT scan is more widely available and is quicker to perform so is often the preferred imaging.

MRI will not always be performed first. The images generated from MRI and CT are different. MRI may require the patient to be sedated.

REFERENCES

Allen, K., & Leslie, S. (2022). Autonomic dysreflexia. *Stat pearls for the National Institute of Health*. https://www.ncbi
.nlm.nih.gov/books/NBK482434/

American Psychiatric Association. (2013). *Diagnostic and statistical manual of mental disorders* (5th ed.).
https://doi.org/10.1176/appi.books.9780890425596

American Academy of Pediatrics. (2021, July 13). *Meningitis in infants and children*. https://www.healthychildren.org
/English/health-issues/conditions/head-neck-nervous-system/Pages/Meningitis.aspx

American Academy of Pediatrics & Committee on Genetics. (1999). Folic acid for the prevention of neural tube
defects. *Pediatrics, 104*(2 Pt. 1), 325–327. https://doi.org/10.1542/peds.104.2.325

American Academy of Pediatrics Subcommittee on Febrile Seizures. (2011). Neurodiagnostic evaluation of the child
with a simple febrile seizure. *Pediatrics, 127*(2), 389–394. https://doi.org/10.1542/peds.2010-3318

Annegers, J. F., Hauser, W. A., Elveback, L. R., & Kurland, L. T. (1979). The risk of epilepsy following febrile convul-
sions. *Neurology, 29*(3), 297–303. https://doi.org/10.1212/WNL.29.3.297

Baker, C., Kadish, H., & Schunk, J. E. (1999). Evaluation of pediatric cervical spine injuries. *American Journal of
Emergency Medicine, 17*(3), 230–234. https://doi.org/10.1016/s0735-6757(99)90111-0

Bale, J. F., Jr. (2015). Virus and immune-mediated encephalitides: Epidemiology, diagnosis, treatment, and prevention.
Pediatric Neurology, 53(1), 3–12. https://doi.org/10.1016/j.pediatrneurol.2015.03.013

Bernson-Leung, M. E., & Rivkin, M. J. (2016). Stroke in neonates and children. *Pediatrics in Review, 37*(11), 463–477.
https://doi.org/10.1542/pir.2016-0002

Caceres, J. A., & Goldstein, J. N. (2012). Intracranial hemorrhage. *Emergency Medicine Clinics of North America, 30*(3),
771–794. https://doi.org/10.1016/j.emc.2012.06.003

Centers for Disease Control and Prevention. (2020a). *Congenital malformations of the nervous system: Neural tube defects*.
https://www.cdc.gov/ncbddd/birthdefects/surveillancemanual/chapters/chapter-4/chapter4-2.html#:~:text=
The%20most%20prevalent%20types%20of,and%20exposure%20of%20neural%20tissue

Centers for Disease Control and Prevention. (2020b, October 27). *Muscular dystrophy*. https://www.cdc.gov/ncbddd
/musculardystrophy/data.html

Children's Hospital of Philadelphia. (2022). *Pediatric brain tumors*. https://www.chop.edu/conditions-diseases
/pediatric-brain-tumors

Copley, P. C., Tilliridou, V., Kirby, A., Jones, J., & Kandasamy, J. (2019). Management of cervical spine trauma in children. *European Journal of Trauma and Emergency Surgery: Official Publication of the European Trauma Society, 45*(5),
777–789. https://doi.org/10.1007/s00068-018-0992-x

Czeizel, A. E., & Dudás, I. (1992). Prevention of the first occurrence of neural-tube defects by periconceptional vitamin supplementation. *New England Journal of Medicine, 327*(26), 1832–1835. https://doi.org/10.1056/
NEJM199212243272602

Denke, N., Normandin, P., & Spann, D. (2020). *Neurologic emergencies in ENA's emergency nursing pediatric course* (5th
ed.). Jones & Bartlett.

Di Pentima, C. (2021, January 19). Viral meningitis in children: Clinical features and diagnosis. *UpToDate*. https:
//www.uptodate.com/contents/viral-meningitis-in-children-clinical-features-and-diagnosis?search=viral%20
meningitis&source=search_result&selectedTitle=2~150&usage_type=default&display_rank=2

El-Ghanem, M., Kass-Hout, T., Kass-Hout, O., Alderazi, Y. J., Amuluru, K., Al-Mufti, F., Prestigiacomo, C. J., &
Gandhi, C. D. (2016). Arteriovenous malformations in the pediatric population: Review of the existing literature.
Interventional Neurology, 5(3–4), 218–225. https://doi.org/10.1159/000447605

Ferriero, D. M., Fullerton, H. J., Bernard, T. J., Billinghurst, L., Daniels, S. R., DeBaun, M. R., deVeber, G., Ichord,
R. N., Jordan, L. C., Massicotte, P., Meldau, J., Roach, E. S., Smith, E. R., & American Heart Association Stroke
Council and Council on Cardiovascular and Stroke Nursing. (2019). Management of stroke in neonates and
children: A scientific statement from the American Heart Association/American Stroke Association. *Stroke, 50*(3),
e51–e96. https://doi.org/10.1161/STR.0000000000000183

Fine, A., & Wirrell, E. C. (2020, July). Seizures in children. *Pediatrics in Review, 41*(7), 321–347. http://publications.aap
.org/pediatricsinreview/article-pdf/41/7/321/827897/pedsinreview_20190134.pdf

Finkel, R. S., Mercuri, E., Meyer, O. H., Simonds, A. K., Schroth, M. K., Graham, R. J., Kirschner, J., Iannaccone, S. T.,
Crawford, T. O., Woods, S., Muntoni, F., Wirth, B., Montes, J., Main, M., Mazzone, E. S., Vitale, M., Snyder, B.,
Quijano-Roy, S., Bertini, E., . SMA Care group. (2018). Diagnosis and management of spinal muscular atrophy:
Part 2: Pulmonary and acute care; medications, supplements and immunizations; other organ systems; and eth-
ics. *Neuromuscular Disorders: NMD, 28*(3), 197–207. https://doi.org/10.1016/j.nmd.2017.11.004

Fraley, C. E., Pettersson, D. R., & Nolt, D. (2021). Encephalitis in previously healthy children. *Pediatrics in Review,
42*(2), 68–77. https://doi.org/10.1542/pir.2018-0175

Francoeur, C., Weiss, M. J., Macdonald, J. M., Press, C., Greer, D. M., Berg, R. A., Topjian, A. A., Morrison, W.,
& Kirschen, M. P. (2021). Variability in pediatric brain death determination protocols in the United States.
Neurology, 10.1212/WNL.0000000000012225. Advance online publication. https://doi.org/10.1212
/WNL.000000000001

Ghofrani, M., Tonekaboni, H., Karimzadeh, P., Nasiri, J., Pirzadeh, Z., Ghazzavi, M., & Yghini, O. (2018). Risk factors
of pediatric arterial ischemic stroke; A regional survey. *International Journal of Preventive Medicine, 9*(1), 69.
https://doi.org/10.4103/ijpvm.IJPVM_262_17

Glauser, T., Shinnar, S., Gloss, D., Alldredge, B., Arya, R., Bainbridge, J., Bare, M., Bleck, T., Dodson, W. E.,
Garrity, L., Jagoda, A., Lowenstein, D., Pellock, J., Riviello, J., Sloan, E., & Treiman, D. M. (2016). Evidence-based
guideline: Treatment of convulsive status epilepticus in children and adults: Report of the Guideline Committee
of the American Epilepsy Society. *Epilepsy Currents, 16*(1), 48–61. https://doi.org/10.5698/1535-7597-16.1.48

Greenham, M., Gordon, A., Anderson, V., & Mackay, M. T. (2016). Outcome in childhood stroke. *Stroke, 47*(4), 1159–1164. https://doi.org/10.1161/STROKEAHA.115.011622

Haspolat, S., Mihçi, E., Coşkun, M., Gümüslü, S., Ozben, T., & Yeğin, O. (2002). Interleukin-1beta, tumor necrosis factor-alpha, and nitrite levels in febrile seizures. *Journal of Child Neurology, 17*(10), 749–751. https://doi.org/10.1177/08830738020170101501

Hofmeister, C., Stapf, C., Hartmann, A., Sciacca, R. R., Mansmann, U., terBrugge, K., Lasjaunias, P., Mohr, J. P., Mast, H., & Meisel, J. (2000). Demographic, morphological, and clinical characteristics of 1289 patients with brain arteriovenous malformation. *Stroke, 31*(6), 1307–1310. https://doi.org/10.1161/01.str.31.6.1307

Horne, J. P., Flannery, R., & Usman, S. (2014). Adolescent idiopathic scoliosis: Diagnosis and management. *American Family Physician, 89*(3), 193–198.

Kalvas, L. B., & Harrison, T. M. (2020). State of the science in pediatric ICU delirium: An integrative review. *Research in Nursing and Health, 43*(4), 341–355. https://doi.org/10.1002/nur.22054

Khandaker, G., Jung, J., Britton, P. N., King, C., Yin, J. K., & Jones, C. A. (2016). Long-term outcomes of infective encephalitis in children: A systematic review and meta-analysis. *Developmental Medicine and Child Neurology, 58*(11), 1108–1115. https://doi.org/10.1111/dmcn.13197

Kuznia, A. L., Hernandez, A. K., & Lee, L. U. (2020). Adolescent idiopathic scoliosis: Common questions and answers. *American Family Physician, 101*(1), 19–23.

Lanni, G., Catalucci, A., Conti, L., Di Sibio, A., Paonessa, A., & Gallucci, M. (2011). Pediatric stroke: Clinical findings and radiological approach. *Stroke Research and Treatment, 2011.* https://doi.org/10.4061/2011/172168

Lau, C., & Teo, W-Y. (2020, September 29). *Clinical manifestations and diagnosis of central nervous system tumors in children.* UpToDate. https://www.uptodate.com/contents/clinical-manifestations-and-diagnosis-of-central-nervous-system-tumors-in-children?search=cns%20tumors&source=search_result&selectedTitle=1~150&usage_type=default&display_rank=1

Laws, J. C., Jordan, L. C., Pagano, L. M., Wellons, J. C., & Wolf, M. S. (2022). Multimodal neurologic monitoring in children with acute brain injury. *Pediatric Neurology, 129,* 62–71. https://doi.org/10.1016/j.pediatrneurol.2022.01.006

Leonard, J. R., Jaffe, D. M., Kuppermann, N., Olsen, C. S., & Leonard, J. C. (2014). Emergency Care Applied Research Network (PECARN) Cervical Spine Study Group. Cervical spine injury patterns in children. *Pediatrics, 135*(5), e1179–e1188. https://doi.org/10.1542/peds.2013-3505

Lewis, A. (2022). The uniform determination of death act is being revised. *Neurocritical Care, 36*(2), 335–338. https://doi.org/10.1007/s12028-021-01439-2

Lo, W. D., Lee, J., Rusin, J., Perkins, E., & Roach, E. S. (2008). Intracranial hemorrhage in children: An evolving spectrum. *Archives of Neurology, 65*(12), 1629–1633. https://doi.org/10.1001/archneurol.2008.502

Lovett, M. E., O'Brien, N. F., & Leonard, J. R. (2019). Children with severe traumatic brain injury, intracranial pressure, cerebral perfusion pressure, what does it mean? A review of the literature. *Pediatric Neurology, 94,* 3–20. https://doi.org/10.1016/j.pediatrneurol.2018.12.003

Mack, E. (2013). Neurogenic shock. *Open Pediatric Medicine Journal, 7,* 16–18. https://doi.org/10.2174/1874309901307010016

Mandadi, A. R., Koutsogiannis, P. & Waseem, M. (2022, August 8). Pediatric spine trauma. In *StatPearls* [Internet]. StatPearls Publishing. https://www.ncbi.nlm.nih.gov/books/NBK442027/

Manworren, R. C., & Stinson, J. (2016). Pediatric pain measurement, assessment, and evaluation. *Seminars in Pediatric Neurology, 23*(3), 189–200. https://doi.org/10.1016/j.spen.2016.10.001

Marks, J., & Eschbach, K. (2021). Seizures. In B. N. Bolick, K. Reuter-Rice, M. A. Madden, & P. M. Severin (Eds.), *Pediatric acute care: A guide for interprofessional practice* (2nd ed., pp. 860–867). Elsevier.

Mathur, M., & Ashwal, S. (2015). Pediatric brain death determination. *Seminars in Neurology, 35*(2), 116–124. https://doi.org/10.1055/s-0035-1547540

McKinney, S. M., Magruder, J. T., & Abramo, T. J. (2018). An update on pediatric stroke protocol. *Pediatric Emergency Care, 34*(11), 810–815. https://doi.org/10.1097/PEC.0000000000001653

Mild Traumatic Brain Injury Committee, A. C. R. M. (1993). Definition of mild traumatic brain injury. *Journal of Head Trauma Rehabilitation, 8*(3), 86–87. https://doi.org/10.1097/00001199-199309000-00010

Minardi, C., Minacapelli, R., Valastro, P., Vasile, F., Pitino, S., Pavone, P., Astuto, M., & Murabito, P. (2019). Epilepsy in children: From diagnosis to treatment with focus on emergency. *Journal of Clinical Medicine, 8*(1), 39. https://doi.org/10.3390/jcm8010039

MRC Vitamin Study Research Group. (1991). Prevention of neural tube defects: Results of the Medical Research Council Vitamin Study. *Lancet (London, England), 338*(8760), 131–137. https://doi.org/10.1016/0140-6736(91)90133-A

National Conference of Commissioners on Uniform State Laws. (1981). Uniform determination of death act. Uniform Law Commission. https://www.uniformlaws.org/committees/community-home/librarydocuments?communitykey¼155faf5d-03c2-4027-99ba-ee4c99019d6c&tab¼librarydocuments

National Institute of Neurological Disorders and Stroke. (2021, April 23). *Stroke information page.* https://www.ninds.nih.gov/Disorders/All-Disorders/Stroke-Information-Page#disorders-r1

National Institute of Neurological Disorders and Stroke. (2022a, May 4). *Meningitis and encephalitis.* National Institutes of Health. https://www.ninds.nih.gov/Disorders/All-Disorders/Meningitis-and-Encephalitis-Information-Page#:~:text=Definition-,Meningitis%20is%20an%20infection%20of%20the%20meninges%2C%20the%20membranes%20that,inflammation%20of%20the%20brain%20itself

National Institute of Neurological Disorders and Stroke. (2022b, April 25). *Myasthenia gravis fact sheet.* https://www.ninds.nih.gov/health-information/patient-caregiver-education/fact-sheets/myasthenia-gravis-fact-sheet#:~:text=Myasthenia%20gravis%20is%20a%20chronic,including%20the%20arms%20and%20legs

O'Neil, M. E., Carlson, K., Storzbach, D., Brenner, L., Freeman, M., Quiñones, A., Motu'apuaka, M., Ensley, M., & Kansagara, D. (2013 January). *Complications of mild traumatic brain injury in veterans and military personnel: A systematic review.* Department of Veterans Affairs (US). https://www.ncbi.nlm.nih.gov/books/NBK189784/

Ozga, D., Krupa, S., Witt, P., & Mędrzycka-Dąbrowska, W. (2020). Nursing interventions to prevent delirium in critically ill patients in the intensive care unit during the COVID19 pandemic-narrative overview. *Healthcare, 8*(4), 578. https://doi.org/10.3390/healthcare8040578

Parsons, J. A. (2021). Current updates and advances in diagnosis and treatment of spinal muscular atrophy. *Journal of Managed Care Medicine, 24*(2), 20–25. https://doi.org/10.www.namcp.org

Leonard, J. R., Jaffe, D. M., Kuppermann, N., Olsen, C. S., Leonard, J. C., & Pediatric Emergency Care Applied Research Network (PECARN) Cervical Spine Study Group. (2014). Cervical spine injury patterns in children. *Pediatrics, 133*(5), e1179–e1188. https://doi.org/10.1542/peds.2013-3505

Rekate, H. L. (2009). A contemporary definition and classification of hydrocephalus. *Seminars in Pediatric Neurology, 16*(1), 9–15. https://doi.org/10.1016/j.spen.2009.01.002

Rekate, H. L., & Blitz, A. M. (2016). Hydrocephalus in children. In J. C. Masdeu & R. G. Gonzalez (Eds.), *Handbook of clinical neurology 3rd series*. Elsevier.

Ridderbusch, K., Spiro, A. S., Kunkel, P., Grolle, B., Stücker, R., & Rupprecht, M. (2018). Strategies for treating scoliosis in early childhood. *Deutsches Ärzteblatt International, 115*(22), 371–376. https://doi.org/10.3238/arztebl.2018.0371

Schwimmbeck, F., Voellger, B., Chappell, D., & Eberhart, L. (2021). Hypertonic saline versus mannitol for traumatic brain injury: A systematic review and meta-analysis with trial sequential analysis. *Journal of Neurosurgical Anesthesiology, 33*(1), 10–20. https://doi.org/10.1097/ANA.0000000000000644

Shi, J., Tan, L., Ye, J., & Hu, L. (2020). Hypertonic saline and mannitol in patients with traumatic brain injury: A systematic and meta-analysis. *Medicine, 99*(35), e21655. https://doi.org/10.1097/MD.0000000000021655

Silverberg, N. D., Iaccarino, M. A., Panenka, W. J., Iverson, G. L., McCulloch, K. L., Dams-O'Connor, K., Reed, N., McCrea, M., & American Congress of Rehabilitation Medicine Brain Injury Interdisciplinary Special Interest Group Mild TBI Task Force (2020). Management of concussion and mild traumatic brain injury: A synthesis of practice guidelines. *Archives of Physical Medicine and Rehabilitation, 101*(2), 382–393. https://doi.org/10.1016/j.apmr.2019.10.179

Sutherly, L. J., & Malloy, R. (2020). Risk factors of pediatric stroke. *Journal of Neuroscience Nursing: Journal of the American Association of Neuroscience Nurses, 52*(2), 58–60. https://doi.org/10.1097/JNN.0000000000000489

Swanson, D. (2015). Meningitis. *Pediatrics in Review, 36*(12), 514–526. https://doi.org/10.1542/pir.36-12-514

Sweeney, A. (2020). *Spinal cord and vertebral trauma in ENA's emergency nursing pediatric course* (5th ed.). Jones & Bartlett.

Tunkel, A. R., Glaser, C. A., Bloch, K. C., Sejvar, J. J., Marra, C. M., Roos, K. L., Hartman, B. J., Kaplan, S. L., Scheld, W. M., Whitley, R. J., & Infectious Diseases Society of America. (2008). The management of encephalitis: Clinical practice guidelines by the infectious diseases society of America. *Clinical Infectious Diseases: An Official Publication of the Infectious Diseases Society of America, 47*(3), 303–327. https://doi.org/10.1086/589747

Venkatesan, A., Tunkel, A. R., Bloch, K. C., Lauring, A. S., Sejvar, J., Bitnun, A., Stahl, J.-P., Mailles, A., Drebot, M., Rupprecht, C. E., Yoder, J., Cope, J. R., Wilson, M. R., Whitley, R. J., Sullivan, J., Granerod, J., Jones, C., Eastwood, K., Ward, K. N., . . . & International Encephalitis Consortium. (2013). Case definitions, diagnostic algorithms, and priorities in encephalitis: Consensus statement of the international encephalitis consortium. *Clinical Infectious Diseases, 57*(8), 1114–1128. https://doi.org/10.1093/cid/cit458

Vernon-Levett, P. (2019). Neurologic system. In M. C. Slota (Ed.), *AACN core curriculum for pediatric high acuity, progressive, and critical care nursing* (3rd ed., pp. 349–444). Springer Publishing Company.

Viscidi, E., Wang, N., Juneja, M., Bhan, I., Prada, C., James, D., Lallier, S., Makepeace, C., Laird, K., Eaton, S., Dilley, A., & Hall, S. (2021). The incidence of hydrocephalus among patients with and without spinal muscular atrophy (SMA): Results from a US electronic health records study. *Orphanet Journal of Rare Diseases, 16*, 207. https://doi.org/10.1186/s13023-021-01822-4

Weinberg, G. A. (2022, Septembe). Meningitis in children. In Merck & Co, Inc, *Merck manual: Consumer version*. https://www.merckmanuals.com/home/children-s-health-issues/bacterial-infections-in-infants-and-children/meningitis-in-children

Woods, K. S., Horvat, C. M., Kantawala, S., Simon, D. W., Rakkar, J., Kochanek, P. M., Clark, R., & Au, A. K. (2021). Intracranial and cerebral perfusion pressure thresholds associated with in hospital mortality across pediatric neurocritical care. *Pediatric Critical Care Medicine: A Journal of the Society of Critical Care Medicine and the World Federation of Pediatric Intensive and Critical Care Societies, 22*(2), 135–146. https://doi.org/10.1097/PCC.0000000000002618

World Health Organization. (2022, February 9). *Epilepsy*. https://www.who.int/news-room/fact-sheets/detail/epilepsy

Wright, Z., Larrew, T. W., & Eskandari, R. (2016). Pediatric hydrocephalus: Current state of diagnosis and treatment. *Pediatrics in Review, 37*(11), 478–490. https://doi.org/10.1542/pir.2015-0134

Behavioral and Psychosocial Review

Kimberly Garcia and Maryann Godshall

Children and adolescents are facing unprecedented psychosocial stressors, manifesting in complex behavioral symptoms. Pediatric critical care nurses will encounter patients whose behavioral or emotional disorders will lead to or result from an acute medical illness. It has been estimated that one in five children in the United States will develop a mental health disorder such as depression, anxiety, behavioral problem, or substance abuse (Gilbert, 2012). Prompt identification and intervention will allow the patient and healthcare team to focus on the medical consequences of the illness rather than the psychiatric symptoms that may impede care.

▶ ABUSE AND NEGLECT

As mandatory reporters, it is essential for the pediatric critical care nurse to accurately screen for the signs of abuse and neglect. Abuse may come in sexual, physical, verbal, or emotional forms. The abuse assessment requires the nurse to compare the reported mechanism of injury to the objective exam findings.

ABUSE: SIGNS AND SYMPTOMS

Children who are being physically abused may present with behavioral and/or physical symptoms of abuse. Behavioral symptoms of abuse may include fear, phobias, night terrors, or sleeping or eating difficulties. Infants may cry excessively or experience developmental delays. Developmental regression may be noted in young children. For school age children, social withdrawal, reduced concentration, and decreased school performance may be evident. School attendance may be affected, and it is important to inquire about the number and duration of absences, as children may not be sent to school if there are overt signs of physical abuse. Observing the interactions between the child and caregivers can provide important clues. The child may appear overly compliant and agreeable or hypervigilant, withdraw to touch, or appear afraid of their caregivers. The caregiver may present as overly protective or controlling and may attempt to oversee the child's contact with hospital staff, limiting time alone to disclose the abuse.

Characteristics of the abuser may include:

- exhibits little concern for the child
- has little interaction with the child
- blames the child
- is demanding
- sees the child as a burden to them
- wants the child to fulfill parental needs (like loving them)
- may be overly protective or controlling

When assessing for the physical indicators of abuse, it is necessary to consider if the reported mechanism of injury is consistent with the clinical presentation. Explanations may change and the caregiver may assign responsibility to the child or their siblings.

Children who are being abused often present with:

- somatic complaints that are vague or have no identifiable underlying etiology. Examples may include abdominal pain, headaches, or sore throat.
- unexplained burns, bites, bruises, or broken bones. Providers should screen carefully for these signs and note the presence of fading bruises.
- bald spots on their head
- injuries to the ears
- torn frenulum (from caregiver shoving a bottle in child's mouth forcefully)

When a child presents with burn injuries, it is essential for the critical care nurse to evaluate the burn pattern. Most accidental burns are scald burns that occur due to spillage and are located on the anterior body surfaces. These burns tend to be asymmetrical and may have obvious splash marks. Accidental contact burns occur when a hot object is touched, burning the palmar surface of the hand. Burns accidentally occurring due to falls tend to result in multiple irregular falls.

Burns that are highly suggestive of abuse include:

- immersion scald burns, particularly if symmetric and well-demarcated. Burns in a sock or glove pattern must be carefully assessed for abuse.
- symmetrically burned buttocks or genitalia
- contact burns in clear patterns may be caused by hot objects (cigarettes, clothing iron, curling irons, or hot cooking tools)

When a child presents with a fracture, detailed information regarding the injury must be obtained. **Fractures** that are suggestive of physical abuse include:

- posterior ribs
- scapula
- ribs
- sternal
- hand
- foot
- face
- various state of previous fracture healing

A long bone fracture is particularly concerning in a child <6 months old in that their bones are very pliable. It takes great force to break a young child's bones. The presence of a subdural hematoma, retinal hemorrhage, or an unexplained traumatic brain injury should cause significant concern.

Signs of sexual abuse must be thoroughly investigated. The child may have difficulty walking or sitting. Female children may experience recurrent urinary tract or yeast infections. Younger children may present with sophisticated knowledge of sexual activities. Sexually transmitted infections or pregnancy should elicit concern as well, especially in females younger than age 14.

NEGLECT: SIGNS AND SYMPTOMS

The physical clues of neglect may include:

- poor hygiene
- dental decay/carries
- failure to thrive
- poor weight gain
- malnutrition

Failure to thrive is an inadequate growth or growth failure. They typically fall below the fifth percentile. In this instance the nurse needs to:

- weigh the child
- take a dietary intake history
- conduct a home environment assessment
- observe attachment issues
- use increased calorie formulas
- vitamin supplementation
- provide for consistency in care

Failure to follow through on prior medical recommendations is an important consideration, including immunizations and vision/dental exams. The child may not be sent to school due to caregiver apathy, lack of initiative, addiction, or underlying psychiatric or medical pathology. Observing the appropriateness of the child's clothing for the season can provide important clues as well.

NURSING IMPLICATIONS AND TREATMENT

As mandatory reporters of abuse and neglect, it is essential that pediatric critical care nurses carefully observe for concerning symptoms. The interdisciplinary team should be involved in advocating for the child's physical and emotional well-being, ensuring that all concerns are investigated before the child returns to the home environment. For those families with limited resources to meet their child's needs, it is important to facilitate their access to community resources.

Clinical Pearl

The evaluation of possible child abuse or neglect requires the nurse to use critical thinking skills. Asking detailed questions about the mechanism of injury can provide important details that the nurse can compare to the available physical evidence.

▶ AGGRESSION AND AGITATION

Children and adolescents requiring critical nursing care may present with behavioral symptoms, including aggression and agitation. The cause for these outbursts may include such pathology as an underlying conduct disorder, mood disorder, drug use, or intellectual/neurodevelopmental disability. The overstimulating environment of the emergency department or critical care unit may trigger behavioral episodes. Further, the child may experience fear or panic and, with immature coping skills, may result to primitive coping mechanisms that are emotion focused. Regardless of the etiology, these episodes jeopardize the safety of the patient and hospital staff, disrupt medical care, and may necessitate the use of restraints.

AGGRESSION AND AGITATION IN CHILDREN ON THE SPECTRUM

Children with autism spectrum disorder (ASD) can be particularly sensitive to over-stimulation. Aggression can be triggered by anxiety. They may present with increased sensitivity to bright lights and may have reduced tolerance for the active hospital environment. The child on the spectrum is at higher risk for elopement and additional oversight may be necessary to assure their safety.

NURSING IMPLICATIONS AND TREATMENT

There are no universally accepted guidelines for the treatment of agitation and aggression in children. However, the pediatric critical care nurse should strive for using the least restrictive options for managing the symptoms, such as using medications to manage the symptoms rather than restraints or seclusion. Strive to understand the root cause of the episode. By identifying the antecedents, the nurse can implement strategies to reduce further exposure to the trigger. Modifying the environment, when possible, may be helpful. Reducing stimuli while displaying care and comfort for the child can offer positive benefits. Protecting the patient, hospital staff, family members, and other patients remains the highest priority when responding to a behavioral emergency.

De-escalation techniques can be particularly useful when a child is experiencing acute aggression or agitation. Strategies such as respecting personal space; maintaining neutral tone and body language; remaining calm, rational, and professional; and focusing on the thoughts behind the feelings may be helpful. Remind the patient that the nurse is there to help, and encourage the patient, when possible, to articulate their needs (Gerson et al., 2019).

For children who are on the autism spectrum, the pediatric critical care nurse must consider whether the patient's basic needs are being met, including providing adequate food and fluids. Treatment interventions directed at reducing the patient's anxiety level may be very effective. Providing sensory stimulation can offer a therapeutic distraction that may reduce anxiety and the associated behavioral symptoms.

Clinical Pearl

Physical restraints should be utilized only when necessary as they are particularly dangerous when used with children. Emphasis should be placed on reducing the restraints as quickly as possible, while maintaining the safety of the patient and the medical milieu.

▶ ANXIETY

Anxiety disorders are among the most common psychiatric disorders in children and adolescents. While observable behaviors of anxiety are considered normal in infants, anxiety symptoms in children predict a range of psychological difficulties in adolescence, including anxiety disorders, panic disorders, and depressive disorders.

SIGNS AND SYMPTOMS

Anxiety is characterized by recurrent emotional and physiologic arousal in response to perceived dangers or threats. Children may experience separation anxiety, which is thought to have survival value and, therefore, is a natural human response. However, these symptoms should diminish by 2 and 1/2 years of age. Thereafter, children may present with intense or persistent fear, shyness, or social withdrawal when faced with unfamiliar people or places. The physical symptoms of anxiety include higher than average resting heart rate, higher than average morning cortisol levels, and low heart rate variability. Separation anxiety disorder is associated with developmentally inappropriate and excessive anxiety related to separation from the primary caregiver.

In comparison, children with generalized anxiety disorder experience significant distress in their activities of daily living, often focused on the child's fear of perceived incompetence in social or academic settings. Additional symptoms may include restlessness, fatigue, thought blocking, irritability, muscle tension, or sleep disturbances. Physical indicators may include tachycardia, shortness of breath, or dizziness. The child may report feelings of becoming diaphoretic while experiencing nausea and/or loose stools. Children with anxiety tend to worry excessively about potential natural disasters and may seek excessive reassurance regarding their performance in activities such as academics or sports.

Children may present with social anxiety disorder, also known as social phobia. Affected children experience intense discomfort or even distress while in social situations. They often report an intense fear of scrutiny or humiliation. Children may demonstrate their distress in the form of crying, tantrums, avoidance, freezing, or even becoming mute (Kodish et al., 2011).

NURSING IMPLICATIONS AND TREATMENT

It is important for the nurse to recognize anxiety. Unmanaged and untreated anxiety can lead to agitation in the patient or family. Parents and children may have different anxiety triggers. In some families, parents and children may provoke an anxiety reaction in each other. If escalating anxiety is not recognized or managed, it can lead to increased agitation. Oftentimes, agitation is the precipitant to aggression. Anxiety is much easier to manage and treat than overt aggression. If anxiety is repeated and not treated, they can go on to develop an anxiety disorder (Gilbert, 2012).

Due to the similarities in the various anxiety disorders, the treatment approach is consistent. Typically, a multimodal approach is necessary, which includes psychotherapy, family psychosocial interventions, and pharmacologic interventions. Research supports the efficacy of combining cognitive behavioral therapy with a selective serotonin reuptake inhibitor (SSRI). To date, there are no medications specifically approved for anxiety disorders by the U.S. Food and Drug Administration (FDA). Regardless, SSRIs are still considered the first line treatment for anxiolysis. Three SSRIs are FDA-approved for use in obsessive-compulsive disorder in children, including sertraline (Zoloft), fluoxetine (Prozac), and fluvoxamine (Luvox). Thus, these agents are frequently used in pediatric anxiety disorders (Kodish et al., 2011).

Antidepressants, including SSRIs, have a black box warning indicating an increased risk of suicidality in children and adolescents. This warning is based on a meta-analysis of 372 randomized clinical trials involving nearly 100,000 participants. Suicidal thinking or suicidal behavior was reported in 4% of patients receiving an antidepressant versus 2% of patients in the control group. Thus, it is essential for the pediatric critical care nurse to monitor for any symptoms of suicidality when treating a patient who is taking an SSRI (Friedman, 2014).

Clinical Pearl

The black box warning associated with all antidepressants has caused concern for patients, families, and healthcare providers. While the risk for suicidal thoughts or behaviors is low, it is essential to monitor for suicidality and report symptoms promptly if present.

▶ SELF-HARM

Self-harm occurs when an individual hurts themselves on purpose. This may first occur when a child transitions into adolescence. At this time, the child thinks more about their feelings, pays more attention to their peers, and worries about "fitting in." Self-harm is a symptom of distress for young people, and it has been on the rise in the past 20 years in the United States. Young girls or women are more likely than boys to self-harm. When boys self-harm the behavior is more consistent and severe.

Forms of self-harm include:

- cutting, scratching, carving, branding, or making marks on the body
- picking at scabs so they do not heal
- pulling hair out
- burning or grazing oneself
- biting, bruising, or hitting oneself
- hitting a part of the body on something hard

Some children may try to hide their self-harm as they are often ashamed of their behavior. They also worry that people will be angry with them or reject them. Sometimes, they don't really understand why they are harming themselves.

SIGNS AND SYMPTOMS

BEHAVIORAL SIGNS

- changes in sleep or eating patterns
- loss of interest in activities they used to enjoy
- isolating and no longer seeing friends
- avoiding activities like swimming where their legs, arms, or torso can be seen. They often wear clothes to cover their arms and legs.
- skipping school or their performance declines at school
- hiding objects like razor blades, knives, lighters, and matches

EMOTIONAL SIGNS

- mood swings
- exhibiting irritability
- having temper tantrums or outbursts
- feeling sad, empty, or hopeless

PHYSICAL SIGNS

- having injuries they can't or won't explain
- being agitated
- seeming slow and lethargic or lacking energy to do things

NURSING IMPLICATIONS AND TREATMENT

The pediatric critical care nurse is in a prime situation to notice this behavior. If noticed the nurse should approach the child in a calm, nonthreatening manner. Be respectful, don't judge, and use active listening. This may help to gain insight into the child's thoughts and feelings. Provide medical care for the cuts or injuries. Some of the things you might say to the child are:

- "I noticed scars on your arms. Can you tell me how you got them?"
- "I can see you are very upset. You might be scared. Together we can figure this out."
- "The fact that you are self-harming tells me you are very upset. I'm not going to ask you many questions, but I do want to help you when you are ready."

Some teens may need help from psychological services. A consult and counseling can help to uncover underlying issues in the child and their home environment. Nurses are at a prime place to notice or screen for unnatural marks on the body and get children and adolescents the help they so desperately need (Raising Children Network AU, 2022).

Self-harm occurs in the context of many psychiatric disorders. In adolescents, the most common comorbid disorders are major depressive disorder (MDD) and borderline personality disorder (BPD).

▶ DEPRESSION

Depressive disorders in children and adolescents represent a significant public health concern, with significant impact on their cognitive, social, and psychological development. It is estimated that approximately 2% to 3% of children and up to 8% of adolescents experience a depressive disorder. As such, early identification and treatment are essential. Depressive disorders are thought to have a genetic and environmental component. While most children with depression never attempt or complete suicide, suicide remains a significant risk and is a primary concern for healthcare providers.

SIGNS AND SYMPTOMS

In prepubescent children, a major depressive episode is often associated with somatic complaints, psychomotor agitation, and hallucinations. Anhedonia, the inability to experience enjoyment, is possible in children but is more commonly seen in adolescents. Both children and adolescents may present with irritability. Adolescents are prone to social withdrawal, isolation from peers, and increased school difficulties. They may become less attentive to their appearance and may demonstrate increased sensitivity to rejection by peers or romantic interests.

Depressed children may struggle to articulate their symptoms. Specifically, rather than endorsing sadness, they may describe anger or frustration. In general, children may report, or caregivers may observe, difficulty concentrating, slowed thinking, lack of interest or motivation, fatigue, ruminations, and preoccupations. Depressive disorders may be misdiagnosed as learning disorders if a careful history is not obtained.

Suicidal ideations, gestures, and attempts are sometimes, but not always, associated with depressive disorders. The risk is highest in children and adolescents with severe mood disorders. Suicide attempts are more likely to be made by females; however, males are more likely to complete suicide. Adolescents who are impulsive are at particularly high risk for attempting suicide.

NURSING IMPLICATIONS AND TREATMENT

Children with a history of depression should be comprehensively evaluated for the presence of suicidal ideations or an increase in depressive symptoms. Typically, the treatment of choice involves a combination of cognitive behavioral therapy and an antidepressant. Currently, only fluoxetine (Prozac) is FDA-approved for the treatment of pediatric depression age 8 and older. Escitalopram (Lexapro) is approved for use in children age 8 and older (U.S. FDA, 2004). Sertraline (Zoloft), fluvoxamine (Luvox), and clomipramine (Anafranil) are often used because they are FDA-approved for use in children for obsessive-compulsive disorder (U.S. FDA, 2004). Psychiatric hospitalization is indicated for patients experiencing increased depressive symptoms with suicidal or homicidal ideations.

Clinical Pearls

Screening for suicidality is essential in the critical care environment. It is important to document the presence or absence of suicidal ideations, particularly for children who have a history of a psychiatric disorder. Having an existing psychiatric disorder (including substance abuse) is the single most important factor associated with increased suicide risk.

▶ SUBSTANCE USE DISORDERS

Substance use disorder is a growing public health concern. Children and adolescents are most likely to use tobacco, alcohol, or marijuana. However, there are many additional substances that may be abused, including cocaine, heroin, club drugs, and lysergic acid diethylamide (LSD), among others. There is an association between early antisocial behavior, conduct disorder, and substance abuse. It is hypothesized that early intervention for children with social deviance or antisocial behavior may reduce the risk for subsequent substance use.

SIGNS AND SYMPTOMS

The diagnostic criteria for substance use disorders are the same for children and adults. However, making the diagnosis can be challenging in children due to the vague symptom presentation. The symptoms pointing to substance use are often nonspecific, making the diagnosis more challenging for healthcare providers. Substance use exists along a continuum, ranging from episodic to routine use, experimentation to dependence. It is important for the critical care nurse to investigate suspicions before reaching conclusions.

Symptoms suggestive of possible substance use include changes in academic performance, nonspecific somatic or physical complaints, changes in familial relationships, changes in peer group, unexplained phone calls, or changes in personal hygiene. Because these symptoms overlap with those seen in depressive disorders, additional exploration is necessary. Adolescents with subpar social skills may use substances as a modality to enhance their comfort with their peer group.

NURSING IMPLICATIONS AND TREATMENT

Before treatment can be implemented, effective screening and identification is necessary. Utilizing the Screening, Brief Intervention, and Referral to Treatment (SBIRT) framework has been recommended, particularly for school-based programming. SBIRT is based on the premise of motivational interviewing, serving to motivate the individual to make changes.

Adolescents with drug or alcohol use disorders may seek treatment in inpatient units, residential treatment facilities, halfway houses, group homes, partial hospitalization programs, or outpatient treatment centers. For those adolescents with a co-occurring psychiatric disorder, dual-diagnosis treatment may be most beneficial.

The treatment of adolescent substance users is evolving. Typically, treatment is approached from a similar paradigm to that used for adults. Buprenorphine is FDA-approved for use in adolescents age 16 years and older who have opiate use disorder. Adolescent treatment typically adopts a multimodal approach, including addressing both substance use and underlying psychiatric symptoms (Stahl, 2021).

Clinical Pearl

Observe for subtle changes in behavior and academic performance. Family members often express concern that the child is depressed since the presenting symptoms are similar.

▶ POST-INTENSIVE CARE DISORDER/SYNDROME

The first dedicated pediatric ICU (PICU) was established in Europe in 1955, and pediatric critical care has only been established as a specialty since 1981. Since that time, major contributions have been made with significant improvements in mortality. As more children survive critical illnesses the focus is changing on their functionality, quality of life, and post-discharge survival. This evolving PICU landscape and advancing technology has coincided with an increasing number of critically ill children with underlying chronic illnesses who sometimes require a prolonged PICU admission. Research has shown that these children experience effects for years after their PICU admission, some more than a decade. This has been described as Post-Intensive Care Disorder or Post-Intensive Care Syndrome (PICS). Residual morbidity in children after a PICU admission can affect four domains:

- physical
- cognitive
- emotional
- social

These domains can be influenced by how the child was pre-admission at their baseline status, the PICU experience itself, and their caregiver, parent, or family unit. See Table 11.1 for examples in each of these domains. This should make PICU caregivers aware of their impact they have on multiple aspects of the lives of the children they care for daily.

Table 11.1 Post-Intensive Care Syndrome Domains and Examples

Domains	Examples
Physical health	Technology dependence Chronic pain Generalized weakness or fatigue Anxiety Sleep disorders Feeding disorders
Cognitive health	Reduced attention ability Memory issues Decreased or alternate communication methods Altered school achievement
Emotional health	Anxiety Depression Abnormal memories/heightened fear Posttraumatic stress disorders symptoms Behavioral problems, acting out
Social health	Loss of friends/peer relationships Loss of social identity Social anxiety School absenteeism Strained family ties and relationships Decreased interest in participation in things
PICS (family issues)	Parent, caregiver, sibling stress and psychiatric complications Job loss Financial strain and instability Food or housing instability Strained personal and family relationships

PICS, Post-Intensive Care Syndrome.
Source: Table adapted from Woodruff, A. G., & Choong, K. (2021). Long-term outcomes and the post-intensive care syndrome in critically ill children: A North American perspective. *Children, 8*, 254. https://doi.org/10.3390/children8040254

Screening and recognition of PICS is evolving in pediatrics. Much research has been done in adults. The ABCDEF bundle is a harm-reduction tool initially used in adults to promote ICU liberation and limit chronic morbidity. This bundle of interventions includes **a**ssessing, preventing, and managing pain; **b**oth spontaneous breathing and awakening trials; **c**hoice of analgesia and sedation; assessing, preventing, and managing **d**elirium; **e**arly mobility and exercise; and **f**amily engagement and empowerment. This worked well in adults and in pediatrics, the evidence is accumulating. Several recent and ongoing studies evaluating early mobilization, delirium prevention, and sedation protocols reveal promising results (Woodruff & Choong, 2021).

Another promising outcome is having PICU patients write "PICU diaries." Patients, along with their family, provide a daily journal or diary, along with photographs and drawings by the child about the child's condition while in the PICU. Having these diaries allow the child to recall events and help them process what they have experienced. In adults, this has helped with decreasing symptoms of posttraumatic stress disorder (PTSD), depression, and anxiety post-ICU experience (Woodruff & Choong, 2021).

POSTTRAUMATIC STRESS DISORDER

As medical technology increases, a growing number of children are surviving critical illness' in the PICU. These children, and their caregivers, are developing severe psychiatric disorders afterward. Some of these include PTSD, depression, and anxiety. This can impair a complete recovery after their PICU stay. Acute stress disorder (ASD) is usually diagnosed **within 30 days** of an overwhelming traumatic event. These children experience symptoms in four domains. They are:

- feelings of dissociation
- reexperiencing the trauma
- avoidance
- hyperarousal

PTSD is diagnosed when these symptoms last for **more than a month** and cause significant functional impairment. PTSD has been associated with serious morbidity and all-cause mortality in larger population studies. Previous research has found that acute and posttraumatic stress (PTS) reactions among PICU families is associated with circumstances surrounding the child's hospitalization and demographic factors.

According to Erçin-Swearinger et al. (2022), hospital-related factors include:

- long length of stay
- unexpected admission
- having prior admissions

Bronner et al. (2008) suggest three components and what may contribute to the development of PTSD in children after a PICU admission.

1. Characteristics of the medical event
   - an unexpected life-threatening event
   - if they are exposed to a high number of invasive procedures
   - stay for a longer duration of time
2. Characteristics of the child
   - female sex
   - younger at the age of trauma
   - psychological vulnerability
   - history of exposure to stressful events and having premorbid problems
3. Characteristics of the family
   - parental stress reaction
   - coping style

One study looked at psychiatric outcomes of children and parents following a PICU admission. They found that 21% of children and 27% of the parents developed PTSD symptoms at 6 to 12 months after discharge as compared with 0% for both after being discharged from a general pediatric unit. A British study found that a significant minority of parents and children had persistent posttraumatic stress symptoms 12 months after discharge (Bronner et al., 2008). One thing found to help them was parental support and guidance. A program called Creating Opportunities for Parent Empowerment (COPE) is an intervention that is started during the hospital admission. Information was given on the anticipated range of behaviors and emotions that children typically display during and after hospitalization. Therapeutic play techniques were taught to the parents to help their child process what was happening. This provided parents with emotional support and empowered them to deal with a potential developing psychopathology.

By helping children process their traumatic experience, COPE has helped patients develop ways of coping through use of puppet play, therapeutic medical play, and social stories. These interventions were found to address a key factor in anxiety that caused children to avoid situations and circumstances perceived as a threat or uncomfortable to them, which they may have perceived as a "life threatening" danger (Baker & Gledhill, 2017). This, along with the use of child life therapists who can facilitate these interventions, is vital in helping a child deal with a critical care experience. It is also helpful if child psychotherapy is instituted particularly for the child who witnessed a traumatic event.

NURSING IMPLICATIONS AND TREATMENT

Nursing implications for PICS and PTSD are first to provide atraumatic care as much as possible so there is no source of stress. The nurse must advocate for adequate sedation for procedures and treatments. Then, perhaps after the fact, screen for it and recognize it. Then implement multidisciplinary treatment using psychological services where available. The following are therapies often utilized:

- start with a child life therapist and work with art, music, and journaling or narratives
- **cognitive therapy**: talking with a mental health expert
- **exposure therapy (ET)**: Mental health experts help patients deal with frightening events in a safe environment. Exposure can be real or imagined. Virtual reality is helping in this realm.

■ **eye movement desensitization and reprocessing (EMDR):** used in conjunction with exposure therapy, EDMR uses a series of guided eye movements that help patients process traumatic events and assist them in managing their reactions. Light therapy may also be implemented with this.

■ **psychopharmacotherapy**: utilizing medications for anxiety and/or depression to help cope

The nurse's primary role is to recognize and coordinate care, then facilitate strategies recommended by psychiatric services.

▶ RESPONDING TO BEHAVIORAL EMERGENCIES

The nurse responding to behavioral aggression, "acting out," or patients attempting to self-harm can be very stressful. The nurse should first remain calm and make sure all people are safe, including themselves. Call for assistance from peers and/or security. Many institutions have behavioral response teams (BERTS) or call a rapid response team (RRT). The key with these teams is first to de-escalate the situation. According to Choi et al. (2019), one might use:

■ good verbal communication

■ calming techniques

■ a change in the environmental/milieu

■ **Establish a rapport with the child and family**. Rapport facilitates communication, builds trust, builds respect, increases cooperation, and reduces anxiety. General strategies for building rapport are:

  ● avoid being judgmental

  ● avoid authoritarian techniques

  ● avoid direct confrontation with the child or the parent

  ● give choices and explain options

  ● provide a comfortable environment and allow the family a sense of control

  ● avoid taking sides with either the parent of the child

  ● avoid power struggles or placing restrictions on the child

  ● set clear boundaries

  ● check back with the child and family to keep them informed (Gilbert, 2012)

The team might recommend:

■ medication administration

■ medication changes (if the reaction was precipitated by a medication reaction/interaction)

Last resort should be:

■ physical restraints (physical hold, violent or nonviolent restraints). Restraints can lead to further functional decline.

■ seclusion

■ transfer to a psychiatric unit if the patient is unresponsive to other interventions (Gaynes et al., 2016)

CASE STUDY 1

A 4-year-old boy is admitted to the critical care unit, where he has a prolonged stay. He has a history of autism spectrum disorder. At the time of his admission, he was extremely withdrawn and would only use gestures to make his needs known. He would not seek comfort when he experienced painful medical interventions. Previously, when the nurses would call his name, he rarely responded. In time, he appears more engaged and starts quietly speaking to the nurses using short sentences. He starts looking to the nursing staff for comfort and has even asked for assistance.

1. The pediatric critical care nurse suspects that which of the following is the most likely explanation?
   A. He has a moderately low intelligence quotient (IQ).
   B. He may have been neglected prior to admission.
   C. He has fetal alcohol syndrome rather than autism.
   D. His autistic symptoms will wax and wane throughout his illness.

2. A child goes into cardiac arrest. The pediatric ICU (PICU) has numerous healthcare providers who arrived to assist. Alarms are sounding loudly. The environment is chaotic. Meanwhile, the 4-year-old boy previously described proceeds to start screaming. He is observed with his hands covering his ears while he is rocking forward and back in the hospital bed. Which of the following actions taken by the nurse next is most appropriate?
   A. Administer a low dose benzodiazepine.
   B. Request an as-needed dose of olanzapine.
   C. Provide the patient with a fidget spinner and partially close his door.
   D. Recommend the patient receive a combination of medication and therapy.

3. Meanwhile, during the code and while the 4-year-old patient is experiencing increased symptoms, a new admission arrives on the unit. This patient, age 14, has a history of a conduct disorder and is detoxing from opiates after receiving naloxone (Narcan) in the ED. The patient refuses to stay in his bed. He proceeds to knock down the intravenous (IV) pole and throws his water cup across the room. He threatens to hit the nurse if she approaches him again. Which of the following actions taken next by the nurse are most appropriate?
   A. Prepare intramuscular (IM) olanzapine and lorazepam.
   B. Approach the patient using de-escalating techniques.
   C. Administer his scheduled dose of oral olanzapine early.
   D. Request security come to the unit prior to approaching the patient.

(See answers next page.)

ANSWERS TO CASE STUDY QUESTIONS

1. B) He may have been neglected prior to admission.
In this case, the child was likely neglected prior to admission. Due to neglect, he was developmentally delayed and was not accustomed to receiving caregiver comfort. Once he was in a more supportive environment, he started to progress. He was playing with the other children and seeking comfort from select staff, which is not usual for a child with autism. Autistic symptoms do not tend to wax and wane, especially with that degree of improvement. There is no indication of a moderately low IQ.

2. C) Provide the patient with a fidget spinner and partially close his door.
In this example, the child is experiencing overstimulation. Rather than treating his symptoms pharmacologically, the nurse should reduce stimulation by partially closing the door and providing sensory stimulation, such as a fidget spinner, to serve as a distraction from the chaotic healthcare environment.

3. D) Request security come to the unit prior to approaching the patient.
Safety is always the highest priority. If the nurse approaches the patient with IM injections currently, he is likely to further escalate, placing the patient and the nurse in jeopardy. Oral medications will not become effective quickly and approaching the patient with medication may exacerbate the episode. De-escalation techniques should not be implemented until the environment has been secured.

CASE STUDY 2

1. A 5-year-old girl is admitted to the burn center. According to the girl's mother, the patient was running around the kitchen while the mother was cooking. The girl bumped into her mother while her mother was taking a large pot of boiling water off the stove. The contents of the pot proceeded to spray across the room, burning the girl. Which of the following injury presentations is most consistent with the mother's report?
   A. Burns appearing in a circumferential "sock" pattern
   B. Symmetrical immersion burns to both hands
   C. Asymmetrical burns with evidence of splash marks
   D. Symmetrical, well-demarcated burns to both palmar surfaces

2. Upon reviewing the girl's past medical records, the nurse notices a concerning history of fractures. Which of the following injuries would most likely be considered accidental rather than due to abuse?
   A. Facial fracture after falling down the steps
   B. Anterior rib fractures after falling off her bike
   C. Long bone fracture at age 3 months after rolling off couch
   D. Subdural hematoma at age 2 after the car seat malfunctioned

(*See answers next page.*)

ANSWERS TO CASE STUDY QUESTIONS

1. C) Asymmetrical burns with evidence of splash marks

Accidental burns tend to present with asymmetrical patterns. Additionally, given the description provided by the patient's mother, the nurse would anticipate splash marks. Symmetrical, well-demarcated, and stocking pattern burns are inconsistent with the reported mechanism of injury.

2. B) Anterior rib fractures after falling off her bike

In this question, the injury that is most likely to be considered accidental is the fracture of anterior ribs after calling off her bike. Facial fractures are unlikely to be sustained while falling down the stairs. Long bone fractures at age 6 months or younger are highly suggestive of abuse. A subdural hematoma would be considered suspicious as well.

KNOWLEDGE CHECK: CHAPTER 11

1. A 10-year-old has presented with an abrupt change in academic performance, which has elicited concern from their teacher. Prior to this semester, the child was considered an ideal student. Now, they appear distracted, have not been completing homework assignments, and have come to school without their books. The teacher has observed the student daydreaming in class and, upon approaching them, the child is easily startled. The child's presentation is most consistent with which of the following explanations?
   A. The child has an undiagnosed depressive disorder.
   B. The child has attention deficit hyperactivity disorder (ADHD), inattentive-type.
   C. The child is experiencing an acute stressor that warrants further investigation.
   D. The child is possibly the victim of bullying and a meeting with their caregiver should be scheduled immediately.

2. The nurse receives a phone call from the mother of a 7-year-old who is receiving treatment for autism spectrum disorder. The mother indicates that her child's behavioral symptoms were increased and, as a result, she kept them home from school for the past week. The mother needs a note authorizing the child's absence and permitting their return to school. Which of the following actions made by the nurse is most appropriate in this situation?
   A. Recommend the patient be evaluated prior to getting the note.
   B. Recommend the patient's medications be adjusted before they return to school.
   C. Provide the patient's mother with the contact information for the crisis hotline and review the child's crisis plan with her in detail.
   D. Instruct the mother that in the future, she is to contact the psychiatrist when the symptoms start, not when they have resolved.

3. Which of the following statements regarding symptoms of sexual abuse in children is most accurate?
   A. Sexual abuse is not associated with eating disorders.
   B. A child touching their own genitalia is considered abnormal.
   C. Children who have been sexually abused may imitate sexual acts.
   D. Somatic symptoms are not characteristic of sexual abuse in children.

4. Compared to older adolescents, younger children with major depressive disorder (MDD) may be more likely to experience which of the following symptoms?
   A. Insomnia
   B. Depressed mood
   C. Somatic complaints
   D. Lack of concentration

5. A 5-year-old boy is admitted to the pediatric ICU (PICU). The nurse notices several bruises on his arms that are in various stages of healing. The nurse asks the boy about his bruises and the boy responded, "Sometimes he (meaning the stepfather) needs to teach me a lesson." Which of the following statements made next by the nurse is most appropriate?
   A. "No adult should ever harm you."
   B. "What does it mean to be taught a lesson?"
   C. "Are there other children at home who are being taught a lesson, too?"
   D. "I am contacting protective services so they can come to your home to speak with your stepfather."

6. While all burns observed in children and adolescents are concerning, certain burn patterns are more suspicious for abuse. Of the following scenarios, which pattern is considered least suspicious for abuse?
   A. Symmetrically burned buttocks
   B. Asymmetrically burned anterior body surface
   C. Bilateral hand/foot burns in a stocking/glove distribution
   D. Small round burns covering the posterior buttocks or back

(See answers next page.)

1. C) The child is experiencing an acute stressor that warrants further investigation.
In this example, the child is experiencing an abrupt change. ADHD symptoms are not abrupt in their onset, and the diagnosis require specific details regarding the timing of symptoms. The fact that the child is startled upon approach may be suggestive of an underlying stressor. The child's presentation may be consistent with depression; however, no associated symptoms are reported that are specific for depression. The assumption that the child is being bullied is inconsistent with the information provided in the scenario and, therefore, should be considered a "reach." Instead, this abrupt change, coupled with the child's startled, stressed/anxious appearing reaction, is suggestive that they are experiencing an acute stressor.

2. A) Recommend the patient be evaluated prior to getting the note.
In this example, all options are technically appropriate; however, the MOST appropriate action is to insist the child is seen/visualized before authorizing a return to school. Children who are absent from school for a week could be recovering from bruises or other signs of abuse. Authorizing a 1-week long absence without visualizing the child may result in physical abuse going unrecognized.The fact that the parent did not seek a medication adjustment or treatment intervention at the onset of the issue warrants further consideration and concern. A medication change may be very appropriate. The nurse should also address the patient's crisis plan. However, this parent was not looking for an intervention when she made the decision to not send the child to school for 1 week, which is very suspicious. Authorizing the child's return to school without seeing them is a disservice to the child and could be considered negligence on the part of the nurse.

3. C) Children who have been sexually abused may imitate sexual acts.
One of the most compelling signs of sexual abuse is a child imitating sexual acts. Sexual abuse in children often present with somatic complaints and/or eating disorders. A child touching their own genitalia is considered normal growth and development, within reason.

4. C) Somatic complaints
Children with MDD are more likely to present with somatic complaints. The younger child's inability to express feelings of depression may contribute. Insomnia, depressed mood, and lack of concentration are reported in older adolescents as well.

5. B) "What does it mean to be taught a lesson?"
In this example, the child has not disclosed what it means to be "taught a lesson." In an abuse investigation, it is very important to not draw conclusions based on one's own perception. Ask the child to explain what that means, especially since the concept of "teaching him a lesson" is likely one he has heard an adult use. The other options are based on the conclusion that the child is being abused before this information is disclosed. The needs more details before assuming the child is being abused and, therefore, at this time it is not appropriate to contact proactive services, tell the child he should not be harmed, or to assess whether other children are being abused in the home.

6. B) Asymmetrically burned anterior body surface
The burns that are symmetrical, including those in a sock/glove distribution (e.g., hands held in scalding water) or posteriorly burned buttocks are highly suspicious for abuse. A series of small burns is suggestive of cigarette burns. It is important to look at placement. Posterior body surface burns are rarely self-inflicted. Instead, an asymmetrically burned anterior body surface area could be indicative that a child spilled something on themselves.

7. Which of the following strategies is most likely to reduce behavioral symptoms associated with autism spectrum disorder?
   A. Providing minimal stimulation
   B. Providing diversity in their routine and schedule
   C. Providing opportunities to socialize with other children
   D. Providing activities that provide both auditory and sensory stimulation

8. A child during the admission phase begins "acting out." The parents become very agitated with the child's behaviors. Which of the following responses would be best by the nurse?
   A. "This is a hospital, that type of behavior will not be tolerated here."
   B. "Mr. and Mrs. X, can't you get your child under control?"
   C. "Why don't we turn on the television and divert their attention."
   D. "Hey, I see that you are upset, can you tell me what you are thinking about?"

9. Which of the following represents the best thing to do in establishing a rapport with a child?
   A. Always take sides with the child during a confrontation.
   B. Directly confront the child when they exhibit bad behavior.
   C. Avoid being judgmental.
   D. Give specific instructions, allowing for no choices.

10. Which of the following would be symptoms exhibited by a child who has Post-Intensive Care Syndrome (PICS)?
   A. Anxiety and depression
   B. Having a large social circle of friends
   C. Consistent attendance at school
   D. Focused and high achievement at school

(See answers next page.)

7. A) Providing minimal stimulation

Behavioral symptoms associated with autism spectrum disorder are often due to the child being over-stimulated. Adherence to a routine and schedule is often therapeutic and differing from the usual routine can exacerbate behavioral episodes. Providing the opportunity to socialize with other children during a behavioral outburst is likely to exacerbate the situation, not improve it. Thus, providing minimal stimulation is most likely to reduce behavioral symptoms associated with autism.

8. D) "Hey, I see that you are upset, can you tell me what you are thinking about?"

The most therapeutic response is to validate child by acknowledging that they are upset and then asking them questions to explore their feelings. Telling a child their behavior is unacceptable for a hospital or asking parents why they cannot control their child would not lead to establishing a rapport or therapeutic relationship. Those responses are insensitive and accusatory. Ignoring the child's behavior is not therapeutic.

9. C) Avoid being judgmental.

Of the provided responses, avoiding being judgmental will lead to establishing rapport with the child and family. A nurse should never take sides or be confrontational. This will escalate the situation. By not allowing for no choices, the nurse hurts the chances of forming a therapeutic relationship.

10. A) Anxiety and depression

Anxiety and depression are symptoms of PICS. Social isolation, and not having a large circle of friends would also be a symptom. The child would not be focused and have frequent absences from school. They would also not be a high achiever at school and may struggle.

REFERENCES

Baker, S., & Gledhill, J. (2017). Systematic review of interventions to reduce psychiatric morbidity in parents and children after PICU admissions. *Pediatric Critical Care Medicine, 18*, 343–348. https://doi.org/10.1097/PCC.0000000000001096

Bronner, M., Knoester, H., Bos, A., Last, B., & Grootenhuis, M. (2008). Posttraumatic stress disorder (PTSD) in children after Paediatric intensive care treatment compared to children who survived a major fire disaster. *Child and Adolescent Psychiatry and Mental Health, 2*(9). https://doi.org/10.1186/1753-2000-2-9

Choi, K. R., Omery, A. K., & Watkins, A. M. (2019). An integrative literature review of psychiatric rapid response teams and their implementation for de-escalating behavioral crises in nonpsychiatric hospital settings. Journal of Nursing Administration, *49*(6), 297–302. https://doi.org/10.1097/NNA.0000000000000756

Erçin-Swearinger, H., Lindhorst, T., Curtis, J. R., Starks, H., & Doore, A.Z. (2022). Acute and posttraumatic stress in family members of children with a prolonged stay in a PICU: Secondary analysis of a randomized trial. *Pediatric Critical Care Medicine, 23*(4), 306–314. https://doi.org/10.1097/PCC.0000000000002913

Friedman, R. A. (2014). Antidepressants' black-box warning—10 years later. *New England Journal of Medicine, 371*, 1666–1668. https://doi.org/10.1056/NEJMp1408480

Gaynes, B. N., Brown, C., Lux, L. J., Brownley, K., Van Dorn, R., Edlund, M., Coker-Schwimmer, E., Zarzar, T., Sheitman, B., Weber, R. P., Viswanathan, M., & Lohr, K. N. (2016). *Strategies to de-escalate aggressive behavior in psychiatric patients*. Agency for Healthcare Research and Quality. https://www.ncbi.nlm.nih.gov/books/NBK379388/

Gerson, R., Malas, N., Feuer, V., Silver, G. H., Prasad, R., & Mroczkowski, M. M. (2019). Best practices for evaluation and treatment of agitated children and adolescents (BETA) in the emergency department: Consensus statement on the American Association for Emergency Psychiatry. *Western Journal of Emergency Medicine: Integrating Emergency Care With Population Health, 20*(2), 409–418. https://doi.org/10.5811/westjem.2019.1.41344

Gilbert, S. (2012). Beyond acting out: Managing pediatric psychiatric emergencies in the emergency department. *Advanced Emergency Nursing Journal, 34*(2), 147–163. https://doi.org/10.1097/TME.0b013e318251a2ea

Kodish, I., Rockhill, C., & Varley, C. (2011). Pharmacotherapy for anxiety disorders in children and adolescents. *Dialogues in Clinical Neuroscience, 13*(4), 439–452. https://doi.org/10.31887/DCNS.2011.13.4/ikodish

Raising Children Network AU. (2022). *Self-harm and teenagers*. The Australian Parenting Website. https://raisingchildren.net.au/teens/mental-health-physical-health/mental-health-disorders-concerns/self-harm

Stahl, S. (2021). *Stahl's essential psychopharmacology* (5th ed.). Cambridge.

U.S. Food and Drug Administration. (2004). *Suicidality in children and adolescents being treated with antidepressant medications*. https://www.fda.gov/drugs/postmarket-drug-safety-information-patients-and-providers/suicidality-children-and-adolescents-being-treated-antidepressant-medications

Woodruff, A. G., & Choong, K. (2021). Long-term outcomes and the post-intensive care syndrome in critically ill children: A North American perspective. *Children, 8*, 254. https://doi.org/10.3390/children8040254

Multisystem Review

Katherine Thompson and Stephanie Morgenstern

 ACID–BASE IMBALANCE

Acid–base imbalance is observed with many different disorders and disease states in pediatric patients. The balance of acids and bases within the body is largely maintained by the respiratory and renal systems via excretion of carbon dioxide and nonvolatile acids, respectively (Emmett & Palmer, 2020). Maintenance of acid–base balance is essential for numerous physiological processes including regulating electrolyte levels, cardiovascular autonomic regulation, and function of the endocrine system (Curley & Moloney-Harmon, 2001).

There are two types of acid–base derangements: acidosis (pH <7.35) or alkalosis (pH >7.45). The pH of blood is determined by the relationship of the partial pressure of carbon dioxide (PCO_2) and serum bicarbonate (HCO_3; Emmett & Palmer, 2020). Further categorization of acidosis and alkalosis is based on primary causes, metabolic or respiratory, with four cardinal acid–base imbalances (Table 12.1).

Table 12.1 Blood Gas Interpretation

	pH	CO_2 (mmHg)	HCO_3 (mEq/L)
Normal	7.35–7.45	35–45	22–26
Respiratory acidosis	↓	↑	NORMAL
Metabolic acidosis	↓	NORMAL	↓
Respiratory alkalosis	↑	↓	NORMAL
Metabolic alkalosis	↑	NORMAL	↑

Abbreviations: CO_2, carbon dioxide; HCO_3, serum bicarbonate.
Source: Curley, M. A., & Moloney-Harmon, P. A. (Eds.). (2001). *Critical care nursing of infants and children* (2nd ed.). Saunders Company.

- metabolic (reflected in the HCO_3 level)
  - metabolic acidosis
  - metabolic alkalosis
- respiratory (reflected in the PCO_2 level)
  - respiratory acidosis
  - respiratory alkalosis

The body uses compensatory mechanisms to restore normal pH levels, when possible. The respiratory and renal systems respond to the four types of acid–base imbalances by raising or lowering levels of PCO_2 or HCO_3 to attempt to maintain a normal pH (Emmett & Palmer, 2020). Chronic disorders that result in acid–base imbalance allow more time for compensation to occur whereas acute insults do not allow time for the compensation response (Curley & Moloney-Harmon, 2001).

In some patients with multisystem problems, there may be more than one type of acid–base imbalance occurring simultaneously. Mixed acid–base disorders occur when there are two types of acid–base imbalance present at once (e.g., respiratory alkalosis and metabolic acidosis). If the two disorders drive the pH in the same direction (respiratory acidosis and metabolic acidosis), it may result in more severe consequences for the patient, as compensation is not possible (Curley & Moloney-Harmon, 2001).

Accurate assessment of acid–base imbalances is critical in anticipating patient needs and implementing interventions to improve outcomes. Identifying the underlying etiology of the imbalance(s) is necessary to mitigate further derangements and clinical complications (Table 12.2).

Table 12.2 Associated Causes of Acid–Base Imbalances

Respiratory Acidosis	Respiratory Alkalosis	Metabolic Acidosis	Metabolic Alkalosis
Croup	Alcohol intoxication	Cardiovascular collapse	Vomiting
Asthma	Salicylate toxin	Diabetic ketoacidosis	Gastrointestinal
Bronchiolitis	Meningitis	Lactic acidosis	suctioning
Chronic lung disease	Neurovascular accidents	Congenital enzymatic	Diuretics
Pneumonia	Encephalitis	defects	Excessive steroid use
Massive pulmonary embolus	Pulmonary edema	Renal failure	Renal failure
Pneumothorax	Pneumonia	Hepatic failure	Extracellular volume
Myasthenia gravis	Hyperthyroidism	Diarrhea	depletion
Guillain-Barré syndrome	Sepsis	Acetazolamide use	Cushing syndrome
Brainstem injury	Anemia	Extracellular volume	Hyperaldosteronism
Cerebral trauma	High altitude	expansion	Laxative use disorder
Opioids	Hyperventilation	Adrenal disorders	Hypokalemia
Cardiac arrest	Anxiety	Intake of chloride	Hypochloremia
Inadequate mechanical	Mechanical ventilation	containing compounds	Hypocalcemia
ventilation	Hepatic failure	Hyperalimentation	Cystic fibrosis
Hyperalimentation with high carbohydrate content	Congestive heart failure with hypoxemia		

Source: Curley, M. A., & Moloney-Harmon, P. A. (Eds.). (2001). *Critical care nursing of infants and children* (2nd ed.). Saunders Company.

▶ RESPIRATORY ACIDOSIS

Respiratory acidosis is an imbalance in which:
- ↓ pH
- ↑ PCO_2
- HCO_3 may be normal or elevated when compensation from the renal system is present (Curley & Moloney-Harmon, 2001).

PATHOPHYSIOLOGY

Hypoventilation and **carbon dioxide (CO_2) retention** are the driving forces of respiratory acidosis. There are several different conditions that result in decreased ventilation including acute/chronic obstructive airway disorders, restrictive pulmonary disorders, neuromuscular disorders, central nervous system depressants, and iatrogenic causes (Curley & Moloney-Harmon, 2001).

SIGNS AND SYMPTOMS

Symptoms of respiratory acidosis vary greatly depending on the severity. They include:
- dyspnea
- shallow respirations
- tachycardia
- headache
- altered level of consciousness
- nausea and vomiting
- **seizures**
- Hypoxemia is a late sign of respiratory acidosis and is a warning sign of impending respiratory failure (Curley & Moloney-Harmon, 2001).

    Additional effects of CO_2 retention include cerebral vasodilation, which can precipitate headaches, and pulmonary vasoconstriction, which can impede pulmonary blood flow and worsen the respiratory condition (Curley & Moloney-Harmon, 2001).

NURSING IMPLICATIONS AND TREATMENT

LABS AND DIAGNOSTICS

- blood gas (arterial, venous, or capillary) analysis
- Supporting lab work may include serum chemistries.

TREATMENT AND MANAGEMENT

- Immediate treatment includes **supporting ventilation and clearance of CO_2** (Curley & Moloney-Harmon, 2001). Identification of the causative factor is essential to completely treat respiratory acidosis. Treating the underlying disorder causing hypoventilation and CO_2 retention is the most effective method to restore acid–base balance (Patel & Sharma, 2021).
- **Compensation mechanism:** An increase in serum bicarbonate will increase the pH and attempt to restore the blood to a normal physiological range (González et al., 2018).

COMPLICATIONS

- There are several complications associated with respiratory acidosis including poor cardiac contractility, decreased threshold for ventricular fibrillation, seizure, respiratory failure, and cardiac/respiratory arrest (Patel & Sharma, 2021).

▶ RESPIRATORY ALKALOSIS

Respiratory alkalosis is an acid–base imbalance in which:

- ↑pH
- ↓ PCO_2
- HCO_3 may be normal or decreased when compensation from the renal system is present (Curley & Moloney-Harmon, 2001).

PATHOPHYSIOLOGY

Hyperventilation and **CO_2 deficit** are the driving forces of respiratory alkalosis. There are several different conditions that result in hyperventilation including:

- intoxications
- increased intracranial pressure
- hypoxia
- pulmonary embolism
- pneumothorax
- increased metabolic demand
- sepsis
- anxiety
- high altitude (Brinkman & Sharma, 2022)

SIGNS AND SYMPTOMS

Symptoms of respiratory alkalosis include:

- cardiac dysrhythmias
- hypotension
- syncope
- confusion
- hyperreflexia
- twitching
- seizures (Curley & Moloney-Harmon, 2001)

There can be paresthesias throughout the body, particularly in distal extremities, caused by vasoconstriction related to hypocapnia. Neurologic concerns can arise in the setting of cerebral vasoconstriction as a result of the hypocapnia. Seizures, syncope, and decreased level of consciousness may occur. The alkalotic state encourages binding of calcium and resultant hypocalcemia. This hypocalcemia can manifest as muscle cramping, twitching, and tetany (Curley & Moloney-Harmon, 2001).

NURSING IMPLICATIONS AND TREATMENT

LABS AND DIAGNOSTICS

Clinical assessments of hyperventilation and associated neurological or musculoskeletal symptoms can be interpreted in real time as manifestations of respiratory alkalosis (Curley & Moloney-Harmon, 2001).

Confirmatory laboratory testing would be in the form of blood gas (arterial, peripheral, or capillary) analysis.

TREATMENT AND MANAGEMENT

- Correcting respiratory alkalosis requires restoring a normal breathing pattern and treating the causative factor. Interventions targeting the hyperventilation alone include sedation and breathing exercises (Curley & Moloney-Harmon, 2001). Instructing the patient to breathe into a paper bag allows for the rebreathing of exhaled CO_2 and can also slow the respiratory rate. As with all forms of acid–base imbalance, treatment of the underlying cause is imperative to resolving the derangement. In severe cases, intubation and mechanical ventilation with the addition of CO_2 can be used to correct the acid–base imbalance.
- Compensation mechanism: A decrease in serum bicarbonate will decrease the pH and attempt to restore the blood to a normal physiological range. This happens over the course of days and is not effective for acute respiratory alkalosis events (Brinkman & Sharma, 2022).

COMPLICATIONS

Complications include neurological damage related to seizures and injuries sustained due to syncope or altered levels of consciousness (Curley & Moloney-Harmon, 2001).

▶ METABOLIC ACIDOSIS

Metabolic acidosis is an acid–base imbalance in which:

- ↓ pH
- PCO_2 may be normal or decreased when compensation from the respiratory system is present (Curley & Moloney-Harmon, 2001).
- ↓ HCO_3

PATHOPHYSIOLOGY

There are **four main mechanisms that result in bicarbonate deficiency**:

- increased production of acid
- decreased excretion of acid
- ingestion of an acid
- bicarbonate losses from the renal or gastrointestinal (GI) systems (Burger & Schaller, 2021)

The serum pH falls as the bicarbonate cannot balance the acidic environment due to excess acid or continued loss of HCO_3 (Curley & Moloney-Harmon, 2001). Some etiologies of **increased acid** include:

- diabetic ketoacidosis
- lactic acidosis
- toxins
- starvation
- hepatic failure
- renal failure (Curley & Moloney-Harmon, 2001)

Some etiologies of **bicarbonate loss** include:

- diarrhea
- hyperalimentation
- acetazolamide use
- adrenal disorders resulting mineralocorticoid deficiencies (Curley & Moloney-Harmon, 2001)

SIGNS AND SYMPTOMS

Patients in metabolic acidosis present in various ways. Some common findings include:

- increased respiratory rate
- tachycardia
- poor perfusion
- altered level of consciousness
- nausea and vomiting
- abdominal discomfort (Curley & Moloney-Harmon, 2001)

In cases of severe metabolic acidosis, signs and symptoms include:

■ Kussmaul respirations
■ bradycardia
■ seizures (Curley & Moloney-Harmon, 2001)

NURSING IMPLICATIONS AND TREATMENT

LABS AND DIAGNOSTICS

■ blood gas (arterial, peripheral, or capillary) analysis
■ electrolyte assessment, including anion gap (Burger & Schaller, 2021)

Further investigation into the causative disorder is required to identify intervention strategies. An important step in diagnosing this acid–base imbalance is obtaining a thorough history to determine if the patient has any recent/chronic history of conditions with predisposition to metabolic acidosis (Burger & Schaller, 2021).

TREATMENT AND MANAGEMENT

Treatment is focused on addressing the underlying cause of metabolic acidosis.

■ correcting fluid balance and electrolytes
■ providing adequate ventilation (Curley & Moloney-Harmon, 2001)
■ Administration of sodium bicarbonate can be used with caution in severe acidosis (pH <7.0 to 7.2), and when there is worsening cardiac function evidenced by poor perfusion and hypotension (Curley & Moloney-Harmon, 2001). Sodium bicarbonate is metabolized into H_2O and CO_2; therefore, supporting ventilation is necessary to avoid further increase to the carbon dioxide levels in the body (Senewiratne et al., 2021).
■ **Compensation mechanism**: A decrease in PCO_2 will increase the pH and attempt to restore the blood to a normal physiological range. The increased respiratory rate compensatory mechanism is activated quickly in the setting of metabolic acidosis to eliminate CO_2 (Curley & Moloney-Harmon, 2001).

COMPLICATIONS

There are several complications that are associated with metabolic acidosis. They include:

■ poor cardiac contractility
■ decreased threshold for ventricular fibrillation
■ decreased cerebral perfusion
■ respiratory distress (Curley & Moloney-Harmon, 2001)

▶ METABOLIC ALKALOSIS

Metabolic alkalosis is an acid–base imbalance in which:

■ ↑pH
■ PCO_2 may be normal or increased when compensation from the respiratory system is present (Curley & Moloney-Harmon, 2001).
■ ↑ HCO_3

PATHOPHYSIOLOGY

Mechanisms that can result in an excess of serum HCO_3 include:

■ processes that cause intracellular shifts of hydrogen ions (e.g., hypokalemia)
■ GI loss of hydrogen
■ renal loss of hydrogen
■ retention of bicarbonate
■ contraction alkalosis (Brinkman & Sharma, 2021)

Examples of these mechanisms include:

■ vomiting
■ suctioning gastric contents
■ diuretic use
■ hypokalemia
■ hypocalcemia
■ exogenous bicarbonate administration

- excess mineralocorticoid syndromes
- renal failure
- laxative overuse (Curley & Moloney-Harmon, 2001)

SIGNS AND SYMPTOMS

Symptoms of metabolic alkalosis include:
- altered level of consciousness
- hypotension
- hyperreflexia
- muscle twitching
- decreased perfusion
- seizures (Curley & Moloney-Harmon, 2001)
- GI distress is typically indicative of the cause of the alkalosis rather than a symptom (Brinkman & Sharma, 2021).

Monitoring of neurologic status, fluid balance, and perfusion are key assessments in patients with metabolic alkalosis (Curley & Moloney-Harmon, 2001).

NURSING IMPLICATIONS AND TREATMENT

LABS AND DIAGNOSTICS

Pertinent laboratory values in metabolic alkalosis are blood gas (arterial, peripheral, or capillary) analysis and electrolyte assessment (Curley & Moloney-Harmon, 2001).

Further investigation into the causative disorder is required to identify intervention strategies. An important step in diagnosing this acid–base imbalance is obtaining a thorough history to determine if the patient has any recent/chronic history of conditions with predisposition to metabolic alkalosis (Curley & Moloney-Harmon, 2001).

TREATMENT AND MANAGEMENT

Treatment is focused on addressing the underlying cause of the metabolic alkalosis. General principles include:
- correcting fluid balance and electrolytes
- supporting renal excretion of bicarbonate
- providing comfort measures for GI distress (Curley & Moloney-Harmon, 2001)
- **Compensation mechanism:** An increase in PCO_2 will decrease the pH and attempt to restore the blood to a normal physiological range. The decreased respiratory rate compensatory mechanism is activated quickly in the setting of metabolic acidosis to eliminate CO_2, though is not effective in correcting the alkalosis and presents additional concerns of hypoxia (Curley & Moloney-Harmon, 2001).

SHOCK

Shock is a general term encompassing the failure of oxygen delivery to the body's cells and tissues (**decreased perfusion**). When patients experience shock, their *oxygen consumption exceeds the delivery, resulting in anaerobic metabolism*. Oxygen delivery depends both on blood flow and oxygenation and thus any condition that affects either can result in shock (Nichols & Shaffner, 2016).

Shock can be classified based on the mechanism of derangement:
- **hypovolemic** (loss of intravascular blood volume)
- **cardiogenic** (due to heart problems). See Chapter 2.
- **distributive**
  - **septic** (due to infections)
  - **anaphylactic** (due to an allergic reaction)
  - **neurogenic** (caused by damage to the autonomic nervous system; the parasympathetic system is unregulated). See Chapter 10.
- **obstructive** (physical obstruction of blood circulation and inadequate blood oxygenation). See Chapter 2.

Shock can present as **compensated** or **uncompensated** with the distinguishing feature being the body's ability to achieve adequate blood pressure for tissue perfusion and oxygen delivery. Once this balance is unable to be maintained uncompensated shock is present (Slota, 2019). Regardless, prompt recognition and treatment are essential to preventing morbidity and mortality.

▶ ANAPHYLACTIC SHOCK

Anaphylaxis results from an acute and systemic allergic or hypersensitivity reaction to a substance (e.g., plant, food, toxin) with an associated inflammatory response (Nichols & Shaffner, 2016). Varied presentations are common, including within different episodes for the same patient (Sicherer & Simons, 2017).

PATHOPHYSIOLOGY

Following exposure to the trigger, inflammatory mediators (immunoglobin E [IgE]), histamine, serotonin, prostaglandin, and bradykinin) begin to circulate. This inflammation causes venous and arterial dilation, increased capillary permeability, and pulmonary vasoconstriction (Slota, 2019). Ultimately, the maldistribution of blood and oxygen results in poor perfusion of the cells and tissues (Nichols & Shaffner, 2016).

SIGNS AND SYMPTOMS

Symptoms of anaphylaxis will usually begin within 5 to 10 minutes of exposure (Slota, 2019) but can take up to several hours (Sicherer & Simons, 2017). Symptoms include:
- anxiety
- agitation
- nausea
- vomiting
- hives
- angioedema
- Stridor or wheezing with associated shortness of breath can be early signs (Slota, 2019).

Defining features of anaphylaxis include:
- skin and/or mucosal involvement with itching
- flushing
- urticaria
- swelling of the lips/tongue/uvula with potential respiratory compromise and/or reduced blood pressure (Sicherer & Simons, 2017)

During the **compensated phase** of anaphylactic shock, vasoconstriction increases peripheral and systemic vascular resistance to maintain adequate blood pressure. Additional assessment findings include mottled, pale, and cool skin; delayed capillary refill; diaphoresis; tachycardia; and decreased urine output. Alterations in mental status may be seen in the compensated phase as restlessness or lethargy, and in the uncompensated phase as loss of consciousness.

Uncompensated shock reveals low blood pressure and low central venous pressure (CVP) and may result in myocardial ischemia detectable on electrocardiogram. If shock goes untreated, multiorgan ischemia may occur with additional assessment findings associated with the affected organ or organ system (Slota, 2019).

NURSING IMPLICATIONS AND TREATMENT

LABS AND DIAGNOSTICS

Diagnosis for anaphylaxis is based on the clinical features.

TREATMENT AND MANAGEMENT

Initial management is focused on maintaining oxygenation and ventilation.
- maintained airway
- supplemental oxygenation
- intravenous (IV) access
- epinephrine (EpiPen®)
- antihistamines

■ corticosteroids

■ Bronchial dilators can be used to relax the smooth muscles of the airway and reduce laryngeal edema.

Edema can progress quickly, warranting frequent assessment and prompt endotracheal intubation and mechanical ventilation may be indicated (Slota, 2019). In more severe cases, emergent tracheostomy placement may be needed to secure a patent airway. As with other shock types, circulation should be supported with fluid, as indicated by the patient's perfusion.

Intramuscular Epinephrine

Intramuscular (IM) injection of epinephrine is the foundation of treatment for anaphylaxis. There is no contraindication to the administration of epinephrine and the preferred route is IM (Ferdman, 2021).

■ 0.01 mg/kg/dose (0.01 mL/kg/dose of 1 mg/mL concentration epinephrine)

■ max 0.3 mg/dose for infants and children, 0.5 mg/dose for adolescents

■ Administer as soon as possible and repeat every 5 to 15 minutes.

■ Administer via the anterolateral aspect of the thigh (Lee, 2021).

AutoInjector

A prepared, single dose of epinephrine (such as EpiPen®, EpiPen Jr®, AUVI-Q®, and generics):

■ **infants and children 15 to 30 kg:** 0.15 mg prefilled syringe IM (EpiPen Jr®)

■ **infants and children 7.5 to 15 kg:** 0.1 mg prefilled syringe IM (AUVI-Q®)

■ **children and adolescents ≥30 kg:** 0.3 mg prefilled syringe IM (EpiPen®)

■ Administer as soon as possible and repeat every 5 to 15 minutes.

■ Administer via the anterolateral aspect of the thigh, through clothing if necessary (Prescribers Digital Reference, (2022).

Intravenous Epinephrine

IV epinephrine is, although effective, not preferred over IM epinephrine. Consider IV epinephrine for cardiac arrest or severe hypotension unresponsive to IM epinephrine (Ferdman, 2021).

■ 0.01 mg/kg/dose (0.1 mL/kg/dose of a 0.1 mg/mL concentration epinephrine)

■ max 0.3 to 0.5 mg/dose

■ Administer as soon as possible and may repeat every 3 to 5 minutes (Lee, 2021).

Close monitoring for rebound symptomatology is required as 6% to 19% require second doses and up to 11% experience biphasic reactions with symptoms recurring hours after an initial exposure (Sicherer & Simons, 2017). Additional supportive medications include antihistamines to counter the effect of histamine release and corticosteroid for the anti-inflammatory effects (Slota, 2019).

COMPLICATIONS

Complications of anaphylactic shock are consistent with those seen in other shock presentations including multiorgan failure, disseminated intravascular coagulation (DIC), and loss of limb or life (Slota, 2019).

▶ SEPSIS/SEPTIC SHOCK

Sepsis definitions have evolved over time. In pediatrics, the 2005 international pediatric sepsis consensus conference published stages as sepsis, severe sepsis, and septic shock based on adult criteria at the time (Table 12.3). Despite the 2016 update to the adult guidelines (Sepsis-3) moving to a two-tiered sepsis and septic shock categorization, most pediatric literature continued to refer to the prior stages defined in 2005. However, with the most recent Surviving Sepsis guidelines for children published in 2020 the categories were defined as septic shock (severe infection leading to cardiovascular dysfunction including hypotension, need for vasoactive medications, or impaired perfusion) and "sepsis-associated organ dysfunction" (severe infection leading to cardiovascular and/or noncardiovascular organ dysfunction).

In other recent publications, sepsis has been defined as a life-threatening organ dysfunction caused by severe infection. Septic shock has been differentiated from sepsis based on cardiovascular dysfunction that persists despite fluid resuscitation (Hilarius et al., 2020). As the leading cause of morbidity, mortality, and healthcare utilization in the world, appropriate and timely sepsis treatment is paramount. The mortality rates range significantly (4%–50%), with many deaths occurring in the first 48 to 72 hours. Geography, severity of illness, and risk factors weigh considerably in these numbers (Weiss et al., 2020).

Table 12.3 Sepsis Categories

International Pediatric Sepsis Consensus Conference (2005)	
SIRS	Two or more of the following: ■ Core temperature >38.5°C (101°F) or <36°C (96.8°F) ■ Tachycardia, >2 *SD* above age-specific norms not otherwise explained OR bradycardia defined as a heart rate in the 10th percentile for age in children <1 year old not otherwise explained ■ Respiratory rate (mean) >2 *SD* above age-specific norms or acute need for mechanical ventilation ■ Leukocyte count elevated or depressed for age (unrelated to chemotherapy) OR >10% immature neutrophils
Sepsis	SIRS in the presence of confirmed or suspected infection
Severe sepsis	Sepsis plus one of the following: ■ Cardiovascular dysfunction ■ Acute respiratory distress syndrome ■ Two or more other organ dysfunctions
Septic shock	Sepsis and cardiovascular organ dysfunction
Surviving Sepsis Campaign International Guidelines for Management of Septic Shock and Sepsis-Associated Organ Dysfunction in Children (2020)	
Sepsis-associated organ dysfunction	Severe infection leading to cardiovascular and/or noncardiovascular organ dysfunction
Septic shock	Severe infection leading to cardiovascular dysfunction (hypotension, need for vasoactive therapies, impaired perfusion)

SD, standard deviation; SIRS, systemic inflammatory response syndrome.

PATHOPHYSIOLOGY

Systemic inflammatory response syndrome (SIRS) can occur due to infection, large **trauma** or **surgical interventions, hypoperfusion states,** or **thermal injuries**. In each of these instances, a systemic release of inflammatory mediators (cytokines) from the body (endogenous), and/or the invading organism (exogenous) occurs. While the body attempts to fight the infection, or heal from the injury, pro-inflammatory mediators circulate resulting in:
■ vasodilation
■ endothelial damage with resulting capillary leak
■ hypovolemia
■ cardiac dysfunction
■ maldistributed blood and oxygen delivery
■ alterations in the coagulation cascade (hyper- or hypo-coagulable states may occur leading to DIC; Slota, 2019)

Septic shock, like other forms of shock, includes a maldistribution of blood and oxygen resulting in poor perfusion of the cells and tissues (Nichols & Shaffner, 2016). In sepsis/septic shock, the causative agent is severe infection from a bacteria, virus, mycoplasma, or fungus. In children, sepsis is most often attributed to gram-positive or gram-negative bacteria (Weiss et al., 2020); however, it is notable that the causative agent is often never isolated (Hilarius et al., 2020).

SIGNS AND SYMPTOMS

Prompt recognition of sepsis is necessary to enable appropriate and timely treatment. Frequent and thorough physical assessment and strict measurement of intake and output is critical prior to and throughout treatment for sepsis. Symptomology is often nonspecific and may vary based on the age or developmental status of the child (Hilarius et al., 2020).

Presenting symptoms may include:
■ fever or hypothermia (<36°C/96.8°F)
■ rigors
■ tachypnea

- tachycardia (or less commonly, bradycardia in neonates/infants)
- delayed capillary refill
- mottled and cool or flushed and ruddy skin
- weak or bounding pulses
- decreased oral intake
- altered mental status (e.g., irritability, confusion, lethargy, etc.)

Patients may be hypotensive or, in compensated shock, normotensive (Balamuth et al., 2017; Hilarius et al., 2020).

In pediatrics, it is particularly important to evaluate vital signs against age-specific normal values to identify derangements (Tables 12.4 and 12.5).

Table 12.4 Normal Vital Signs by Age

Age	Heart Rate	Blood Pressure	Respiratory Rate
Premie	120–170	55–75/35–45*	40–70
0–3 months	110–160	65–85/45–55	30–60
3–6 months	100–150	70–90/50–65	30–45
6–12 months	90–130	80–100/55–65	25–40
1–3 years	80–125	90–105/55–70	20–30
3–6 years	70–115	95–110/60–75	20–25
6–12 years	60–100	100–120/60–75	14–22
>12 years	60–100	100–120/70–80	12–18

*Gestational age approximates normal mean airway pressure (MAP).
Source: Kleinman, K., McDaniel, L., & Molley, M. (2021). *The Harriet Lane handbook* (22nd ed.). Elsevier.

Table 12.5 Estimated Blood Pressure Percentiles by Age

Measurement	50%	5%
Systolic	90 + (age × 2)	Neonate: 60
		1 month–1 year: 70
		2–10 years: 70 + (age × 2)
		>10 years: <90
MAP	55 + (age × 1.5)	40 + (age × 1.5)

MAP, mean airway pressure.
Source: Kleinman, K., McDaniel, L., & Molley, M. (2021). *The Harriet Lane handbook* (22nd ed.). Elsevier.

Assessment of past medical history and risk factors for sepsis is critical. Patients at high risk for sepsis may be predisposed to more rapid deterioration. These include patients with immunocompromising conditions (i.e., asplenia, oncologic diagnosis, post bone marrow transplant), or those with chronic disease or recent hospitalization. Patients with open wounds or those with invasive catheters (e.g., central venous catheters, urinary catheters, peritoneal dialysis catheters) require assessment of these sites for signs of localized infection such as redness, drainage, or warmth. It is important to note that severely neutropenic patients may not show these typical signs of local infection (Balamuth et al., 2017; Hilarius et al., 2020).

Ongoing assessment should include continuous assessment for responsiveness to treatment and signs of associated complications. Special attention should be given to cardiovascular and respiratory assessments including heart rate and rhythm, perfusion (capillary refill, pulse, skin color), blood pressure, heart sounds, lung sounds, respiratory rate and work of breathing, and oxygenation. Urine output is often used as a surrogate marker of end organ perfusion and should be monitored closely.

NURSING IMPLICATIONS AND TREATMENT

LABS AND DIAGNOSTICS

Laboratory and diagnostic studies should not significantly delay treatment. **Blood cultures** are the gold standard for identification of pathogens in the bloodstream and should be obtained as early as possible after sepsis is suspected. Additional cultures may be indicated based on risk factors, and may include urine cultures, wound cultures, or tracheal aspirate. *Ideally, all cultures are obtained prior to antibiotic initiation, but they should not delay treatment* (Weiss et al., 2020).

Blood **lactate levels** may be useful as a marker of maldistribution of blood flow or oxygen. In children, most studies support levels of >2 to 4 mmol/L as clinically significant (Weiss et al., 2020). This is not a diagnostic value but may be useful in understanding the severity of shock, and in guiding resuscitation.

Additional laboratory values can be used to identify organ dysfunction or further support the diagnosis of sepsis. Complete blood counts (CBC) with differential may show an immune system response such as increased white blood cells; however, this alone is not a strong predictor of sepsis (Hilarius et al., 2020). Metabolic panels, liver function panels, blood urea nitrogen (BUN), and creatinine can identify organ dysfunction.

TREATMENT AND MANAGEMENT

Antimicrobial therapy should be administered within *1 hour* of sepsis recognition for those presenting in shock, and within *3 hours* for those without shock. As mentioned, cultures can assist with antimicrobial type and duration selection, but initial therapy should have broad pathogen coverage. More than one antimicrobial is often used to cover all possible pathogens until blood culture sensitivities result. Once the pathogen(s) is identified, therapy should be narrowed. If no pathogen is identified, a patient's presentation and current condition should be considered by the multidisciplinary team to determine if narrowing or stopping antimicrobial therapy is appropriate (Box 12.1; Weiss et al., 2020). If the source of infection is one that can be controlled via a procedure, it should be conducted as soon as possible (Weiss et al., 2020). Examples may include debridement of wounds, or removal of an infected invasive catheter.

Box 12.1 Septic Shock Hour 1 Interventions

- Initiate fluid resuscitation (10–20 mL/kg increments, to a total of 40–60 mL/kg in the first hour)
- Measure lactate level to allow trend to guide fluid resuscitation
- Obtain blood cultures
- Initiate broad-spectrum antibiotics
- Initiate vasoactive medications if age-specific hypotension or evidence of abnormal perfusion persists despite fluid resuscitation

Source: Weiss, S., Peters, M. J., Alhazzani, W., Agus, M. S. D., Flori, H. R., Inwald, D. P., Nadel, S., Schlapbach, L. J., Tasker, R. C., Argent, A. C., Brierley, J., Carcillo, J., Carrol, E. D., Carroll, C. L., Cheifetz, I. R., Choong, K., Cies, C. J., Cruz, A. T., De Luca, D., . . . Tissieres, P. (2020). Surviving sepsis campaign international guidelines for the management of septic shock and sepsis-associated organ dysfunction in children. *Pediatric Critical Care Medicine, 21*(2), e52–e106. https://doi.org/10.1097/PCC.0000000000002197

Fluid resuscitation should be initiated immediately following recognition of sepsis and concurrent to the previously mentioned therapies. The **rapid administration of isotonic crystalloid fluid (Lactated Ringer's [LR] or normal saline solution [NSS]) in increments of 10 to 20 mL/kg up to 40 to 60 mL/kg in the initial hour is recommended.** Recent studies support the use of buffered isotonic IV fluids, such as LR, over 0.9% saline for the initial fluid resuscitation of septic shock. Albumin has not been found to improve patient outcomes and is not recommended during initial resuscitation. Fluid administration should be titrated to clinical end points of cardiac output such as blood pressure (typically the 5%–50% for age), heart rate, and urine output (0.5–1.0 mL/kg/hr). If signs of fluid overload develop fluid administration should be halted. In areas where critical care is unavailable, more conservative fluid administration is recommended (no more than 40 mL/kg; Weiss et al., 2020).

Patients experiencing septic shock should have continuous blood pressure monitoring via arterial catheter, and where available, ancillary modalities of cardiac output measurement/estimation (ultrasound Doppler, pulse contour analysis, ScvO2 measurement). Most patients in septic shock will require a central venous catheter (CVC) for administration of fluids and/or vasoactive medications, but treatment may be initiated or completed via peripheral venous access if a CVC is not available (Weiss et al., 2020).

Vasoactive infusions should be used when fluid resuscitation alone is unable to achieve adequate cardiac output or age-appropriate blood pressures. **Epinephrine** or **norepinephrine** are recommended as first-line vasoactive medications. In patients requiring high doses of the first-line agent, addition of another catecholamine or a vasopressin infusion is indicated. Heart rate, blood pressure, pulse quality, capillary refill, and urine output should be monitored closely throughout treatment (Weiss et al., 2020). For a summary of first-line treatments to be completed in the first hour following septic shock identification, see Box 12.1.

> **Clinical Pearl**
>
> SvO2 vs. ScvO2: Venous oxygenation measurements taken at the pulmonary artery are called mixed venous oxygen saturation, or SvO2, while measurements taken at the superior vena cava are called central venous oxygen saturation, or ScvO2.

For patients with refractory shock despite antimicrobial therapy, adequate fluid resuscitation, and vasoactive infusions, additional treatment and management strategies include intubation and mechanical ventilation to reduce metabolic demand and intravenous corticosteroids to treat adrenal insufficiency. **Extracorporeal membrane oxygenation (ECMO)** may be used in the treatment of septic shock as rescue therapy for those unresponsive to all treatments (venoarterial [VA] ECMO) or for of sepsis-induced acute respiratory distress syndrome (venovenous [VV] ECMO; Weiss et al., 2020).

Other care considerations during treatment of septic shock include:
- targeting normal **blood calcium** levels to optimize myocardial contractility
- use of **antipyretics** to reduce the metabolic demand associated with fever
- **early enteral nutrition** for those without contraindications
- **red blood cell administration** for patients with hemoglobin concentrations ≤7 g/dL
- **Continuous renal replacement therapy** (CRRT) may be indicated to treat renal failure or fluid overload that is unresponsive to diuretic therapies.

COMPLICATIONS
- organ or multiorgan failure
- DIC
- loss of limb or life

Complications from treatment may also occur and can include allergic reactions to medications and/or fluid overload.

▶ HYPOVOLEMIC SHOCK

Hypovolemic shock is the most common cause of shock in children and is characterized by poor perfusion related to decreased intravascular volume (Pomerantz, 2022). There are two main categories of fluid loss that can lead to a hypovolemic state, and at extreme deficits, can lead to shock.
- **Intravascular losses** that can lead to hypovolemia include hemorrhage, third-space losses, nephrotic syndrome, and capillary leak syndrome (Curley & Moloney-Harmon, 2001).
- **Extravascular losses** that can result in hypovolemia occur in the form of GI losses such as diarrhea and vomiting (Pomerantz, 2022).

PATHOPHYSIOLOGY

In a low flow, low volume state there is decreased venous return to the heart, decreased preload, and thereby stroke volume (Curley & Moloney-Harmon, 2001). With a reduced stroke volume, compensatory tachycardia and increase in systemic vascular resistance (SVR) develop to maintain cardiac output and shunt blood to vital organs (Curley & Moloney-Harmon, 2001). This compensation often maintains an adequate blood pressure until approximately 25% of the intravascular volume has been lost (Curley & Moloney-Harmon, 2001). When the body can no longer compensate for the volume loss, perfusion decreases to the body, organs and tissues are deprived of oxygen, resulting in a shock state (Pomerantz, 2022).

NURSING IMPLICATIONS AND TREATMENT

ASSESSMENT

Symptoms of hypovolemic shock vary based on the progression of shock and can present in all body systems. Obtaining a thorough history is necessary to identify causative factors. Symptoms include:
- tachycardia
- hypotension

- Neurologic signs include a spectrum of findings from confusion and agitation, to obtunded or unresponsive (Curley & Moloney-Harmon, 2001).
- Skin may be dry, cool, and pale or mottled.
- Peripheral pulses will be diminished.
- Capillary refill time will be >*2 seconds* (Curley & Moloney-Harmon, 2001).
- Decrease in urine output may be one of the earliest notable signs of a hypovolemic state (Curley & Moloney-Harmon, 2001). Low urine output is classified as <0.5 to 1 mL/kg/hr for infants and <2 mL/kg/hr for children (Curley & Moloney-Harmon, 2001). Of note, hypovolemic shock caused by dehydration presents with several classic assessment findings including sunken fontanel, poor skin turgor, and dry mucous membranes (Curley & Moloney-Harmon, 2001).

The initial compensatory response is tachycardia. The increase in SVR (afterload) results in a vasoconstriction, which elevates blood pressure and may show a narrowed pulse pressure (Curley & Moloney-Harmon, 2001). Over time, the body cannot compensate for the volume loss, and hypotension will develop. It is important to note that **hypotension is a late sign of hypovolemic shock** (Curley & Moloney-Harmon, 2001).

LABS AND DIAGNOSTICS

Laboratory studies helpful in evaluating hypovolemic shock secondary to GI losses include:
- electrolyte levels
- blood gas
- lactate level
- blood glucose
- urinalysis including specific gravity (Pomerantz, 2022)

Laboratory studies helpful in evaluating hypovolemic shock secondary to hemorrhage include:
- hemoglobin and hematocrit level
- coagulation studies
- blood gas measurements (Pomerantz, 2022)
- Diagnostic imaging may be indicated in cases of suspected traumatic hemorrhagic shock (Pomerantz, 2022).

NURSING IMPLICATIONS AND TREATMENT

Treatment targets replacing the intravascular volume, improving preload and stroke volume, and restoring oxygen delivery to the tissues (Pomerantz, 2022).

As with all types of shock, **administration of oxygen is a first-line treatment to help support oxygen delivery to tissues**. If there are obvious signs of volume loss those should be addressed in the appropriate manner (e.g., pressure held on bleeding wounds, antiemetics administered to address vomiting; Pomerantz, 2022). Obtaining stable vascular access is essential in the treatment and resuscitation of a hypovolemic patient.

Fluid resuscitation is the hallmark treatment for hypovolemic shock. The primary initial action for nonhemorrhagic and hemorrhagic shock is rapid administration of isotonic crystalloid at volumes of 10 to 20 mL/kg (Pomerantz, 2022). Boluses should be given over 5 to 10 minutes and repeated up to three times, with focused assessments after each bolus to evaluate for signs of fluid overload including rales, worsening respiratory distress, or hepatomegaly (Pomerantz, 2022). Hypovolemia caused by hemorrhagic sources should also be treated with 10 mL/kg replacement of blood and blood components, as indicated (Pomerantz, 2022).

COMPLICATIONS

Major complications of hypovolemic shock include cardiovascular collapse and death (Curley & Moloney-Harmon, 2001).

▶ SUBMERSION INJURIES

Submersion injuries, otherwise known as drowning, occur when a person is submerged under any liquid medium (such as water or cleaning solutions). These injuries are categorized as drowning death, drowning with morbidity, and drowning without morbidity. Drowning is the leading cause of death in children under 5 years old, thus critical care nurses must be prepared to care for this population (Migliaccio, 2021). Risk factors include:

- overestimating swimming abilities
- risk taking behavior
- lack or supervision (especially toddlers)
- seizure disorder
- underlying cardiac dysrhythmias

SIGNS AND SYMPTOMS

Symptomology is most often respiratory in nature and can vary from mild coughing and shortness of breath to pulmonary edema and respiratory failure. Common findings include:

- adventitious breath sounds (rales, wheezing, crackles, rhonchi)
- tachypnea and increased work of breathing

Subacute respiratory symptoms can occur and may progress to acute respiratory distress syndrome (ARDS). Additional symptoms may occur as a result of hypoxia and exposure including:

- altered mental status
- hypothermia
- arrhythmias
- organ failure

PATHOPHYSIOLOGY

The hypoxic insult can produce:

- **cerebral edema** and increased intracranial pressure due to neuronal cell death from hypoxia
- **renal failure** secondary to acute tubular necrosis
- **Hypoxia induced cardiomyopathy** may be present, with associated **hypotension** (Migliaccio, 2021).

NURSING IMPLICATIONS AND TREATMENT

ASSESSMENT

Frequent physical assessment of the drowning victim is necessary. Focused assessments should include hourly neurological exam, thorough respiratory evaluation, monitoring for development of arrhythmias, and end organ assessments such as urine output. Neurologic assessments may reveal deficits secondary to hypoxia and should assess pupil reactivity, strengths, mental status, and the presence of cough and gag. Neurologic assessment may worsen as cerebral edema develops; thus, the keen identification of evolving alterations will allow prompt treatment. If the Glasgow Coma Scale (GCS) drops to 8 or lower, mechanical respiratory support is indicated (Migliaccio, 2021).

LABS AND DIAGNOSTICS

Chest radiographs and laboratory studies such as blood gases will help to identify the severity of respiratory injury and guide treatment. Typical radiographic findings include patchy opacities, perihilar markings, and diffuse pulmonary edema. Additional laboratory studies should seek to evaluate end-organ function (Migliaccio, 2021).

TREATMENT AND MANAGEMENT

Initial management is focused on resuscitation and follows standard assessment of airway, breathing, and circulation. Depending on the mechanism of injury, **cervical spine immobilization** may be indicated until further evaluation of injuries is possible. Any abnormal cardiac rhythms should be treated according to standard pediatric advanced life support protocols (Migliaccio, 2021).

Respiratory support shall be provided, as needed, based on the severity of injury, ranging from supplemental oxygen to noninvasive positive pressure ventilation to intubation and mechanical ventilation. Intubation is indicated if arterial partial pressures of oxygen, obtained via arterial blood gas (ABG) specimens, are consistently below 80 mmHg or if oxygen saturations are below 90% despite noninvasive ventilation strategies. Intubation may also be indicated, as mentioned previously, for neurologic compromise with resulting inability to support respiratory needs (Migliaccio, 2021).

Temperature management may be necessary depending on weather and submersion time. Depending on the severity of hypothermia, patients may be warmed by removal of wet clothing and use forced air blankets (i.e., Bair Hugger™), warmed IV fluids, and warm water lavage. In severe cases, extracorporeal warming (ECMO) may be used (Table 12.6; Migliaccio, 2021). The goal rate of warming depends on the severity of hypothermia, but generally controlled warming at a rate of 0.25°C to 0.5°C per hour is targeted to avoid the effects of rapid vasodilation such as hypotension and cerebral edema (Verger & Lebet, 2008).

Table 12.6 Hypothermia Categories, Presentation, and Associated Warming Techniques

Patient Temperature	Categorization	Usual Presentation	Warming Techniques
32°C–35°C	Mild	Intact mental status Shivering Intact organ function	Passive (removal of wet clothes) Forced Air blanket
28°C–31.9°C	Moderate	Altered mental status (+/-) Shivering Atrial dysrhythmias	Passive Forced air blanket Warmed IV fluids Warm water lavage
<28°C	Severe	Obtunded Absent reflexes Ventricular dysrhythmias/Asystole No response to defibrillation or resuscitation drugs	Passive Forced air blanket Warmed IV fluids Warm water lavage Extracorporeal warming

IV, intravenous.
Source: Migliaccio, D. (2021). Pediatric drowning. *Trauma Reports, 22*(2), 1–16.

Hypotension may occur as the body warms and vasodilation occurs. Cardiomyopathy or cold-induced diuresis may produce or worsen hypotension. Treatment should include IV fluids and vasoactive medications (Migliaccio, 2021).

Management of increased intracranial pressure includes hypertonic saline, mannitol, and loop diuretics. Ongoing monitoring, assessment, and treatment of neurologic, respiratory, and end organ injury continues through a patient's inpatient stay (Migliaccio, 2021) to reduce secondary injury from cellular death-mediated complications (i.e., cerebral edema, acute tubular necrosis). Treatment with antibiotics may be indicated for signs of pulmonary infection, or if submersion occurred in overtly contaminated liquid (Migliaccio, 2021).

COMPLICATIONS

Complications from submersion injuries include sustained neurologic deficits, secondary brain swelling from anoxia, organ failure, and death.

▶ HYPOTHERMIA AND HYPERTHERMIA

Critically ill children are at increased risk for poor thermoregulation related to both physiologic and environmental factors (Curley & Moloney-Harmon, 2001). Some causes of **hyperthermia** in pediatric patients include:
- infectious fever
- endocrine disorders
- traumatic brain injury
- congenital nervous system malformations
- drug induced hyperthermia
- environmental factors (Curley & Moloney-Harmon, 2001)

Causes of **hypothermia** in pediatric patients include:
- environmental factors
- neonatal sepsis
- anesthetics
- neuromuscular blockades
- water submersions
- therapy induced hypothermia (Curley & Moloney-Harmon, 2001)

PATHOPHYSIOLOGY

The most common cause of hyperthermia in pediatric patients is fever (Curley & Moloney-Harmon, 2001). The mechanism for development of fever is pyrogen mediated increase to the body's "set" temperature in the hypothalamus (Curley & Moloney-Harmon, 2001). Those pyrogens can originate from bacteria, proteins, or protein byproducts (Curley & Moloney-Harmon, 2001). Oxygen consumption increases by 10% for every 1°C-temperature elevation; this increase in metabolic demand can lead to metabolic acidosis if there is inadequate oxygen delivery (Curley & Moloney-Harmon, 2001).

The three stages of hypothermia include:
- **Mild (32°C–35°C):** The body attempts to create heat by shivering and increasing metabolism. Circulation is reduced.
- **Moderate (28°C–32°C):** The mechanism of shivering fails to generate heat. The pulse becomes slow and weak. Breathing slows, and confusion or sleepiness begins.
- **Severe (<28°C):** Essential body systems, including cardiac, respiratory, and neurological systems, begin to slow, become weaker, or cease to function (Corneli & Kadish, 2021). Unlike the slowing of other essential body systems, the renal system experiences an increase in urine output in a phenomenon called "cold diuresis" (Curley & Moloney-Harmon, 2001). This diuresis decreases preload and further worsens cardiac output (Corneli & Kadish, 2021).

NURSING IMPLICATIONS AND TREATMENT

ASSESSMENT

Signs and symptoms of **hyperthermia** in the pediatric patient include:
- chills
- discomfort
- tachypnea
- tachycardia
- oral temperature >37.8°C
- shivering (Curley & Moloney-Harmon, 2001)

The nurse should assess for obvious signs of infection and obtain a thorough history to identify possible sources of elevated temperature.

Signs and symptoms of **hypothermia** vary greatly based on the degree of hypothermia. Some indicators include:
- core body temperature <35°C
- mental status changes
- cardiac dysrhythmias
- shivering
- paradoxical flushed cheeks
- muscle rigidity (Corneli & Kadish, 2021)

As hypothermia progresses and worsens, the patient will present unresponsive with fixed and dilated pupils (Corneli & Kadish, 2021).

LABS AND DIAGNOSTICS

Diagnosis of hyperthermia is confirmed by obtaining an *oral temperature >37.8°C or a rectal temperature >38.8°C.* More important than the diagnosis of hyperthermia is determining the etiology of the hyperthermia, so as to guide treatment.

Hypothermia diagnostics include:
- electrocardiograms
- invasive blood pressure monitoring
- blood gas analysis
- electrolyte evaluation
- coagulation studies
- blood glucose level (Curley & Moloney-Harmon, 2001)

TREATMENT AND MANAGEMENT

Hyperthermia

It is recommended to treat fevers in patients who are at risk for febrile seizures, have underlying chronic disease, temperatures >40°C, and anytime there is concern for concomitant environmental hyperthermia plus fever (Curley & Moloney-Harmon, 2001). Antipyretic drugs such as ibuprofen (Advil, Motrin) and acetaminophen (Tylenol) are effective at reducing fever. Aspirin may be used but is *not recommended* in children because of risk of Reye's syndrome and decreased platelet functioning (Curley & Moloney-Harmon, 2001). Tepid sponge baths are an effective treatment option either alone, or in tandem with antipyretic agents (Curley & Moloney-Harmon, 2001). If fever is suspected to be infectious in nature, blood cultures should be obtained and IV antibiotics administered in addition to antipyretics (Curley & Moloney-Harmon, 2001).

Hypothermia

Hypothermic patients should be rewarmed in a controlled manner. There are several different methods that facilitate rewarming including:

- radiant warmers
- heated blankets
- warmed IV fluids
- warmed gastric lavage (Curley & Moloney-Harmon, 2001)
- There should be a warming gradient of approximately 10°C between the patient and the temperature of the warming device (Curley & Moloney-Harmon, 2001). Electrolyte derangements should be treated as necessary to optimize metabolic function (Curley & Moloney-Harmon, 2001). Of note, if a patient presents severely hypothermic in an arrest state, rewarming efforts should continue throughout the resuscitation as some essential physiologic mechanisms are unable to function at extremely low temperatures. Hypothermic patients are not declared deceased until the core temperature is at least 32°C (Curley & Moloney-Harmon, 2001).

COMPLICATIONS

Major complications of hyperthermia include metabolic acidosis and death (Curley & Moloney-Harmon, 2001). Major complications of hypothermia include respiratory depression, circulatory collapse, and death (Corneli & Kadish, 2021).

▶ TOXIN AND DRUG EXPOSURE/INGESTION

Compared to adults, human toxin exposures occur disproportionately in children. Specifically, in 2019 children <3 years old accounted for nearly a third of exposures, with children ≤5 years old accounting for 42.8% (Gummin et al., 2021). Development should be considered when evaluating a pediatric patient's potential toxin exposure. Toddlers or young children are far more likely to be involved with unintentional ingestions than a nonmobile infant (Toc & Burns, 2017), and likewise adolescents are more likely to have intentional overdoses or illicit drug exposure. In young children, toxin exposure is more prevalent in males, while teen and adult exposures are predominantly female (Gummin et al., 2021).

PATHOPHYSIOLOGY

The pathophysiology of toxic exposure varies considerably such as:

- the toxin
- the type of exposure (ingestion, inhalation, etc.)
- the dose
- quantity
- Preparation: Each type may produce different effects.

One of the most common toxic exposures/ingestions is **acetaminophen (Tylenol)**, which when consumed in supratherapeutic doses results in accumulation of the toxic metabolite, N-acetyl-p-benzoquinoneimine (NAPQI). With accumulation of NAPQI, liver inflammation and cellular death occur, resulting in oxidative stress, rising liver enzymes, and potential liver failure (Toce & Burns, 2017). Supratherapeutic doses will vary based on patient age and condition, but the **minimal toxic dose for children is 150 mg/kg or 7.5 to 10 g for an adult**. Nearly *all* patients with single ingestions >350 mg/kg will experience liver toxicity, but repeated excess dosing is associated with increased morbidity and mortality (Heard & Dart, 2022). The *maximum recommended oral doses* to avoid toxicity are:

- 75 mg/kg/day in infants, the lesser of 100 mg/kg/day OR
- 1,625 mg/day in children, or 3,250 mg/day in adolescents (Micromedex, 2022)

Another common toxicity is from **salicylate (aspirin)** exposure. Large salicylate exposures result in a stimulation of the medulla that causes tachypnea with resulting respiratory alkalosis. Subsequent fatty acid and glucose metabolism derangements from alteration in oxidative phosphorylation then produce metabolic acidosis, hyperthermia, and hypoglycemia (Toce & Burns, 2017).

Other toxicities may result in cellular asphyxiation, as is seen with **carbon monoxide (CO)** and **cyanide poisoning**. When CO exposure occurs, oxygenation of cells is inhibited. CO has a higher affinity for and binds to heme of the hemoglobin molecule, displacing oxygen molecules. Ultimately, anaerobic metabolism occurs, resulting in lactic acid accumulation, metabolic acidosis, and cellular inflammation and death. As a result of this, pulse oximetry is not a valid measurement of respiratory status. Carboxyhemoglobin levels should be monitored.

NURSING IMPLICATIONS AND TREATMENT

LABS AND DIAGNOSTICS

Diagnosis of toxic exposure is often a combination of toxidrome identification and supportive laboratory studies. *Toxicology panels* may be obtained via *urine* and *blood serum* studies and can indicate the presence of certain toxins; however, these studies are not all inclusive. Specific serum drug levels are available for some drugs and may be indicated based on the presenting symptoms or history. Other illicit substances may not show on these panels. Acid–base balance assessment via blood gas will identify derangements, which are present in many toxidromes and may help guide both diagnosis and treatment. Depending on the toxin, renal and liver function may be affected, warranting evaluation of electrolytes, BUN, creatinine, aspartate aminotransferase (AST), alanine aminotransferase (ALT), and coagulation studies (partial thromboplastin time [PTT], prothrombin, international normalized ratio). Electrolyte and blood gas studies will also assist in the identification of an anion gap metabolic acidosis. The acronym "MUDPILES" is used when evaluating differential diagnoses for anion gap metabolic acidosis (Table 12.7).

Table 12.7 MUDPILES: Causes of Anion Gap Metabolic Acidosis

M	Methanol, metformin
U	Uremia
D	Diabetic ketoacidosis
P	Propylene glycol, paracetamol (acetaminophen), paraldehyde, phenformin
I	Iron, isoniazid, ibuprofen
L	Lactate (carbon monoxide, cyanide, hydrogen sulfide)
E	Ethylene glycol (antifreeze, coolant)
S	Salicylates (aspirin)

Source: Toce, M. S., & Burns, M. M. (2017). The poisoned pediatric patient. *Pediatrics in Review, 38*(5), 207–220. https://doi.org/10.1542/pir.2016-0130

Electrocardiograms should be used to identify dysrhythmias, signs of myocardial ischemia, or other conduction abnormalities for all patients with suspected or confirmed ingestion or exposure.

TREATMENT AND MANAGEMENT

Collecting the history of events leading up to the presentation will aid in identifying the toxic exposure. In the absence of a clear history, assessment should seek to identify risk for exposure and symptomology that can be attributed to a specific toxin/group of toxins, otherwise known as a toxidrome. Risk can be associated with age and developmental abilities, but also availability of toxins, thus it is important to determine the medications and products (e.g., gardening, cleaning, medications left on the counter and in reach of children) available in the home. Clinical presentation can evolve as toxins are absorbed, metabolized, or excreted, warranting thorough and frequent physical assessments and monitoring.

Abnormalities common with **toxin exposure** and point to exposures that *stimulate the sympathetic nervous system or anticholinergic activity* include fever and tachycardia. Abnormalities common with **sedatives, calcium channel blockers**, or **acetylcholinesterase inhibitors** include hypothermia, bradycardia, and hypotension.

■ **Respiratory patterns** should be closely evaluated as some toxins may blunt respiratory drive and produce hypopnea, while other toxins may induce metabolic acidosis requiring respiratory compensation as tachypnea. Age-appropriate norms should be used to identify derangements (Slota, 2019; Toce & Burns, 2017). Respiratory assessment may reveal coarse breath sounds due to excess secretions or wheezing in some exposures. Airway assessment, administration of supplemental oxygen, and intubation are key for this patient.

Neurologic assessments should focus on:
■ mental status
■ eye examination including pupillary size and accommodation
■ nystagmus evaluations
■ reflexes
■ possible seizure activity

Neurologic impairment may progress over time, starting with agitation or irritability and advancing to coma and seizures, thus frequent serial assessments are imperative.

■ **Skin and mucous membranes** should be inspected for flushing, diaphoresis, moisture level, or ulcerations.

■ **GI affects** like the presence of hypo- or hyperactive bowel sounds as well as the presence of increased urine output, stool, and emesis should be noted. Strict intake and output measurement is indicated (Toce & Burns, 2017; Slota, 2019).

■ **Electrolyte and glucose abnormalities** are common following toxin exposure requiring assessment for signs of such abnormalities like dysrhythmias, altered reflexes, irritability, diaphoresis, or dizziness (Toce & Burns, 2017).

TREATMENT AND MANAGEMENT

Treatment and management will depend heavily on the toxin, the time from exposure, and symptomology. Initial treatment should focus on supporting airway, breathing, and circulation and obtaining IV access. After initial stabilization, the focus is on prevention of absorption (gastric decontamination, ocular irrigation, dermal irrigation), antidote administration, and symptom control.

Gastric decontamination can be used following early identification of ingestions, and most often is completed using activated charcoal. The use of ipecac syrup, gastric lavage, or whole bowel irrigation are *no longer considered a standard of care*. Multiple doses of activated charcoal may be indicated in the setting of certain life-threatening ingestions (e.g., salicylates, phenobarbital). Salicylate (aspirin) does not have an available antidote, and thus treatment is based on symptom management, prevention of further absorption, and/or increased drug clearance. Decontamination therapy with activated charcoal is often used in conjunction with urine alkalinization with sodium bicarbonate fluids to improve renal tubular reabsorption of the drug. Hemodialysis may also be indicated depending on how much time has passed since ingestion of the toxic substance. Frequent monitoring of salicylate levels will guide treatment.

One common toxicity with an available antidote is acetaminophen. Acetaminophen toxicity may be treated with the antidote, N-acetylcysteine (NAC), which detoxifies the body of the toxic metabolite, NAPQI, and generates glutathione, which further assists with NAPQI metabolism. The decision to use NAC is based on the Rumack–Matthew nomogram that depends on the patient's serum acetaminophen levels at least 4 hours from ingestion. If the serum acetaminophen level at that time is above the treatment line per the nomogram, antidote therapy is initiated. Without knowledge of the time of ingestion treatment will depend on liver function values and the serum drug level. A summary of first-line treatments and/or antidotes for common drug toxicities can be found in Table 12.8.

Table 12.8 Drug Toxicities, Symptoms, and First-Line Treatments

Category	Examples	Symptoms	Treatment/Antidote
Anticholinergics	Atropine Diphenhydramine	Altered mental status, agitation, dilated and sluggish pupils, increased heart rate and blood pressure, fever, flushed, dry skin, decreased bowel sounds	Symptom control: Benzodiazepines for agitation, antihypertensive medications Physostigmine (rare)

(continued)

Table 12.8 Drug Toxicities, Symptoms, and First-Line Treatments (*continued*)

Category	Examples	Symptoms	Treatment/Antidote
Sympathomimetics	Albuterol, cocaine	Agitation, tremor, seizure, dilated but reactive pupils, increased HR, BP, and RR, fever, diaphoresis, increased bowel sounds	Benzodiazepines, antihypertensive medications
Serotonergics	Methylphenidate, MDMA, SSRI	Agitation, confusion, increased HR and BP. Dilated but reactive pupils, muscle rigidity and/or twitching	Benzodiazepines, cyproheptadine
Cholinergics	Acetylcholine, nicotine, organophosphates	Coma, delirium, seizures, constricted pupils, decreased HR, increased BP and RR, diaphoresis, increased bowel sounds/diarrhea, salivation, urination, N/V	Atropine
Sedatives	Benzodiazepines, opioids, clonidine	Coma/lethargy, decreased HR, RR, BP, constricted pupils (opioids), decreased bowel sounds (opioids)	Flumazenil (benzodiazepine) Naloxone (opioid)
Calcium Channel Blockers	Verapamil, nifedipine	Coma, decreased HR and BP	Atropine, glucagon, calcium chloride
Beta Blockers	Metoprolol	Coma, seizure, decreased HR and BP	Glucagon, beta agonists
Hypoglycemics	Insulin, sulfonylureas	Coma, seizure, increased HR, hypothermia, hypoglycemia, diaphoresis	Activated charcoal (acute), dextrose, sodium bicarbonate
Acetaminophen	Tylenol	Coma, delirium, N/V, right upper quadrant tenderness	N-acetylcysteine
Salicylates	Aspirin	Agitation, delirium, seizure, increased HR and RR, N/V	Activated charcoal (acute), sodium bicarbonate

BP, blood pressure; HR, heart rate; MDMA, methylenedioxy; N/V, nausea/vomiting. RR, respiratory rate; SSRI, selective serotonin reuptake inhibitors.

Sources: Slota, M. (2019). *AACN core curriculum for pediatric high acuity, progressive and critical care nursing* (3rd ed.). Springer Publishing Company; Toce, M. S., & Burns, M. M. (2017). The poisoned pediatric patient. *Pediatrics in Review, 38*(5), 207–220. https://doi .org/10.1542/pir.2016-0130

Symptom-based treatment may be indicated, even if the toxin is not identified. Rhythm disturbances such as QTc prolongation or QRS widening are common with certain drugs and are usually attributed to an alteration in sodium channel dependent ventricular depolarization. Treatment is aimed at increasing available sodium and decreasing the blockade of sodium channels with IV sodium bicarbonate bolus and infusion. Bradycardia may also be seen as a result of calcium channel blocker or beta blocker ingestion. Treatment for both includes glucagon, which drives serum calcium into the cells, resulting in increased contractility and atrial-ventricular (AV) node conduction.

COMPLICATIONS

Complications of toxic exposure are many, including organ dysfunction or failure, and death.

Clinical Pearl

Depending on the time of ingestion of toxic substances, if systemic absorption has already occurred, typical treatments may not be an option. Hemodialysis may be the only form of treatment to remove these toxins from the blood. (This applies to only certain toxins.)

▶ POST-TRANSPLANT COMPLICATIONS

Organ and stem cell transplantation carries many risks; some of those risks are universal and others are specific to the organ/cell being transplanted. Three universal post-transplant complications are:

- **rejection** of the transplanted organ and risk for infection
- **malignancy** related to immune suppression (Curley & Moloney-Harmon, 2001)
- **graft-versus-host disease (GVHD),** which occurs in higher incidence in stem cell transplantation and intestinal or multi-visceral transplantation (Curley & Moloney-Harmon, 2001)

PATHOPHYSIOLOGY

Organ rejection is a result of the *host immune system recognizing antigens on the donor organ as foreign*. This causes an activation of the host immune system to attack the donor organ resulting in lymphocyte infiltration, edema, cellular necrosis, and loss of the graft (Curley & Moloney-Harmon, 2001). GVHD is, in effect, the opposite of rejection as discussed previously. GVHD occurs when the immune cells from the donor recognize the host cells as foreign and initiate an immune attack on the host (Zeiser, 2022).

Risk for infection is related to immune suppression therapy required to protect the donor organ from being attacked by the host immune system. Many immune suppression drugs inhibit T and B cell proliferation and activity (Curley & Moloney-Harmon, 2001). (See Table 12.9 for common immune suppression medications.) Inhibition of these lymphocytes weakens the response of the immune system to recognize threats (Curley & Moloney-Harmon, 2001).

Table 12.9 Common Immune Suppression Medications and Nursing Indications

Drug	Mechanism	Nursing Considerations
Antithymocyte globulin	T cell depletion	▦ Monitor vital signs frequently during infusion ▦ Premedicate with acetaminophen and diphenhydramine ▦ Can cause cytokine-release syndrome
Rituximab	B cell depletion	▦ Monitor for infusion reactions ▦ May experience first dose effect of anaphylactic like reaction ▦ Monitor for pulmonary edema
Azathioprine	Reduced T cell proliferation	▦ Monitor CBC and platelet levels ▦ Observe for signs of liver dysfunction ▦ Administer with food
Mycophenolate mofetil	Inhibit T and B cell proliferation	▦ Cannot take with antacids ▦ Capsules should not be open or crushed ▦ Must be renally dosed in patients with renal dysfunction
Cyclosporine	Calcineurin inhibitor	▦ Observe for CNS symptoms ▦ Monitor renal function ▦ Monitor drug levels
Tacrolimus	Calcineurin inhibitor	▦ Monitor BUN and creatinine ▦ No not mix with $NaHCO_3$ in IV form ▦ Adheres to plastic surfaces, give nearest patient ▦ Monitor Tacrolimus trough levels
Sirolimus	Decrease in T cell proliferation	▦ Oral solution only ▦ Prolonged half-life, 7–10 days ▦ Should be diluted before administration
Corticosteroids	Reduces number of circulating lymphocytes	▦ May increase glucose levels ▦ Monitor electrolytes

BUN, blood urea nitrogen; CBC, complete blood count; CNS, central nervous system; IV, intravenous.
Source: Claeys, E., & Vermeire, K. (2019). Immunosuppressive drugs in organ transplantation to prevent allograft rejection: Mode of action and side effects. *Journal of Immunological Sciences, 3*(4), 14–21. https://doi.org/10.29245/2578-3009/2019/4.1178

Post-transplant lymphoproliferative disorders (PTLD) are malignancies that occur secondary to immune suppression (Friedberg & Aster, 2021). The primary pathway for development of PTLD is via an Epstein-Barr virus (EBV) B cell proliferation in the setting of suppressed T cell surveillance activity (Friedberg & Aster, 2021). Without the full function of T cells to recognize EBV and destroy the affected B cells, the B cells are left to proliferate into lymphoblastoid cells (Friedberg & Aster, 2021).

NURSING IMPLICATIONS AND TREATMENT

ASSESSMENT

Rejection: Signs and symptoms of rejection vary based on the transplanted organ but generally follow a pattern of symptoms related to dysfunction of that organ/organ system. Patients with heart and lung transplants experiencing rejection may show signs of heart failure, pulmonary edema, and hypoxemia (Curley & Moloney-Harmon, 2001). Patients who have received liver transplantation may have abdominal pain, flushing, distended abdomen, and loss of appetite (Curley & Moloney-Harmon, 2001). Kidney transplant recipients may see a decline in renal function, fever, and hypertension when experiencing organ rejection (Curley & Moloney-Harmon, 2001).

Graft-versus-host disease: GVHD has characteristic signs and symptoms including manifestations on the skin and in the GI tract (Zeiser, 2022). The most common symptom is a maculopapular rash that can range from mild to severe (Zeiser, 2022). The upper and lower GI tracts are involved, and most patients experience abdominal pain and diarrhea (Zeiser, 2022).

Infection: Signs and symptoms of infection vary. General signs and symptoms include fever, malaise, and viral symptoms congruent with the type of illness acquired (Curley & Moloney-Harmon, 2001).

Post-transplant lymphoproliferative disorders: Symptoms of PTLD are nonspecific such as fever, weight loss, fatigue, and lymphadenopathy (Friedberg & Aster, 2021).

LABS AND DIAGNOSTICS

Rejection: Rejection is most decisively diagnosed with a biopsy of the transplanted organ, this is the gold standard (Curley & Moloney-Harmon, 2001). Other pertinent labs include organ specific function studies (e.g., BUN and creatinine, liver enzymes).

Graft-versus-host disease: GVHD is often a diagnosis of exclusion after other diagnoses have been eliminated (Zeiser, 2022). Biopsy of the affected tissue can confirm GVHD with histologic analysis (Zeiser, 2022).

Infection: Blood cultures, viral panels, and other serologies to search for possible infectious sources are required to definitely diagnose an infectious process (Curley & Moloney-Harmon, 2001).

Post-transplant lymphoproliferative disorders: Laboratory studies are essential to diagnose PTLD. Laboratory results that may be seen in patients with PTLD include anemia, thrombocytopenia, leukopenia, hypercalcemia, and hyperuricemia (Friedberg & Aster, 2021). Additionally, biopsy and histological evaluation of tissue are utilized for classification and gene identification of the malignant tissue (Friedberg & Aster, 2021).

TREATMENT AND MANAGEMENT

Rejection: Administration of anti-rejection medication in a timely and consistent manner is imperative to decrease risk of rejection occurring (Curley & Moloney-Harmon, 2001). Once rejection has been identified steroids and increased immunosuppressant medications are deployed to address the rejection (Curley & Moloney-Harmon, 2001).

Graft-versus-host disease: Steroids are the initial treatment for GVHD (Zeiser, 2022). If the patient has a favorable response to the steroid treatment, it may be tapered over time (Zeiser, 2022).

Infection: Treatment of active infection is the same in post transplanted patients as in nontransplant recipient patients. Of note, transplant recipient patients may be on prophylactic medications such as ganciclovir (for cytomegalovirus) and sulfamethoxazole (for pneumocystis carinii) to prevent infections from occurring (Curley & Moloney-Harmon, 2001).

Post-transplant lymphoproliferative disorders: Treatment of PTLD is guided by the same oncologic principles of nontransplant related malignancies (Friedberg & Aster, 2021).

HOSPITAL-ACQUIRED CONDITIONS

Medical errors, including hospital-acquired conditions, are prevalent in the healthcare system. The Institute of Medicine's seminal paper *To Err is Human* (1999) states that an estimated 44,000 to 98,000 patients die from preventable medical errors. Specifically, hospital-acquired infections affect 1 in 25 hospitalized patients (Centers for Disease Control and Prevention [CDC], 2017a). Many national and international organizations focus on reducing harm that results from hospitalization. The National Healthcare Safety Network (NHSN), a surveillance system based at the CDC, provides operational definitions and reporting requirements, allowing nationalized effort and attention on harm reduction strategies and accountability of institutions for their associated rate of harm. Pediatric hospital collaboratives, like Solutions for Patient Safety (SPS), work to apply such definitions of harm to the pediatric population and establish applicable evidence-based harm prevention bundles available.

Hospital-acquired harm can manifest as infections related to *hospital-inserted devices* (central-line associated bloodstream infection [CLABSI]), *injuries* due to a lack of adherence to standard care practices (pressure injury or peripheral intravenous catheter infiltration), or *side effects of adverse drug events* (i.e., wrong dose, wrong route). Hospital-acquired infections are associated with increased morbidity, mortality, and length of stay, and have significant cost effects as value-based insurance systems no longer reimburse for care associated with these preventable conditions. In the following sections, you will find a more detailed review of three of the most common and significant hospital-acquired conditions: CLABSIs, catheter-associated urinary tract infection (CAUTI), and hospital-acquired pressure injury.

Clinical Pearl

Both low- and high-tech strategies have been designed to ensure safe medication administration. Low-tech strategies include supporting all nine rights, including the use of standardized communication strategies, independent double check workflows, and patient education. High-tech solutions include bar code technology and smart pumps with technology that inhibits over- and underdosing of titratable drips during pump programming (MacDowell et al., 2021).

▶ CENTRAL LINE-ASSOCIATED BLOODSTREAM INFECTION

CLABSI is defined as a pathogen isolated from a blood culture in a patient with a central catheter (or within the last 48 hours) that is not attributed to any other source. Alternative sources of bloodstream infections in hospitalized children may be related to translocation from mucosal barrier injuries, pneumonia, or intestinal compromise (e.g., necrotizing enterocolitis). CLABSI rates are reported publicly through the Centers for Medicare & Medicaid Services and are calculated as the number of CLABSIs per 1,000 central line days (CDC, 2017a; SPS, 2022).

SIGNS AND SYMPTOMS

Symptoms of CLABSI are consistent with other infections, including hyper- or hypothermia, increased heart rate, and elevated white blood cells (specifically neutrophils). Some patients will progress into sepsis, with associated hypotension and systemic inflammatory response.

NURSING IMPLICATIONS AND TREATMENT

Diagnosis is contingent upon a blood culture with pathogen growth. Treatment for CLABSI includes symptom management with fluids and vasoactive medications, as indicated, along with antibiotics. Antibiotic treatment will usually consist of broad-spectrum coverage until speciation from blood cultures allow a tailored treatment plan. Central lines may be removed or replaced if believed to be colonized with the pathogen.

CLABSI is considered a preventable infection, and hinges largely on appropriate care practices from the nurse. It is important to note that multidisciplinary attention is necessary to prevent CLABSIs, with attention to insertion practices, site selection, and early line removal being particularly important. However, the bedside nurse is predominantly responsible for maintenance of the central line and can largely reduce the risk for CLABSI with strict adherence to evidence-based central line maintenance bundles. While the exact composition of CLABSI prevention/central line maintenance bundles may vary between institutions, organizations like SPS define core components. For insertion, bundle elements include chlorhexidine disinfection, prepackaged insertion kits, full sterile barriers, and insertion by only trained providers. For maintenance, the prevention bundle includes daily discussion of line necessity, functionality and utilization, regular dressing assessments, standardized dressing, cap and tubing changes, standardized dressing change procedures, and daily chlorhexidine skin treatment and linen changes.

▶ CATHETER ASSOCIATED URINARY TRACT INFECTION

CAUTIs are healthcare-associated infections that occur while admitted to a hospital with a urinary device in place. These infections most often originate from endogenous organisms that enter the urinary tract through the urethra (Shuman & Chenoweth, 2018). These infections significantly contribute to healthcare costs, as well as increasing morbidity and lengths of stay. Duration of catheterization is the most significant risk factor for CAUTI, with anatomic variation, insertion, and maintenance practices also affecting total risk.

SIGNS AND SYMPTOMS

CAUTIs will often present without physical symptoms. Polyuria and bacteriuria are not useful in diagnosis, as the presence of an indwelling catheter makes these usual and not necessarily indicative of infection. Patients may or may not present with fever (Shuman & Chenoweth, 2018).

NURSING IMPLICATIONS AND TREATMENT

For the previously noted reasons, diagnosis is challenging. Urine cultures will often reveal bacteria related to biofilm collection, so assessment for clinically significant quantities of bacteria in combination with physical symptoms is necessary to decide if treatment is indicated. Patients with symptomatic infection should receive appropriate antibiotic treatment, but treatment is not recommended for patients without clinically significant symptoms (Shuman & Chenoweth, 2018).

Nursing care is mainly focused on prevention of CAUTI, and, similarly to CLABSI, the standard of care for prevention is defined by organizations like SPS. Prevention bundles include techniques to prevent infection during the insertion and maintenance phases of care. During insertion, the nurse should use aseptic technique, and advocate to avoid unnecessary catheterization. During maintenance, securing the catheter, maintenance of a closed system, routine perineal hygiene, the drainage bag at a level below that of the bladder, maintenance of unobstructed flow of urine, and prompt removal when no longer necessary are essential to CAUTI prevention (SPS, 2021).

A complication of CAUTI can be urosepsis, which may require treatment as described in the sepsis section of this chapter.

▶ VENTILATOR ASSOCIATED EVENTS

Ventilator associated events (VAEs) is a relatively new metric, serving to capture potentially preventable events associated with mechanical ventilation. Historically, ventilator associated pneumonia (VAP) was the only event tracked for surveillance, but inconsistent definitions and a lack of consensus encouraged a different approach. More recently it was noted that additional VAEs such as pulmonary edema, atelectasis, and ARDS may also be preventable. In 2015, the adult VAE definition was modified for application into the pediatric and neonatal population (PedVAE). This new definition was intended as a surveillance metric, and not a clinical diagnosis that drives patient care. PedVAE is defined as a "deterioration in respiratory status after a period of stability or improvement on the ventilator" (NHSN, 2022).

SIGNS AND SYMPTOMS

The specific signs and symptoms of a VAE include an increased mean airway pressure (MAP) or fraction of inspired oxygen (FiO$_2$; Table 12.10) for at least 2 calendar days, following at least 2 calendar days of stability or improvement (SPS, 2022). The designation as a PedVAE is not a clinical diagnosis, and clinical management should be based on physical assessment and radiologic studies.

Table 12.10 PedVAE Worsening Oxygenation Definitions

Indicator	Details
FiO$_2$	2+ days of an FiO$_2$ increase of $\geq$0.25 over the minimum[a] FiO$_2$ on the first day of at least 2 days of stability or improvement
MAP	2+ days of an increased MAP of $\geq$4 cm H$_2$O over the minimum[b] MAP on the first day of at least 2 days of stability or improvement.

[a]minimum FiO$_2$ = lowest value in the calendar day sustained for at least 1 hour.
[b]minimum MAP = lowest value in the calendar day for any duration.
FiO$_2$, fraction of inspired oxygen; MAP, mean airway pressure; PedVAE, pediatric ventilator-associated events.
Source: Solutions for Patient Safety. (2022, January). *Operational definitions.* https://www.solutionsforpatientsafety.org/wp-content/upl oads/sps-operating-definitions_January-2022-1.pdf

NURSING IMPLICATIONS AND TREATMENT

LABS AND DIAGNOSTICS

Diagnostics particularly for VAP is a chest x-ray (CXR). This along with the patient's clinical picture (lung sounds, etc.) would aid in diagnosis.

TREATMENT AND MANAGEMENT

Due to the previously ill-defined definition for pediatric ventilator-associated events, prevention strategies have not been well studied based on the new PedVAE definition. Harm-prevention bundles that exist today are still focused on reducing ventilator associated pneumonia. According to SPS, a daily assessment of readiness to extubate, head of bed elevation of 30° to 45°, minimized ventilator circuit disruptions and oral hygiene at least every 12 hours are recommended components to pneumonia prevention (SPS, 2021).

COMPLICATIONS

Complications of VAP include increased days on mechanical ventilation, increased lengths of stay, development of secondary lung injury, or worsening respiratory status such as ARDS, as well as death.

▶ ICU LIBERATION

The ABCDEF bundle includes six domains focused on optimizing care for critically ill patients by liberating them from mechanical ventilation and the ICU environment. Use of the ABCDEF bundle has many benefits including decreasing in hospital mortality, delirium, use of restraints, and readmissions to the ICU (Society of Critical Care Medicine, 2021).

- **A**: Assess, prevent, and manage pain
  - Utilize age, and developmental level, appropriate pain assessment tools.
  - Nonpharmacologic pain relief methods such as music and nonnutritive sucking should be used to augment analgesia (Smith et al., 2022).
- **B**: Both spontaneous awakening trials and spontaneous breathing trials
- **C**: Choice of analgesia and sedation
  - IV opioids should be used to treat moderate to severe pain (Smith et al., 2022).
  - Validated scales should be used to assess level of sedation in pediatric patients.
- **D**: Delirium: assess, prevent, and manage
  - Validated pediatric scales should be used frequently to assess for delirium in critically ill pediatric patients (Smith et al., 2022).
  - Benzodiazepine use should be minimized when possible to reduce risk of delirium (Smith et al., 2022).
- **E**: Early mobility and exercise
  - Encourage early mobility and exercise within the first 2 to 5 days of critical illness.
  - Utilize a standardized early mobility protocol that includes inclusion criteria, contraindications, age/developmental specific goals, and criteria for stopping mobility (Smith et al., 2022).
  - Mobility goals should be evaluated and prescribed daily to facilitate progressive mobility when possible (Smith et al., 2022).

- **F**: Family engagement and empowerment
  - Parental/family presence throughout an ICU stay can provide comfort for both the patient and the caregivers resulting in decreased levels of anxiety and distress (Smith et al., 2022).

▶ DEATH AND DYING

Death and dying are not infrequent events in the pediatric intensive care environment. There are several factors to consider when caring for the dying patient and their family including consultation with palliative care, patient/family involvement, spiritual support, and use of child life specialists.

DEVELOPMENTAL CONCERNS

The concept of death and one's understanding of death evolves over time. Children begin to have a basic awareness of death around 3 to 5 years of age. Generally, death is thought of as temporary and reversible, and is associated with the elderly, during the preschool age (Curley & Moloney-Harmon, 2001). As the child grows that concept changes to a permanent and personal understanding of the finality of death (Curley & Moloney-Harmon, 2001). The developmental stage must be considered when discussions of death and dying are being had with children (patient or otherwise) and the conversations should be tailored to the understanding of the child.

NURSING IMPLICATIONS AND TREATMENT

Palliative care collaboration can improve the quality of life for patients with life-threatening illness at all stages of care. Particularly in the dying phase, a palliative care team can give recommendations on pain management, reduction of suffering, and bereavement support (Hauer, 2022). Additional resources available to nursing may include child life specialists who are able to support both the patient and family members, particularly siblings, during end-of-life events, and spiritual services such as a religious leaders or meditation resources (Romito et al., 2021).

TREATMENT AND MANAGEMENT

Some physical symptoms of the dying process include pain, agitation, dyspnea, nausea/vomiting, and increased secretions (Suttle et al., 2017). Parents consistently report pain management as a priority intervention for their dying children (Suttle et al., 2017). Management of other distressing symptoms should be tailored to the needs of the patient and family.

Emotional and spiritual needs of the patient and family must be considered. If the patient is able to discuss their death, that should be allowed and not avoided, with care taken to answer only what the child asks and let them lead the conversation (Curley & Moloney-Harmon, 2001). It is important to allow the family to maintain a connection to their dying child by providing opportunities for them to engage with the child, such as brushing their hair and holding their hand (Suttle et al., 2017). Parents should be allowed to remain present during cardiopulmonary resuscitation, if this occurs, as literature shows this is beneficial for their coping and long-term grief (Suttle et al., 2017).

CASE STUDY

Tommy, a 2-year-old with a past medical history of being born at 26 weeks' gestation, chronic lung disease, and baseline oxygen requirement of 2 L via nasal cannula, presents to the pediatric ICU (PICU) after a cardiac arrest at home, with return of spontaneous circulation achieved by emergency medical services. He has been experiencing severe vomiting and diarrhea for more than 2 days. His parents state they were giving him extra fluid through his gastric tube, but that he had not produced any urine for at least 24 hours. They called 9-1-1 when they went to check on him during his nap and he was found to be blue and not breathing. They state they had put him down for a nap about 60 minutes beforehand.

Upon admission, Tommy is tachycardic to the 170s, with a blood pressure of 65/35. His perfusion is poor, with a capillary refill time of 5 seconds and thready peripheral pulses. He is being bag-valve ventilated with 100% FiO_2 and an oxygen saturation of 95%. His temperature is 33°C.

CASE STUDY QUESTIONS

1. The nurse expects the following to be a priority intervention for Tommy:
   A. Initiate antibiotics
   B. Rapid bolus of isotonic fluid
   C. Initiation of vasoactive medication
   D. Send a toxicology laboratory panel

Tommy was successfully intubated. He has received a total of 60 mL/kg of Lactated Ringer's (LR). His heart rate is now in the 160s, with a blood pressure of 68/40. A laboratory panel is sent with the following notable labs:
- Arterial blood gas: pH 6.9, PCO_2 60, PO_2 75, HCO_3 8
- Potassium 2.5 mmol/L
- Sodium 125 mmol/L
- Chloride 80 mmol/L

2. The nurse interprets the blood gas as:
   A. Mixed metabolic/respiratory acidosis
   B. Mixed metabolic/respiratory alkalosis
   C. Metabolic acidosis
   D. Respiratory acidosis

3. Tommy remains hypothermic, with a core temperature of 33.5°C (92.3°F). The nurse knows this is considered ____ hypothermia and anticipates the following intervention:
   A. Moderate; gastric lavage
   B. Mild; gastric lavage and forced air blanket
   C. Severe; gastric lavage, warmed fluids, and possibly extracorporeal warming
   D. Mild; forced air warming

While the nurse is preparing an epinephrine infusion for Tommy's continued hypotension, she notices that Tommy's EKG morphology changes to a wide complex tachycardia. She checks for a pulse and does not feel one. She presses the code bell and initiates compressions. The pediatric ICU (PICU) team completes 60 minutes of CPR without a return of spontaneous circulation.

4. Which of the following interventions should be considered during the active resuscitation?
   A. Escort the family to a designated waiting room with a chaplain.
   B. Allow the family to be present in the room during the resuscitation.
   C. Have the medical team discuss organ donation with family.
   D. Administer pain medication to Tommy.

(See answers next page.)

ANSWERS TO CASE STUDY QUESTIONS

1. B) Rapid bolus of isotonic fluid

Tommy is presenting in hypovolemic shock due to fluid loss from emesis and diarrhea. The priority treatment is to restore his intravascular volume. He does not currently have any indication for antibiotics. Vasoactive medications may be indicated if he is unresponsive to fluid resuscitation but would not be initiated prior to fluid administration. While toxic exposure is technically possible, it is unlikely, and not a priority intervention.

2. A) Mixed metabolic/respiratory acidosis

Tommy is presenting with severe metabolic acidosis due to electrolyte losses as evidenced by his low HCO_3, as well as respiratory acidosis due to his cardiac arrest and chronic lung disease, as evidenced by his elevated CO_2. His arterial blood gas is mixed and uncompensated.

3. D) Mild; forced air warming

A core temperature between 32°C and 35°C is considered mild hypothermia. Warming is usually effectively achieved using forced air warming devices. More invasive measures such as gastric lavage or extracorporeal warming are indicated in moderate and severe hypothermia.

4. B) Allow the family to be present in the room during the resuscitation.

Allowing the parents to be present during resuscitation efforts has been proven to improve coping and long-term grief. The medical team should refrain from discussing organ donation with the family due to the possible conflict of interest. Instead, third party organizations can facilitate these conversations. Pain management is not necessary during active resuscitations.

KNOWLEDGE CHECK: CHAPTER 12

1. A pediatric ICU (PICU) nurse is responding to a rapid response on the acute care floor. The patient was receiving vancomycin for the first time and experienced an anaphylactic reaction. You administered subcutaneous epinephrine per order. They are now calm, breathing easily, with a heart rate and blood pressure that are normal. The nurse should anticipate which of the following will be part of the treatment plan:
   A. Transfer to the PICU
   B. Administration of a low dose epinephrine infusion
   C. Fluid resuscitation
   D. Resuming the vancomycin

2. The nurse is caring for a 5-year-old patient in septic shock. The nurse anticipates the initial intervention will be _____.
   A. Obtaining blood cultures
   B. Administration of broad-spectrum antibiotics
   C. Administration of a rapid bolus of 20 mL/kg Lactated Ringer's (LR)
   D. Initiation of an epinephrine infusion

3. It has been an hour since a patient has been identified to be in septic shock. The nurse has administered a total of 60 mL/kg of Lactated Ringer's (LR) and attempted to obtain blood cultures twice. The nurse's next step should be:
   A. Assist the physician with central venous access device (CVAD) insertion and obtain blood cultures from the CVAD once in place
   B. Have a second nurse attempt to obtain blood cultures
   C. Administer corticosteroids
   D. Notify the provider that they were unable to obtain blood cultures and administer the first dose of antibiotics

4. Acetaminophen toxicity, which occurs due to toxic metabolite accumulation, can be effectively treated based on the Rumack–Matthew nomogram using the following antidote:
   A. Flumazenil
   B. N-acetylcysteine (NAC)
   C. Activated charcoal
   D. Cyproheptadine

5. A 3-year-old boy presents to the ED with the following vital signs: heart rate (HR): 50, blood pressure (BP): 70/30, respiratory rate (RR): 20, temperature 37°C (98.6°F). He is awake and calm. His mother states she briefly left her son unattended in her home while she was unloading her groceries from the car, and when she found him, he was in her bedroom. She noticed her medications were knocked off her bedside table and some of the pills were on the floor. She did not know if any were missing. She states she takes metoprolol for her heart and glipizide for her type 2 diabetes. This happened 4 hours ago, but she is now worried and wants her son evaluated. What does the nurse anticipate will be part of this patient's treatment plan?
   A. Glucagon
   B. Intravenous (IV) dextrose
   C. Activated charcoal
   D. Atropine

6. The priority treatment for a patient presenting post-submersion injury, with a core temperature of 27°C (80.6°F) includes:
   A. Extracorporeal warming
   B. Bolus of 0.9% normal saline
   C. Intubation and mechanical ventilation
   D. Hypertonic saline for treatment of increased intracranial pressure (ICP)

(See answers next page.)

1. A) Transfer to the PICU
Up to nearly 20% of patients may experience rebound symptoms, so transfer to the PICU for close monitoring and available prompt treatment is indicated. Low dose epinephrine is not a treatment for anaphylactic shock and is not otherwise indicated with normal blood pressures. Fluid resuscitation may be needed in uncompensated shock, but this patient was adequately treated and is currently not in uncompensated shock. Resuming the antibiotic that prompted the anaphylactic reaction is not appropriate. An alternative antibiotic would be selected.

2. C) Administration of a rapid bolus of 20 mL/kg Lactated Ringer's (LR)
The initial intervention for a patient in septic shock is rapid fluid resuscitation in increments of 10 to 20 mL/kg. LR is the preferred crystalloid, but normal saline can also be used. Blood cultures and administration of broad-spectrum antibiotics should occur within 1 hour but are not the initial intervention for a patient in shock. Epinephrine infusions may be used for patients who remain hypotensive despite 40 to 60 mL/kg of fluid resuscitation.

3. D) Notify the provider that they were unable to obtain blood cultures and administer the first dose of antibiotics
Antibiotic administration within 1 hour of sepsis identification is the goal. Blood cultures should be obtained prior to antibiotic administration, when possible, but antibiotic administration should not be significantly delayed particularly when the patient is in septic shock. An hour has passed, and thus further attempts to obtain blood cultures should occur after antibiotic administration. Corticosteroids are not recommended for sepsis unless the patient remains hypotensive despite adequate fluid resuscitation and vasoactive infusions.

4. B) N-acetylcysteine (NAC)
NAC is the antidote for acetaminophen toxicity. It works by detoxifying the body of the toxic metabolite, N-acetyl-p-benzoquinoneimine (NAPQI), and generates glutathione, which further assists with NAPQI metabolism. Flumazenil is the antidote for benzodiazepine overdose. Cyproheptadine is a serotonin antagonist used when Serotonin Syndrome is present from drugs such as methylphenidate. Activated charcoal is not an antidote, but rather a decontamination treatment, often used with salicylate poisoning.

5. A) Glucagon
This patient's presentation is consistent with beta-blocker exposure and not glipizide exposure. Glucagon is the first-line treatment for beta-blocker toxicity as it increases heart rate and contractility by driving calcium into the cells. IV dextrose would be used if the patient ingested glipizide and was showing signs of hypoglycemia (i.e., tachycardia, diaphoresis, agitation). Activated charcoal may be used following acute ingestions but is unlikely to be effective this long after exposure. Atropine is not effective in reversing bradycardia following beta-blocker exposure. It is a first-line treatment in calcium channel blocker or cholinergic toxicity.

6. C) Intubation and mechanical ventilation
A patient presenting with a core temperature of 27°C (80.6°F) is severely hypothermic and is likely to require extracorporeal warming. Supportive care inclusive of boluses of normal saline for hypotension secondary to warming-induced vasodilation, and hypertonic saline to reduce ICP increases due to neuronal cell death may be indicated but are later interventions. Initial care will be focused on resuscitation and assessment of airway, breathing and circulation. Patients presenting with such profound hypothermia would be expected to be comatose and without effective breathing, warranting intubation and mechanical ventilation as a priority treatment.

7. A 10-year-old patient with a central venous catheter, urinary catheter, and nasogastric tube has been experiencing fevers of 38.5°C to 38.8°C (101.3°F–101.8°F) for the last 12 hours. Their current vital signs are:

Temperature: 38.9°C (102°F)
Heart rate: 120 bpm
Blood pressure: 75/39
Respiratory rate: 24

This patient is most likely exhibiting symptoms of a:
A. Catheter associated urinary tract infection (CAUTI)
B. Peritonitis
C. Gastric ulcer
D. Central line associated bloodstream infection (CLABSI)

8. Which of the following is not an intervention to prevent catheter associated urinary tract infection (CAUTI)?
A. Keep the urinary drainage bag below the level of the bladder
B. Discuss need for urinary catheter daily and remove promptly when no longer needed
C. Use aseptic technique when inserting indwelling urinary catheters
D. Daily urinary culture surveillance

9. A patient is intubated due to acute respiratory failure. The arterial blood gas after intubation is as follows:

pH: 7.31
PCO_2: 50 mmHg
PO_2: 80 mmHg
HCO_3: 22 mEq/L
SaO_2: 95%

Which of the following acid–base imbalances is present?
A. Respiratory acidosis
B. Respiratory alkalosis
C. Metabolic acidosis
D. Metabolic alkalosis

10. A 2-year-old is admitted the ICU for tachycardia, hypotension, and lethargy. The parents report that the lethargy and diarrhea started 3 days prior when a "stomach bug" affected the patient and their 5-year-old sibling. The medical team orders laboratory studies, including a blood gas. What acid–base imbalance would the nurse expect to discover?
A. Respiratory acidosis
B. Respiratory alkalosis
C. Metabolic acidosis
D. Metabolic alkalosis

11. A 15-year-old, in apparent distress, complains of difficulty breathing and lightheadedness. Upon examination, the nurse observes muscle twitching in the legs and bilateral hands in spasm with a tucked thumb, wrist flexion, and extension of the fingers. Vital signs are as follows:

Heart rate (HR): 120
Respiratory rate (RR): 55
Blood pressure (BP): 108/67
O_2 sat: 97%

Based on the assessment findings, what immediate intervention would the nurse recommend?
A. Administer 20 mL/kg fluid bolus of 0.9% NaCl
B. Obtain electrolyte panel
C. Apply nasal cannula at 2 L/min
D. Instruct the patient to breathe into a paper bag

(See answers next page.)

7. D) Central line associated bloodstream infection (CLABSI)

This patient's hypotension, fever, and tachycardia are consistent with possible infection. While it is possible that this patient is experiencing CAUTI, their symptoms are more consistent with bloodstream infection. Without an invasive peritoneal drain or catheter peritonitis is unlikely. A gastric ulcer would present with pain with eating and is unlikely to cause infection.

8. D) Daily urinary culture surveillance

Daily asymptomatic urinary cultures are not recommended as part of a CAUTI prevention bundle. Keeping the urinary drainage bag below the level of the bladder prevents backflow and possible introduction of bacteria from healthcare providers manipulating the drainage bag. Daily discussion of necessity allows for early removal, which directly prevents catheter-associated infections. Finally, aseptic technique during insertions of urinary catheters reduces the risk of bacterial introduction during catheter placement.

9. A) Respiratory acidosis

The pH is below 7.35 indicating acidosis. The PCO_2 is >45 mmHg, outside the normal limits, indicating hypercarbia. The combination of increased partial pressure of carbon dioxide and decreased pH indicates acidosis secondary to a respiratory process. Alkalosis is when the pH is >7.45. The bicarbonate is within normal limits, indicating the derangement is not primarily from the metabolic system.

10. A) Metabolic acidosis

The patient is exhibiting signs of metabolic alkalosis secondary to gastrointestinal losses. Hypotension, tachycardia, and altered level of consciousness are symptoms of metabolic acidosis. There are no indications of an altered respiratory status for this patient. Metabolic alkalosis is characterized by additional factors such as hyperreflexia and muscle twitching.

11. D) Instruct the patient to breathe into a paper bag

The patient is experiencing symptoms of respiratory alkalosis secondary to hyperventilation. Hypocapnia and resultant decrease in pH causes ionized calcium to be bound to protein. This abrupt decrease in calcium precipitates muscle spasm and tetany. Fluid bolus is not indicated as the patient is not hypotensive. Obtaining an electrolyte panel would be helpful in diagnosing derangements but is not an immediate action while the patient is stable. Nasal cannula is not required for a patient who has an appropriate oxygen saturation.

12. A 10-year-old terminal oncology patient has transitioned to comfort care as their treatment options have been exhausted. The patient's parents, grandparents, and two younger siblings are present. The medical team has just exited the room after explaining the dying process and pain management strategies. Which of the follow would be appropriate actions for the nurse to take?
    A. Avoid eye contact with family
    B. Disclose to the family a clinical trial that just started
    C. Only speak to the parents
    D. Consult a child life specialist to assist the family

13. Which of the following best describes the presentation of hypovolemic shock?
    A. Weak peripheral pulses, dry mucous membranes, oliguria, lethargy
    B. Rash, flushed skin, bounding pulses
    C. Flash capillary refill, confusion, bounding pulses, rigors
    D. Dyspnea, weak peripheral pulses, altered level of consciousness, pale skin

14. A 9-month-old is 1-week postoperative from a liver transplant and is sent to the ED from the clinic after the clinic nurse obtained the following vital signs:

    Heart rate (HR): 180
    Respiratory rate (RR): 32
    Blood pressure (BP): 60/40
    O_2 sat: 94%
    T: 38.2°C

    The nurse assesses the patient as lethargic, with bounding pulses, and warm extremities. Oxygen is administered and an isotonic fluid bolus is ordered. Blood cultures are obtained, and antibiotics initiated. Which of the following is the most likely etiology of this scenario?
    A. Graft-versus-host disease (GVHD)
    B. Acute rejection
    C. Hemorrhage
    D. Infection

15. A 2-year-old presents to the ED after having fallen into a lake while ice fishing. They are shivering, alert but not oriented, and exhibiting first degree heart block. Based on what the nurse knows about the stages of hypothermia, which of the following interventions should be initiated?
    A. Prepare to administer adenosine
    B. Administer warmed intravenous (IV) fluids
    C. Initiate extracorporeal warming
    D. Prepare to administer mannitol

16. A 2-day-old, term neonate requires admission to the pediatric ICU for treatment of a congenital diaphragmatic hernia. They are mechanically ventilated, and the vital signs are as follows:

	0800	1200
Heart rate (HR)	166	125
Respiratory rate (RR)	40	40
Blood pressure (BP)	64/38	60/40
O_2 Sat	97%	94%
Temp	36.7°C	36.4°C

    The nurse appropriately assesses the change in vital signs and anticipates which of the following actions?
    A. Administration of atropine
    B. Obtaining blood cultures and administering antibiotics
    C. Initiation of epinephrine
    D. Obtaining a chest x-ray (CXR)

(See answers next page.)

12. D) Consult a child life specialist to assist the family

The child life specialist can assist the younger siblings in understanding and coping with the impending death of their sibling. The nurse should not avoid methods of communication with the family, including eye contact. It is important for the nurse to facilitate connection and communication as much as possible during the dying process. It is not within the nurse's scope of practice to offer additional medical treatment to patients and families.

13. A) Weak peripheral pulses, dry mucous membranes, oliguria, lethargy

Decreased intravascular volume results in decreased perfusion to the kidneys and decreased preload. Flushed skin and rash are associated with anaphylactic shock. Flash capillary refill, rigors, and bounding pulses are associated with septic shock. Dyspnea, weak peripheral pulses and pale skin are associated with cardiogenic shock.

14. D) Infection

The post-transplant patient is at risk for infection secondary to immune suppression. GVHD is uncommon in liver transplants and presents with cutaneous and gastrointestinal symptoms. Acute rejection does not cause hypotension and fever. Hemorrhage and coagulopathies are possible after liver transplant but there are no data given here to suggest bleeding.

15. B) Administer warmed intravenous (IV) fluids

The patient is experiencing moderate hypothermia and requires aggressive rewarming techniques. Adenosine is administered in supraventricular tachycardic rhythms. Extracorporeal warming is indicated in severe hypothermia (<28°C/82.4°F). The altered mental status the patient is experiencing is not from cerebral edema, and therefore would not require mannitol.

16. B) Obtaining blood cultures and administering antibiotics

Neonatal sepsis often presents with hypothermia. Hypothermia induces bradycardia. Atropine is not indicated as this is not a primary bradycardia. Epinephrine would result in an increase in heart rate, but would not address the causative factor of the physiologic response, which is infection. A CXR will not allow diagnosis of infection or guide antibiotic choice.

REFERENCES

Balamuth, F., Alpern, E. R., Abbadessa, M. K., Hayes, K., Schast, A., Lavelle, J., Fitzgerald, J. C., Weiss, S. L., & Zorc, J. J. (2017). Improving recognition of pediatric severe sepsis in the emergency department: Contributions of a vital sign-based electronic alert and bedside clinician identification. *Annals of Emergency Medicine, 70*(6), 759–768. https://doi.org/10.1016/j.annemergmed.2017.03.019

Brinkman, J. E., & Sharma, S. (2021). Physiology, metabolic alkalosis. In *StatPearls* [Internet]. StatPearls Publishing. https://www.ncbi.nlm.nih.gov/books/NBK482291/

Brinkman, J. E., & Sharma, S. (2022, January). Respiratory alkalosis. In *StatPearls* [Internet]. StatPearls Publishing. https://www.ncbi.nlm.nih.gov/books/NBK482117/

Burger, M., & Schaller, D. J. (2021). Metabolic acidosis. In *StatPearls* [Internet]. StatPearls Publishing. https://www.ncbi.nlm.nih.gov/books/NBK482146/

Centers for Disease Control and Prevention. (2017a, December 5). *Hospital-associated infections: 2017 national and state healthcare-associated infections progress report.* U.S. Department of Health and Human Services. https://www.cdc.gov/hai/data/archive/2017-HAI-progress-report.html

Center for Disease Control and Prevention. (2017b, October). *Intravascular catheter-related infection (BSI): Guidelines for the prevention of intravascular catheter-related infections, 2011.* U.S. Department of Health and Human Services. https://www.cdc.gov/infectioncontrol/guidelines/BSI/index.html

Corneli, H., & Kadish, H. (2021). Hypothermia in children: Clinical manifestations and diagnosis. *UpToDate.* https://www.uptodate.com/contents/hypothermia-in-children-clinical-manifestations-and-diagnosis

Curley, M. A., & Moloney-Harmon, P. A. (Eds.). (2001). *Critical care nursing of infants and children* (2nd ed.). Saunders Company.

Emmett, M., & Palmer, B. (2020). Simple and mixed acid-base disorders. *UpToDate.* https://www.uptodate.com/contents/simple-and-mixed-acid-base-disorders

Ferdman, R. M. (2021). Anaphylaxis. In B. N. Bolick, K. Reuter-Rice, M. A. Madden, & P. M. Severin (Eds.), *Pediatric acute care. A guide for interprofessional practice* (2nd ed., pp. 598–602). Elsevier.

Friedberg, J., & Aster, J. (2021). Epidemiology, clinical manifestations, and diagnosis of post-transplant lymphoproliferative disorders. *UpToDate.* https://www.uptodate.com/contents/epidemiology-clinical-manifestations-and-diagnosis-of-post-transplant-lymphoproliferative-disorders

González, S. B., Menga, G., Raimondi, G. A., Tighiouart, H., Adrogué, H. J., & Madias, N. E. (2018). Secondary response to chronic respiratory acidosis in humans: A prospective study. *Kidney International Reports, 3*(5), 1163–1170. https://doi.org/10.1016/j.ekir.2018.06.001

Gummin, D. D., Mowry, J. B., Beuhler, M. C., Spyker, D. A., Bronstein, A. C., Rivers, L. J., Pham, N. P. T., & Weber, J. (2021). 2020 annual report of the American Association of Poison Control Centers' national poison data system (NPDS): 38th annual report. *Clinical Toxicology (Philadelphia), 59*(12), 1282–1501. https://doi.org/10.1080/15563650.2021.1989785

Hauer, J. (2022). Pediatric palliative care. *UpToDate.* https://www.uptodate.com/contents/pediatric-palliative-care

Heard, K., & Dart, R. (2022). Clinical manifestations and diagnosis of acetaminophen (paracetamol) poisoning in children and adolescents. *UpToDate.* https://www.uptodate.com/contents/clinical-manifestations-and-diagnosis-of-acetaminophen-paracetamol-poisoning-in-children-and-adolescents

Hilarius, K. W. E., Skippen, P. W., & Kissoon, N. (2020). Early recognition and emergency treatment of sepsis and septic shock in children. *Pediatric Emergency Care, 36*, 101–108. https://doi.org/10.1097/PEC.0000000000002043

Institute of Medicine. (1999). *To err is human: Building a safer health system.* The National Academies Press.

Lee, C. K. K. (2021). Drug dosages. In K. Kleinman, L. McDaniel, & M. Molloy (Eds.), *Harriet Lane handbook* (pp. 665–1076). Elsevier.

MacDowell, P., Cabri, A., & Davis, M. (2021, March 12). *Medication administration errors.* Patient Safety Network. https://psnet.ahrq.gov/primer/medication-administration-errors

Migliaccio, D. (2021). Pediatric drowning. *Trauma Reports, 22*(2), 1–16.

National Healthcare Safety Network. (2022, January). *Pediatric Ventilator-Associated Event (PedVAE).* PedVAE Events. https://www.cdc.gov/nhsn/pdfs/pscmanual/pedvae-current-508.pdf

Nichols, D. G., & Shaffner, D. H. (2016). *Roger's textbook of pediatric intensive care* (5th ed.). Wolters Kluwer.

Patel, S., & Sharma, S. (2021). Respiratory acidosis. In *StatPearls* [Internet]. StatPearls Publishing. https://www.ncbi.nlm.nih.gov/books/NBK482430/

Prescribers Digital Reference. (2022). *Epinephrine—drug summary.* https://www.pdr.net/drug-summary/EpiPen-epinephrine-134.6164

Pomerantz, W. (2022). Hypovolemic shock in children: Initial evaluation and management. *UpToDate.* https://www.uptodate.com/contents/hypovolemic-shock-in-children-initial-evaluation-and-management

Romito, B., Jewell, J., Jackson, M., Ernst, K., Hill, V., Hsu, B., Lam, V., Mauro-Small, M., & Vinocur, C. (2021). Child life services. *Pediatrics, 147*(1), 1–10. https://doi.org/10.1542/peds.2020-040261

Senewiratne, N., Woodall, A., & Can, A. (2021). Sodium bicarbonate. In *StatPearls* [Internet]. StatPearls Publishing. https://www.ncbi.nlm.nih.gov/books/NBK559139/

Shuman, E. K., & Chenoweth, C. E. (2018). Urinary catheter-associated infections. *Infectious Disease Clinics of North America, 32*, 885–897. https://doi.org/10.1016/j.idc.2018.07.002

Sicherer, S. H., & Simons, F. E. R. (2017). Epinephrine for first-aid management of anaphylaxis. *Pediatrics, 139*(3), e1–e9. https://doi.org/10.1542/peds.2016-4006

Slota, M. (2019). *AACN core curriculum for pediatric high acuity, progressive and critical care nursing* (3rd ed.). Springer Publishing Company.

Society of Critical Care Medicine. (2021). *ICU liberation bundle (A-F).* https://www.sccm.org/iculiberation/abcdef-bundles

Smith, H. A., Besunder, J. B., Betters, K. A., Johnson, P. N., Srinivasan, V., Stormorken, A., Farrington, E., Golianu, B., Godshall, A., Acinelli, L., Almgren, C., Bailey, C., Boyd, J., Cisco, M., Damian, M., deAlmeida, M., Fehr, J., Fenton, K., Gilliland, F., . . . Berkenbosch, J. W. (2022). 2022 Society of Critical Care Medicine clinical practice guidelines on prevention and management of pain, agitation, neuromuscular blockade, and delirium in critically ill pediatric patients with consideration of the ICU environment and early mobility. *Pediatric Critical Care Medicine, 23*(2), e74–e110. https://doi.org/10.1097/PCC.0000000000002873

Solutions for Patient Safety. (2021, November). *SPS prevention bundle.* https://www.solutionsforpatientsafety.org/wp-content/uploads/SPS-Prevention-Bundles_NOV-2021-1.pdf

Solutions for Patient Safety. (2022, January). *Operational definitions.* https://www.solutionsforpatientsafety.org/wp-content/uploads/sps-operating-definitions_January-2022-1.pdf

Suttle, M. L., Jenkins, T. L., & Tamburro, R. F. (2017). End-of-life and bereavement care in pediatric intensive care units. *Pediatric Clinics, 64*(5), 1167–1183. https://doi.org/10.1016/j.pcl.2017.06.012

Toce, M. S., & Burns, M. M. (2017). The poisoned pediatric patient. *Pediatrics in Review, 38*(5), 207–220. https://doi.org/10.1542/pir.2016-0130

Verger, J. T., & Lebet, R. M. (2008). *AACN procedure manual for pediatric acute and critical care.* Elsevier.

Weiss, S., Peters, M. J., Alhazzani, W., Agus, M. S. D., Flori, H. R., Inwald, D. P., Nadel, S., Schlapbach, L. J., Tasker, R. C., Argent, A. C., Brierley, J., Carcillo, J., Carrol, E. D., Carroll, C. L., Cheifetz, I. R., Choong, K., Cies, C. J., Cruz, A. T., De Luca, D., . . . Tissieres, P. (2020). Surviving sepsis campaign international guidelines for the management of septic shock and sepsis-associated organ dysfunction in children. *Pediatric Critical Care Medicine, 21*(2), e52–e106. https://doi.org/10.1097/PCC.0000000000002197

Zeiser, R. (2022). Treatment of acute graft-versus-host disease. *UpToDate.* https://www.uptodate.com/contents/treatment-of-acute-graft-versus-host-disease

Professional Caring and Ethical Practice

Maryann Godshall

The professional caring and ethical practice content of the pediatric CCRN® exam consists of the following:

- advocacy/moral agency
- caring practices
- response to diversity
- facilitation of learning
- collaboration
- systems thinking
- clinical inquiry

Note: The order of content listed does not necessarily reflect importance.

▶ SYNERGY MODEL

The guiding model for the critical care nurses is the Synergy Model developed in 1995. **Synergy** occurs when individuals work together in mutually enhancing ways toward a common goal. The American Association of Critical-Care Nurses (AACN) is committed to making sure that certified nurses practice based on the needs of their patients and families and puts the patient first and at the center of nursing practice. The integration of the AACN Synergy Model is the basis of care and at the core, integrates patient characteristics and nurse competencies. It views patients in a holistic way as opposed to looking at separate, disconnected body systems. Each patient is unique and brings unique characteristics to each care situation and must be recognized. It is a partnership that will result in optimal outcomes. These characteristics are all connected. A patient is evaluated on each of the following eight characteristics according to their capacity in that category and assigned a number: 1 (very low), 3 (moderate), or 5 (very high; see Table 13.1; Swickard et al., 2014).

Table 13.1 Patient Characteristics

Complexity	Unique entanglement of two or more systems (body, family, friends, support systems therapy, or treatments)
Participation in care	The extent to which the patient can actively participate in their care (patient and family)
Participation in decision-making	Their ability to actively participate in any decision-making about their care (patient and family)
Predictability	How likely one is expected to follow a certain course of events or their illness trajectory
Resiliency	Having the capacity to return to a previous level of health and functioning using their own compensatory/coping mechanisms
Resource availability	Extent of resources (i.e., personal, psychological, and social) the patient/family/caregivers/ community bring to the care situation
Stability	The ability to maintain a constant, steady state of optimal functioning
Vulnerability	Being susceptible to real or perceived stressors that can adversely affect the patient and their response to situations and outcomes

Source: Table adapted from the AACN Resource Handbook, 2021.

Each nurse brings a unique set of skills and competencies to their care. Those characteristics are blending their knowledge, skill set, abilities, and experience needed to meet the needs of patients and families. The nurse characteristics include those in Table 13.2.

Table 13.2 Nurse Competencies

Clinical judgement	The clinical reasoning that includes clinical decision-making, critical thinking, an overall grasp of the situation, combined with nursing skills acquired through integrating their education, experience, and integrating the best evidence-based practice.
Advocacy/moral agency	Speaking or interacting on someone's behalf; representing their beliefs, concerns, and desires for care (moral agent); and trying to resolve ethical and/or clinical concerns within or outside the clinical setting. This includes providing accurate education so one can provide truly informed consent and accurate decision-making.
Caring practices	Nurses creating and exhibiting compassionate care in a therapeutic and supportive environment for patients, families, and staff. With the goal being to promote comfort and healing and preventing unnecessary suffering.
Collaboration	Working together that involves integrating an inter-disciplinary approach to insure optimum care and outcomes for the patient and family. This also includes communication that promotes/encourages each person's contributions toward achieving optimal/realistic patient/family goals.
Clinical inquiry	The ongoing practice of questioning and evaluating what is done in practice. Creating change through evidence-based practice, current research, and individual experiential knowledge. (Not just accepting we do it this way because we have always done it this way).
Facilitation of learning	The ability to facilitate learning for patients, families, the healthcare team, and the community. This includes both formal and informal methods of learning.
Response to diversity	Having the sensitivity and awareness to recognize, appreciate, and incorporate differences into the provision of care. Differences may include, but are not limited to, individuality, cultural, spiritual, gender, race, ethnicity, lifestyle, socioeconomic, age, and values.
Systems thinking	Involves the nurse looking at how environmental and system resources exist for the patient/family and staff are connected to each other within the entity of the healthcare system and non-healthcare system: their interrelationship.

Source: Table adapted from the AACN Resource Handbook, 2021.

An important aspect of the synergy model is to match patient needs to nurse competencies to achieve optimal outcomes. The eight nursing competencies shown in Table 13.2 are evaluated on a five-point scale that ranges from 1 (novice) to 5 (expert). For example, a nurse on level 3 collaboration looks for opportunities to be mentored or coached. A nurse on level 5 would be one who coaches or mentor's others. This mirrors Benner's (1984) theoretical model that explains the acquisition of nursing knowledge and expertise. The five levels possible are:

1. novice
2. advanced beginner
3. competent
4. oroficient
5. expert

Note: Nurses at the novice stage are still in nursing school.

▶ OUTCOMES

Outcomes are measured on a continuum and described as low, medium, or high. Each of these must be viewed based on the following perspectives:

- patient perspective
  - looking at their comfort and quality of life
  - functional and behavioral changes
  - trust and satisfaction
- nursing perspective
  - following a typical pathway and experiencing no complications
  - physiological changes
- system perspective
  - determined by length of stay and complications of treatment if they arise
  - costs, rehospitalizations, resource utilization (Joint Commission International, 2022)

▶ ETHICAL ISSUES

The basic principles of ethics are (Varkaye, 2021):

- autonomy
  - having the power to make rational decisions and moral choices
  - informed decision-making and consent
- beneficence
  - "Do good and prevent harm."
  - Act on behalf of the patient (advocate) to prevent harm, remove conditions that may cause harm, help persons with disabilities, and rescue persons in danger to ensure positive outcomes.
  - Engage in health promotion.
- nonmaleficence
  - obligation to "do no harm"
  - Protect from potential harmful situations.
  - Do not kill, do not cause pain or suffering, do not incapacitate, do not cause offense, and do not deprive others of the goods of life.
- futility
  - Futility means any treatment that, within a reasonable degree of medical certainty, is seen to be without benefit to the patient.
  - The treatment at hand is seen as ineffective and should no longer be given.
  - Advanced directives-expressed wishes of the patient, and they should be followed. These wishes should guide care (Angelucci, 2007).
- justice
  - fair, equitable, and appropriate treatment of persons and health care resources
- truth-telling or veracity
  - full disclosure to the patient, however grave the disease is

KNOWLEDGE CHECK: CHAPTER 13

1. A nurse is doing a physical assessment on an infant. They notice a braided band of threads that is heavily soiled on the infant's wrist. Which action by the nurse is most appropriate?
   A. Leave the band in place and wash it with warm soapy water.
   B. Ask the parent about the band and its significance.
   C. Tell the parent the band must be removed as you want to start an IV in that hand.
   D. Explain to the parent this band is a source of potential infection and it should be removed.

2. A patient is admitted to the pediatric ICU (PICU) with status asthmaticus, and they have chronic asthma. Upon doing the admission database, they mention that they smoke both cigarettes and marijuana on a daily basis. Which of the following statements by the nurse would be most appropriate?
   A. "Well, your secret is out, you better quit smoking now, don't you think?"
   B. "This is your third admission to the PICU for asthma, when do you think quitting smoking might be a good idea?"
   C. "I realize you want to just be normal and fit in, but smoking to do that is going to kill you!"
   D. "This is your third admission for asthma, have you ever explored trying to quit smoking? I can have the social worker talk to you about a smoking cessation program if you are interested."

3. A nurse is caring for a 12-year-old girl who is recovering from a traumatic injury. The injury occurred when her father drove her home from baseball practice while he was intoxicated. Which of the following statements would be most therapeutic and facilitate a trusting relationship with the girl and her family?
   A. "You must be very angry at your dad for driving the car when drunk and causing this to happen to you."
   B. "I hope you are going to remind your dad not to drink the next time he drives you from baseball practice."
   C. "I'm sure you will be just fine when this is all over, now please take your medicine."
   D. "I have some time now if you would like to talk about things or what happened to you."

4. The nurse is caring for an 8-year-old boy who has been physically abused. Which of the following should the nurse include in the plan of care?
   A. Encourage the child to confront the abuser.
   B. Provide a care environment that fosters trust.
   C. Reinforce to the child that not all adults are going to abuse them.
   D. Ask the child questions about the abuse to get facts so the adult can be prosecuted.

5. A dressing change needs to be done on a 15-year-old girl for a burn injury sustained in a house fire. The nurse comes in to change the dressing and the adolescent refuses. Which of the following actions would be the BEST response in this situation?
   A. Tell the patient it is time for the dressing change and to get ready anyway.
   B. Sedate the patient.
   C. Allow the patient the option to do the dressing change now or in 30 minutes.
   D. Tell the child if the dressing does not get changed, the wound will get infected.

6. A child is dying from a terminal brain tumor. The family decides they want comfort care and has made decision to allow the child a natural death. They do not visit often. The nurse is concerned about the high doses of opioids being given to the child as they are unconscious. What is the best course of action or resource for the nurse caring for this child?
   A. Consult the hospital ethics committee.
   B. Tell their friends about this situation to release stress.
   C. Refuse to take care of the patient.
   D. Notify the Joint Commission that the hospital is vigorously assisting death in children.

(See answers next page.)

1. B) Ask the parent about the band and its significance.

In order to display cultural competence, the nurse should inquire as to its meaning and significance before removing. Washing it would address the risk of infection but would not address being culturally sensitive. Demanding for the band to be removed or shaming the caregiver insinuating they are not clean is not culturally sensitive (Mullen & Pate, 2019).

2. D) "This is your third admission for asthma, have you ever explored trying to quit smoking? I can the social worker talk to you about a smoking cessation program if you are interested."

Asking the patient if they have ever explored quitting smoking puts the choice of quitting or not in their hands and gives them control. The nurse offers the patient a choice and a gently suggested solution. This also gives the patient the power to make the decision. The other three statements are very judgmental, sarcastic, and not therapeutic. These statements might build a barrier between the patient and the nurse. There is no reason to assume the patient is smoking to fit in.

3. D) "I have some time now if you would like to talk about things or what happened to you."

"I have some time now if you would like to talk about things or what happened to you" is an open-ended statement and shows that the nurse cares and is available to listen to whatever the girl would like to share. This is the most therapeutic response. The nurse should not make the assumption that the girl is angry. A therapeutic, empathetic relationship allows the girl to talk without the nurse making any judgments about her or her family. It is not the child's responsibility to monitor the dad's drinking. Suggesting that she do so is not kind or therapeutic. Rushing the girl to take medications does not convey interest or a caring practice (Mullen & Pate, 2019).

4. B) Provide a care environment that fosters trust.

The child will need an environment of trust, care, and empathy. This will facilitate a healing environment that will begin the healing process. The child should never be told to confront the abuser. Telling the child that not all adults will abuse him asks the child to believe or assume things that are beyond his age level. The child should never be questioned by healthcare, and it is not the job of the nurse to gather facts for the case. This would not be advocating for the child.

5. C) Allow the patient the option to do the dressing change now or in 30 minutes.

It is important to allow the girl choices to participate in their care and decision-making. Telling the patient that it is time for the dressing change whether she is ready or not is too authoritative and will not develop a trusting relationship. Sedation is not required and not an ethical as an option. Scare tactics and threats will not build a therapeutic relationship.

6. A) Consult the hospital ethics committee.

If a nurse is experiencing moral distress over an end-of-life decision, the ethics committee would be a valuable resource to clarify opioid administration for relieving pain verses over sedating someone to shorten their life. In this situation it is ethically acceptable to use higher than normal doses of pain medication to alleviate pain and anxiety for this child with a terminal brain tumor. The Health Insurance Portability and Accountability Act (HIPAA) prevents the discussion of patient information with others. A nurse cannot refuse to care for the patient. This is not a situation for The Joint Commission (Varkaye, 2021).

7. A nurse is caring for a male patient who recently immigrated to the United States from China. Which of the following indicates a need for correction when delivering culturally competent nursing care?
   A. Ask the patient if he has cultural practices from his country of origin the nurse should be aware of.
   B. Discourage the use of acupuncture and cupping for pain relief.
   C. Ask if he can speak any English.
   D. Inquire if he has any food preferences for meals.

8. An adolescent is admitted to the hospital with an intentional overdose. The medical record indicates the patient is male, but the patient identifies as a female and goes by the name "Rebecca." How should the nurse respond in this situation?
   A. Tell the patient, "I am sorry, but you are listed in the medical record as male, and we will need to follow that."
   B. Designate the patient as a "bisexual" and use the pronouns "they" and "them" or "it" when referring to the patient.
   C. Tell the patient that as a healthcare provider, they need to follow the science.
   D. Address the patient by the name Rebecca and use the pronouns "she," "her," and "hers" when referring to the patient.

9. A nurse manager feels that there has been a significant increase in the number of medication errors made on the unit. What would the most appropriate action for the new nurse manager to take?
   A. Track the number of medication errors that have occurred on the unit.
   B. Send out an email telling the staff to be more careful.
   C. Assign a medication safety learning module to the entire staff.
   D. Do nothing as addressing this may make them look bad in their new role.

10. Which of the following would be the best example of implementing the synergy model in a unit?
   A. Assign a novice nurse with the most complex patient on the unit.
   B. Assign an experienced nurse with the most complex patient on the unit.
   C. Take a nurse on orientation, off orientation and assign them with a newly diagnosed multisystem failure patient who is intubated and on vasopressors because you are short staffed and need the "hole filled" in staffing.
   D. Have an ice-cream party on the unit to create harmony so everyone hopefully gets along when the unit is busy.

(See answers next page.)

7. B) Discourage the use of acupuncture and cupping for pain relief.

Discouraging the use of acupuncture and cupping for pain relief would not be appropriate or practicing cultural competence. Asking the patient kindly if they have cultural practices would enable the nurse to fit them into care. Asking if the patient speaks English would enable communication or let the nurse know if there is a need for an interpreter or a language line needed. Inquiring about food preferences would be beneficial so that the patient gets food he is used to and would eat.

8. D) Address the patient by the name Rebecca and use the pronouns "she," "her," and "hers" when referring to the patient.

Refer to the patient as "she," "her," and "hers" as this is the patient's identity. The nurse telling the patient they must go by what the medical record says or saying they must follow the science will not build a therapeutic and trusting relationship. Bisexual is a sexual orientation to both male and female. This patient has identified as transgender, not bisexual. Using pronouns such as "them" or "it" is not therapeutic to a patient who identifies as a girl.

9. A) Track the number of medication errors that have occurred on the unit.

The new nurse manager should track the actual amount of medication errors to identify if this is a problem that truly exists. The first step of any problem-solving process is to collect data. Sending out an email is general and the actual staff members involved may not perceive themselves as the problem or the one who made the suspected error. Assigning a leaning module would not be the best initial response. First, the new manager needs to verify there is indeed a medication error problem, do a root cause analysis, and then assign a method in which how to address the problem like a learning module. Doing nothing to make sure one does not "look bad" would be the worst inaction and exemplify poor leadership and problem-solving skills (Olender et al., 2020).

10. B) Assign an experienced nurse with the most complex patient on the unit.

Assigning an experienced nurse with the most complex patient would be matching the qualities of the patient's acuity with the abilities of the nurse. This is the best example of synergy. Assigning a novice nurse or taking a novice nurse off orientation to "fill a staffing hole" is not wise, ethical, dangerous, but not synergistic. Having an ice cream party to make staff happy only addresses the nursing side of the nurse–patient relationship. An active partnership between the patient and the nurse is how optimal outcomes are achieved. The needs and characteristics of the patient should influence and drive the competencies of the nurse. You would want an experienced, competent nurse to care for this high acuity patient.

REFERENCES

Angelucci, P. A. (2007). What is medical futility? *Nursing Critical Care, 2*(1), 20–21. https://journals.lww.com /nursingcriticalcare/fulltext/2007/01000/what_is_medical_futility_.4.aspx

Benner, P. (1984). *From novice to expert: Excellence and power in clinical nursing practice.* Addison-Wesley Publication Company, Nursing Division.

Joint Commission International. (2022). *Human factors analysis in patient safety systems.* The Source. https://store .jointcommissioninternational.org/human-factors-analysis-in-patient-safety-systems/

Mullen, J., & Pate, M. F. (2019). Caring for critically ill children and their families. In M. Slota (Ed.), *AACN Core curriculum for pediatric high acuity, progressive and critical care nursing* (3rd ed.). Springer Publishing Company.

Olender, L., Capitulo, K., & Nelson, J. (2020). The impact of interprofessional shared governance and a caring professional practice model on staff's self-report of caring, workplace engagement, and workplace empowerment over time. *Journal of Nursing Administration, 50*(1), 52–58. https://doi.org/10.1097/NNA.0000000000000839

Swickard, S., Swickard, W., Reimer, A., Lindell, D., & Winkelman, S. (2014). Adaptation of the AACN synergy model for patient care to critical care transport. *Critical Care Nurse, 34*(1), 16–29. https://doi.org/10.4037/ccn2014573

Varkaye, B. (2021). Principles of clinical ethics and their application to practice. *Medical Principles & Practice, 30*, 17–28. https://doi.org/10.1159/000509119

Practice Test Questions

1. A 6-month-old patient with a patent ductus arteriosus (PDA) is post cardiac catheterization for coil placement to occlude the PDA. The patient begins to cry and the occlusive dressing covering the catheterization site is now saturated with blood. The most appropriate initial nursing action is to:
   A. Administer a sedative to calm patient
   B. Apply pressure above the insertion site
   C. Notify the physician of the bleeding
   D. Reinforce the pressure dressing

2. A 16-year-old patient presents with fatigue, myalgias, weight loss, low-grade fever, and dyspnea. The patient has a past medical history of severe aortic stenosis requiring aortic valve replacement with a prosthetic valve 3 months prior. A new regurgitant murmur is assessed on auscultation and the patient denies recent illness. The most likely explanation of their symptoms is:
   A. Constrictive pericarditis
   B. Infective endocarditis (IE)
   C. Pericardial effusion
   D. Pulmonary embolus (PE)

3. The critical care nurse is caring for a 17-year-old patient with moderate pulmonary stenosis. The patient is scheduled for a cardiac catheterization intervention with a balloon valvuloplasty in the afternoon. Which physical exam finding can the critical care nurse expect to find on the patient before the scheduled catheterization?
   A. Dyspnea on exertion
   B. Hepatomegaly
   C. Lung crackles on auscultation
   D. Orthopnea

4. A 4-month-old patient with trisomy 21 is recovering from a complete atrioventricular canal defect (CAVC) repair. They have a central venous pressure (CVP) catheter in place with a measurement reading of 15 mmHg. Which of the following statements regarding CVP monitoring is most accurate for this patient?
   A. The decreased CVP is due to blood loss from the surgical intervention.
   B. The elevated CVP measurement may result from pulmonary hypertension.
   C. The CVP measurement indicates postoperative cardiogenic shock.
   D. CVP monitoring is reflective of left atrial pressures within the heart.

5. Which of the following physical examination findings indicate a postoperative complication of an open-heart surgery that required the use of cardiopulmonary bypass (CPB)?
   A. Bradycardia
   B. Diaphoresis
   C. Hypertension
   D. Weak pulses

6. A 3-month-old patient with unrepaired Tetralogy of Flow (TOF) is undergoing phlebotomy to obtain a morning basic metabolic panel (BMP). During the venipuncture, the patient is crying and cyanotic with pulse oximeter measurements of 55%. The nurse suspects the patient is having a tet spell and places the patient in a knee-to-chest position and applies 100% oxygen. Which of the following statements is most accurate?
   A. Administering phenylephrine will decrease systemic vascular resistance (SVR) and promote oxygenation.
   B. It is common for patients to frequently experience tet spells until surgical intervention.
   C. The increase in right ventricle outflow tract (RVOT) obstruction causes right to left shunting.
   D. The knee-to-chest position and oxygen administration aim to decrease pulmonary blood flow.

7. A postoperative patient is recovering from an arterial switch operation. The chest tube output is 2 mL/kg/hr for the first 3 hours. At 4 hours, patient assessment reveals tachycardia, weak pulses, and muffled heart sounds. The nurse anticipates which of the following interventions?
   A. Antibiotic therapy
   B. Antithrombotic therapy
   C. Crystalloid fluid administration
   D. Pericardiocentesis

8. A neonate is recovering from a patent ductus arteriosus (PDA) ligation via a left thoracotomy. The patient is crying and difficult to console. Initial vital signs reveal a temperature of 37.6°C (99.7°F), a heart rate of 180 beats/min, blood pressure (BP) of 80/38 mmHg, a respiratory rate (RR) of 66 breaths/min, and an oxygen saturation of 98% on room air. Which of the following interventions is most appropriate at this time?
   A. Initiate a pharmacologic and nonpharmacologic pain management plan.
   B. Prepare an intravenous crystalloid fluid bolus to treat hypotension.
   C. Suction the patient nares bilaterally to ensure patency.
   D. Warm 3 to 4 ounces of the mothers stored breastmilk to console the patient.

9. A 3-month-old with complete atrioventricular canal (CAVC) presents to the ED with respiratory distress. The patient is tachypneic with moderate increased work of breathing. On auscultation, breath sounds are coarse and chest x-ray reveals increased pulmonary markings. Which of the following medications is most appropriate based on this patient's presentation?
   A. Milrinone (Primacore)
   B. Furosemide (Lasix)
   C. Digoxin (Lanoxin)
   D. Propranolol (Inderel)

10. The critical care nurse has settled a 4-month-old atrioventricular canal (CAVC) patient after return from the operating room (OR). The patient had a long bypass run; is on epinephrine, dopamine, and fentanyl; and has atrial and ventricular epicardial wires in place but not connected to the pacemaker. The patient was warmed to a temperature of 38.1°C (100.6°F) rectal. What initial intervention should the critical care nurse expect to perform for this patient?
   A. Cool and sedate the patient.
   B. Attach the pacemaker.
   C. Assess the patient for low cardiac output syndrome (LCOS).
   D. Obtain an EKG.

11. What noninvasive technology is used following cardiac surgery to monitor regional oxygen saturation to monitor for low cardiac output?
   A. Pulse oximetry
   B. Near infrared spectroscopy
   C. Transcutaneous oxygen monitor
   D. Bispectral index monitoring

12. A common postoperative complication occurs when a patient requires the use of a pacemaker following surgery in the areas of the conduction pathway. Which of the following terms indicate a pacemaker spike without the correlated expected response of a P wave or QRS complex?
   A. Failure to sense
   B. Failure to capture
   C. Failure to pace
   D. Failure to contract

13. A postoperative patient is in a junctional rhythm following open-heart surgery. What is significant of this finding in relation to decreased cardiac output?
    A. Slower heart rate
    B. Poor contractility
    C. Faster heart rate
    D. Loss of atrial kick

14. A 1-month-old is brought to the ED by the parent for crying and poor feeding. The nurse palpates a fast brachial pulse and places the patient on a cardiac monitor, which alarms for a heart rate of 248. A cuff blood pressure is then taken and reads 64/32 (50) mmHg. Which initial intervention should the nurse consider?
    A. Obtaining intravenous (IV) access
    B. Administering acetaminophen
    C. Vagal maneuvers
    D. Obtaining a 12 lead EKG

15. A 3-week-old patient 2 weeks post modified Blalock Taussig Shunt (mBTS)/Norwood procedure for hypoplastic left heart syndrome (HLHS) is crying and is difficult to console. The patient is cyanotic and diaphoretic with a sunken fontanel. Vital signs reveal a temperature of 37.3°C (99.1°F) axillary, a heart rate of 185 beats/min, blood pressure of 54/28 mmHg, a respiratory rate of 64 breaths/min, and an oxygen saturation of 56% on room air, and is unable to auscultate a shunt murmur. Which initial intervention is most appropriate at this time?
    A. Call a code.
    B. Administer sedation.
    C. Apply the bag/valve/mask (BVM).
    D. Start an intravenous (IV) line.

16. A 4-day-old patient is 8-hours post a cardiac surgical procedure requiring bypass. Which electrolyte replacement can improve hypotension?
    A. Potassium
    B. Sodium
    C. Glucose
    D. Calcium

17. The nurse in the critical care unit is caring for a 3-month-old patient 1-week postoperative from a Tetralogy of Fallot (TOF) repair. It is the start of the shift and the initial vital signs reveal a temperature of 36.4°C (97.5°F) axillary, a heart rate of 82 beats/min, arterial blood pressure of 72/36 mmHg, a respiratory rate of 24 breaths/min, and an oxygen saturation of 94% on room air. Which of the following is the most appropriate initial intervention?
    A Get warm blankets for the patient.
    B. Notify the frontline practitioner.
    C. Obtain a blood gas.
    D. Check a rectal temperature.

18. A 6-day-old patient post left thoracotomy has just had a first bottle of maternal breast milk after surgery. When recording input and output (I&O) a few hours later, the nurse notices a change in the chest tube output from serous to off-white with a thicker consistency. What labs can the nurse antici-pate will be ordered after notifying the frontline practitioner?
    A. Blood culture/complete blood count (CBC)
    B. Chest tube culture/CBC
    C. Arterial blood gas (ABG)/ionized calcium (iCal)
    D. Chest tube cell count/triglyceride

19. A 5-day-old infant underwent a Norwood operation earlier in the day for hypoplastic left heart syn-drome. Which assessment would be consistent with low cardiac output syndrome (LCOS)?
    A. Cool, mottled extremities, delayed capillary refill time, and decreased pulses
    B. Warm, flushed extremities, delayed capillary refill time, and decreased pulses
    C. Cool, mottled extremities, increased capillary refill time, and decreased pulses
    D. Cool, mottled extremities, delayed capillary refill time, and increased pulses

20. A 7-month-old patient has been on the unit since birth after having multiple surgeries for a complex congenital heart defect. There are no further interventions that can be done for this patient. The family would like to bring this patient home. This patient is still on inhaled nitric oxide (iNO; Inomax) and milrinone (Primacor) for heart failure. The patient has a tracheostomy and is ventilated and has a G-tube for continuous feeds. Which intervention would be required to get this patient out of the ICU?
   A. Transition off iNO to sildenafil (Revatio).
   B. The family needs to learn trach management.
   C. The family needs to learn G-tube care.
   D. Transition off milrinone (Primacor) to captopril (Capoten).

21. A 2-month-old patient alarms. Upon walking into the room, the nurse notes this rhythm on the monitor. Their vital signs are as follows: heart rate (HR) 180, respiratory rate (RR) 85, blood pressure (BP) 42/28. Capillary refill is 4 seconds. What should the nurse's immediate intervention be?

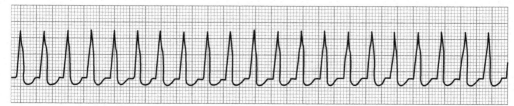

   A. Attempt vagal maneuvers
   B. Give intravenous (IV) amiodarone (Cordarone)
   C. Give intravenous (IV) propranolol (Inderal)
   D. Synchronized cardioversion

22. A patient in the pediatric ICU (PICU) has been consistently not ventilating well. Suddenly, the nurse notices this rhythm on the monitor. The patient has no pulse. After starting CPR, what would the immediate treatment be?

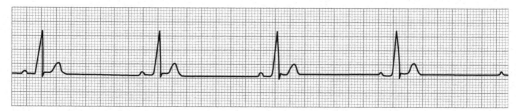

   A. Defibrillate.
   B. Administer atropine.
   C. Administer epinephrine.
   D. Begin atrioventricular (AV) pacing.

23. A 15-year-old patient is in the pediatric ICU (PICU) after a removal of an abscess. They are being treated with intravenous (IV) clindamycin. The patient complains of dizziness and palpations. Within seconds, they lose consciousness. The rhythm on the monitor is as shown. After defibrillation, which of the following medications should be administered next?

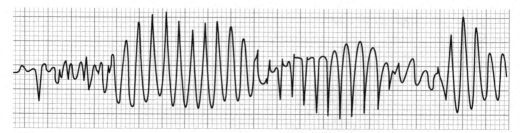

   A. Norepinephrine (Levophed)
   B. Magnesium sulfate
   C. Lidocaine
   D. Atropine

24. A nurse is assisting in the care of an infant following admission to the pediatric ICU (PICU) after cardiac surgery. The infant is hypotensive, has +1 distal pulses, and has delayed capillary refill. The displayed rhythm strip is obtained.

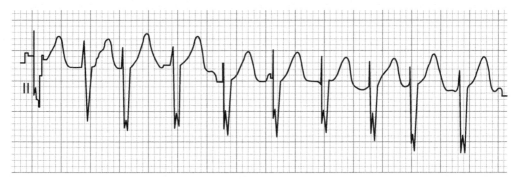

Which of the following interventions for management of this infant do you anticipate?
A. Increase the epinephrine infusion to achieve goal blood pressures and improve perfusion.
B. Do nothing; this rhythm tends to only last 24 to 48 hours.
C. Administer an antiarrhythmic, such as amiodarone.
D. Initiate ventricular pacing to re-establish atrioventricular (AV) synchrony.

25. A 7-day-old infant is admitted to the pediatric ICU (PICU) with a 2-day history of irritability, poor feeding, and vomiting. Which of the following symptoms would indicate this patient is in cardiogenic shock?
A. Increased peripheral pulses and metabolic alkalosis
B. Hypothermia and hypertension
C. Cool, mottled skin and oliguria
D. Polyuria and altered mental status

26. A 2-month-old presents to the ED with a 3-day history of cough, congestion, and low-grade fever. There is a 2-year-old sibling in the home who attends daycare who had similar symptoms last week, but there are no other known sick contacts. The patient's parents brought the 2-month-old to the ED today because they developed respiratory distress with accessory muscle use. Upon exam, the patient has significant nasal congestion and is tachypneic with moderate subcostal retractions, mild wheezing, and rales. What is the most likely diagnosis for this patient?
A. Pneumonia
B. Bronchiolitis
C. Laryngotracheobronchitis
D. Bronchitis

27. A 2-month-old patient presents to the ED with a 2-day history of cough, congestion, and low-grade fever and has developed respiratory distress with accessory muscle use. Their most likely diagnosis is bronchiolitis. Which of the following is the most common etiology of bronchiolitis?
A. *Staphylococcus aureus*
B. *Haemophilus influenza* type b (Hib)
C. Respiratory syncytial virus (RSV)
D. Parainfluenza

28. A 2-month-old with a 2-day history of cough, congestion, and low-grade fever has developed respiratory distress with accessory muscle use. The bedside nurse caring for this patient notes the work of breathing has worsened. The respiratory rate is 80 and moderate to severe intercostal and substernal retractions are present. Interventions to improve the patient's work of breathing would include:
A. Nasal suctioning, high flow nasal cannula, nebulized 3% saline
B. Oropharyngeal suctioning, intubation, racemic epinephrine
C. Oropharyngeal suctioning, nasal cannula, albuterol
D. Nasal suctioning, high flow nasal cannula, albuterol

29. A 15-year-old patient is admitted to the pediatric ICU (PICU) after a 3-day history of fever, chills, body aches, and diffuse rash. The patient was fluid resuscitated in the ED and a vasoactive infusion was initiated. Upon arrival to the PICU, they are noted to be tachypneic and hypoxic, and a blood gas reveals pH 7.21, CO_2 28, HCO_3 15, base deficit of −4, lactate 4.2.
    Which of the following is the most likely cause of the patient's respiratory failure?
    A. Acute respiratory distress syndrome (ARDS)
    B. Air leak syndrome
    C. Pulmonary embolism (PE)
    D. Pneumonia

30. A 15-year-old patient is admitted to the pediatric ICU (PICU). Upon arrival to the PICU, they are noted to be tachypneic and hypoxic, and a blood gas reveals pH 7.21, CO_2 28, HCO_3 15, base deficit of −4, lactate 4.2. Several hours later, the patient develops worsening respiratory distress and hypercarbia and is intubated. Following intubation, a blood gas demonstrates profound hypercarbia with pH 7.1 and CO_2 78, and the decision is made to place the patient on high frequency oscillatory ventilation. They are sedated with midazolam, fentanyl, and rocuronium. The morning after admission, the patient's labs reveal a hemoglobin level of 6.4, hematocrit 18, platelets 147,000. The bedside nurse would anticipate that the physician will order:
    A. Platelet transfusion
    B. Normal saline bolus
    C. 5% albumin bolus
    D. Packed red blood cell (PRBC) transfusion

31. Patients with bronchopulmonary dysplasia are often discharged home dependent on medical technology including tracheostomy and mechanical ventilator. When completing discharge teaching, it is essential that the caregivers understand the need to always have emergency equipment available, including:
    A. Spare trach (same size and one size smaller), spare trach ties, lubricant, normal saline, suction equipment, manual resuscitator bag, and oxygen
    B. Spare trach (same size and one size larger), spare trach ties, lubricant, normal saline, suction equipment, manual resuscitator bag, and oxygen
    C. Spare trach (same size only), spare trach ties, lubricant, normal saline, suction equipment, manual resuscitator bag, and oxygen
    D. Spare trach (same size and one size smaller), spare trach ties, lubricant, normal saline, suction equipment

32. The nurse is caring for a 9-year-old with dilated cardiomyopathy who is awaiting heart transplant. Which of the following is the best way to prepare the patient for their upcoming heart transplant surgery?
    A. Wait until a few hours before surgery to prepare them to reduce their anxiety.
    B. Allow the patient to be part of the decision-making process and encourage them to do as much as possible to increase their cooperation.
    C. Begin discussing the upcoming transplant in advance and support explanations with diagrams, pictures, and models.
    D. Minimize the patient's separation from their parents and implement strategies to reduce parental anxiety.

33. A 2-year-old child presents to the pediatric ED in respiratory distress. On assessment, the child is febrile and tachycardic, with inspiratory stridor, drooling, significant retractions, and diminished breath sounds. After the child is placed on a cardiac, respiratory, and pulse oximetry monitor, which of the following interventions is most appropriate?
    A. Obtain intravenous (IV) access and administer a 20mL/kg normal saline bolus and antibiotics.
    B. Place the child in a supine position and attempt to visualize the airway using a tongue depressor.
    C. Allow the child to assume a position of comfort and immediately notify anesthesiology and otolaryngology.
    D. Accompany the child to radiology to obtain an anterior-posterior chest x-ray.

34. A patient is being supported on high frequency oscillatory ventilation and is receiving sedative and paralytic infusions. The patient is requiring high mean airway pressures to maintain adequate ventilation. The patient's saturations acutely drop to 80% despite the patient receiving 100% FiO_2. What other assessment findings will be important in determining the cause of the acute desaturation?
    A. Chest wiggle
    B. Endotracheal tube (ETT) size
    C. Ventilator circuit connections
    D. Train of four test

35. A patient on high frequency oscillatory ventilation who is adequately sedated is requiring high mean airway pressures to maintain adequate ventilation. The patient's saturations acutely drop to 80% and the chest wiggle is significantly diminished on the right side. The patient's blood pressure is beginning to decrease. What should the nurse anticipate doing next?
    A. Prepare for emergent needle decompression of the right chest.
    B. Sedate the patient.
    C. Turn the patient with the right side down.
    D. Deflate the cuff of the endotracheal tube (ETT).

36. An anesthetic medication that is used for its bronchodilatory effects in patients with asthma is:
    A. Ketamine (Ketalar)
    B. Vasopressin (Pitressin)
    C. Propofol (Diprivan)
    D. Morphine (AVINza)

37. Corticosteroids are commonly used in the treatment of asthma. The nurse caring for this patient population recognizes that the following is a potential side effect from this medication:
    A. Hypotension
    B. Hypoglycemia
    C. Decreased appetite
    D. Increased susceptibility to infections

38. A pediatric ICU (PICU) nurse is providing teaching to a parent whose child will be discharged on oral anticoagulation therapy. Which of the following would not be a key educational point?
    A. "This medication does not require any additional monitoring or follow-up."
    B. "Bleeding is one of the risks of this therapy, and high-impact sports such as basketball, boxing, and gymnastics should be avoided."
    C. "You should notify the primary provider if your child gets sick because illness can increase the risk for bleeding and may require a change in dose."
    D. "Your child should wear a Medi-Alert ID bracelet, and teachers, babysitters, and other family members should be aware that they take this medication."

39. A patient is in hypercapnic respiratory failure. They are being volume ventilated. What is the best treatment for this situation to remove retained CO_2?
    A. Maintain current ventilator settings to allow for permissive hypercapnia.
    B. Start a bicarbonate drip to treat the respiratory acidosis.
    C. Increase the tidal volume on the ventilator.
    D. Decrease the respiratory rate on the ventilator.

40. A 4-month-old former 24-week premature, trached, and ventilator-dependent infant is being admitted to the pediatric ICU (PICU) for acute respiratory failure. The mother reports that this morning the patient acutely became hypoxic. The mother suctioned the patient's tracheostomy tube, provided bag ventilation, and connected the infant back to the ventilator and the patient improved, but since has significant desaturations when they cry. Parents deny any fever, cough, or change in tracheal secretions. The mother also reports that she recently was unable to refill the patient's sildenafil and it has been about 5 days since they have had their medication. The patient's hypoxia is most likely related to:
    A. Mucus plugging of the tracheostomy
    B. Ventilator malfunction
    C. Pulmonary hypertensive crisis
    D. Bacterial tracheitis

41. You receive a child postoperatively that is intubated and on an assist control (AC) mode of ventilation. Their initial blood gas is good. The repeat arterial blood gas (ABG) an hour later is the following:

    pH: 7.49
    PO_2: 143
    PCO_2: 23
    HCO_3: 22

    Which of the following orders would the nurse anticipate?
    A. Increase FiO_2.
    B. Increase the rate.
    C. Decrease the rate.
    D. Increase positive end expiratory pressure (PEEP).

42. The patient undergoes a cardiac catheterization during admission to evaluate their pulmonary hypertension and response to vasodilators. Which catheterization data represents the presence of pulmonary hypertension?
    A. Resting pulmonary artery pressure of <15 mmHg
    B. Resting pulmonary artery pressure of >15 mmHg
    C. Resting pulmonary artery pressure of >25 mmHg
    D. Resting pulmonary artery pressure of <25 mmHg

43. A 5-year-old child is being admitted to the pediatric ICU (PICU) following being struck by a vehicle while riding their bike. The patient initially had a Glasgow Coma Scale (GCS) of 6 and was intubated at the scene of the accident. Upon arrival to the PICU, they develop severe respiratory distress despite being intubated, and frank blood is suctioned from the endotracheal tube.

    Heart rate (HR): 130
    Blood pressure (BP): 80/30
    SpO_2: 88%

    What is the most likely cause of the patient's clinical deterioration?
    A. Rib fractures
    B. Tension pneumothorax
    C. Posttraumatic atelectasis
    D. Hemothorax

44. A 3-year-old child is admitted to the pediatric ICU (PICU) with known aspiration of a miniature toy truck; the patient is awake and alert and with no respiratory distress or hypoxia. The patient is to undergo rigid bronchoscopy and esophagogastroduodenoscopy (EGD) for retrieval of the foreign body. The patient acutely develops chest and back pain, subcutaneous emphysema, and hematemesis. A chest x-ray (CXR) is performed, which reveals pneumomediastinum. The most likely cause of the change in clinical status is:
    A. Esophageal rupture
    B. Traumatic rupture of the diaphragm
    C. Tracheobronchial trauma
    D. Tension pneumothorax

45. The bedside nurse is assessing a 15-year-old following a traumatic crash on their all-terrain vehicle (ATV). The patient has been complaining of right lower chest pain that worsens with movement or when they push down on the area with their hand. The patient's pain is most likely caused by:
    A. Tension pneumothorax
    B. Rib fractures
    C. Spinal fractures
    D. Hemothorax

46. The most common reason for surgical correction of pectus excavatum is:
    A. Respiratory compromise
    B. Cardiac compromise
    C. Delayed growth
    D. Cosmetic concerns

47. A 16-year-old is admitted to the pediatric ICU (PICU) following a video-assisted thoracoscopic surgery (VATS) procedure for recurrent pneumothorax. On postoperative day 2, they are noted to have decreased breath sounds at the base, increased oxygen requirement, and consolidation on chest x-ray (CXR). They are afebrile and remain hemodynamically stable. The most likely cause of these symptoms is:
    A. Pneumonia
    B. Pneumothorax
    C. Atelectasis
    D. Tension pneumothorax

48. The nurse is assessing a 2-week-old patient who was just admitted for increased work of breathing. The parents state that the baby "makes a funny noise" when they cry and that "their neck moves in and out when they breathe." The nurse assesses the patient and notes that the patient has mild suprasternal retractions and a stridorous cry. Which of the following diagnoses is most likely?
    A. Choanal atresia
    B. Tracheomalacia
    C. Pulmonary interstitial emphysema
    D. Pulmonary embolism

49. A 6-year-old intubated patient is admitted to the pediatric ICU (PICU) after being struck by a motor vehicle. The medical team wants to attempt to wean them from mechanical ventilation. Their sedation infusions are decreased and the ventilator rate, tidal volume, and peak end expiratory pressure are decreased. About an hour after the changes were made, the patient begins to have an increased respiratory rate, increasing end tidal carbon dioxide, and subcostal retractions. Which of the following is the most appropriate intervention?
    A. Obtain a chest x-ray (CXR).
    B. Increase the patient's FiO_2 on the ventilator.
    C. Turn the sedation back up to the previous rate.
    D. Turn the ventilator settings back to the previous settings.

50. A nurse monitoring a patient's aldosterone levels knows the primary effect of aldosterone is:
    A. Decreased renal potassium excretion
    B. Increased sodium levels
    C. Increased renal potassium excretion
    D. Increased serum sodium levels

51. A patient is on mechanical ventilation. The respiratory therapist increases the positive inspiratory pressure (PIP). What effect would that have on the arterial blood gas (ABG)?
    A. Decreased $PaCO_2$ and increased PaO_2
    B. Increased $PaCO_2$ and decreased PaO_2
    C. Decreased $PaCO_2$ and decreased PaO_2
    D. Increased $PaCO_2$ and increased PaO_2

52. The nurse should immediately intervene if the child's blood glucose is at what level?
    A. 200 mg/dL
    B. 120 mg/dL
    C. 80 mg/dL
    D. 35 mg/dL

53. A patient is admitted with a pituitary tumor. The nurse knows pituitary tumors inhibit the production of what hormone?
    A. Cortisol
    B. Antidiuretic hormone (ADH)
    C. Adrenocorticotropic hormone (ACTH)
    D. Glucagon

54. A 2-week-old infant is admitted to the pediatric ICU (PICU) following a seizure at home. The parents report the infant has been healthy up until this morning when they would not feed and became lethargic. On the nurse's assessment, they appear to have poor muscle tone and muscle spasms. The nurse notes a smell of "sweet smell" from the patient's urine. Which disease process should the nurse suspect this infant may have?
A. Glucose-6-phosphate-dehydrogenase deficiency (G6PD) deficiency
B. Rhabdomyolysis
C. Diabetic ketoacidosis
D. Maple syrup urine disease

55. A 14-year-old (born at 24 weeks' gestation) was admitted with headaches needing a ventriculoperitoneal (VP) shunt revision. The night following surgery, the patient became febrile and had respiratory distress and was transferred to the pediatric ICU (PICU). They were intubated and placed on volume ventilation. The initial arterial blood gas showed:

pH: 7.27
PCO_2: 39
PO_2: 79,
HCO_3: 17.4
Base deficit: −8.3

The patient was adequately sedated and given a neuromuscular blocker. Repeat arterial blood gas (ABG) was:

pH: 7.07
PCO_2: 55
PO_2: 72
HCO_3: 17
Base deficit: −12

How would these blood gases be interpreted?
A. Respiratory acidosis
B. Respiratory alkalosis
C. Metabolic acidosis
D. Metabolic alkalosis

56. A child was in a motor vehicle crash (MVC) and sustained a subdural hematoma, which was evacuated. They have been stable for about a week in the pediatric ICU (PICU). The nurse notices the child has dry skin and a urine output of 650 mLs in 2 hours. A STAT chemistry panel was ordered, and the sodium was 152 mEq/L, glucose was 90 mg/dL, and potassium was 4.7 mEq/L. Which of the following conditions might this child be exhibiting?
A. Diabetes mellitus
B. Diabetes insipidus (DI)
C. Syndrome of inappropriate antidiuretic hormone (SIADH)
D. Cushing syndrome

57. Which condition can result in the development of acute hypoglycemia?
A. Glucose consumption that exceeds glucose production
B. Development of an insulinoma
C. Use of oral antihyperglycemic agents
D. Acute onset of gastroenteritis

58. A patient is admitted to the pediatric ICU (PICU) with a blood glucose of 1,120 mg/dL, pH of 6.89, and ketoacidosis. An insulin drip was started at 0.1 units/kg/hr. At 1800, the lab results reveal a blood glucose of 580 mg/dL and pH of 7.09. What does the nurse anticipate the next order to be?
A. Hold the insulin and recheck labs in 1 hour.
B. Continue with the current insulin infusion and add dextrose to the intravenous fluid (IVF).
C. Give the patient a 20 mL/kg normal saline solution (NSS) bolus.
D. Continue with the current insulin infusion and continue to monitor.

59. A 4-year-old is admitted to the pediatric ICU (PICU) with new onset diabetes and is in diabetic keto-acidosis (DKA). Admitting blood glucose level is 850 mg/dL. They are placed on intravenous (IV) fluids and an insulin drip. Eight hours after admission, blood sugar levels and electrolytes are normalizing. The patient starts complaining of a headache and appears lethargic, falling asleep as you speak with them. Heart rate (HR) is now 42 and blood pressure (BP) is 148/92. Respiratory rate (RR) is 10. Based on this information, the PICU nurse suspects the child may be developing:
   A. Hyperkalemia
   B. Sepsis
   C. Seizure activity post-DKA
   D. Cerebral edema

60. A 12-year-old presents with fever, increased work of breathing (WOB), and dactylitis. They report increasing fatigue over the last week and new bruising on their arms. Which of the following laboratory findings is expected?
   A. Absolute reticulocyte count of 3.6%
   B. White blood cell (WBC) count of 256,000/µL
   C. Hemoglobin (Hgb) and hematocrit (HCT) of 14 g/dL and 42%
   D. Factor VIII level of 5%

61. Heparin-induced thrombocytopenia is a result of what?
   A. An autoimmune response where platelets are inappropriately identified as foreign and targeted for phagocytosis in the spleen
   B. Systemic microhemorrhages cause chronic bleeding resulting in a continued platelet response
   C. Megakaryocyte suppression within the bone marrow is a rare but known side effect of heparin therapy
   D. Immune-mediated complexes cause platelet activation resulting in thrombus formation and thrombocytopenia

62. The nurse is caring for a 2-year-old patient with sickle cell disease presenting with acute pallor, lethargy, and tachycardia. The nurse finds these symptoms most concerning for:
   A. Splenic sequestration
   B. Acute chest syndrome
   C. Aplastic crisis
   D. Vaso-occlusive pain crisis

63. A child presents with altered gait and paresthesia in bilateral lower extremities. They are found to have a mass compressing their spinal cord. All of the following are likely diagnosis except:
   A. Neuroblastoma
   B. Rhabdomyosarcoma
   C. Ewing sarcoma
   D. Low grade glioma

64. A student nurse observes a 1-year-old child who is hospitalized for bacterial pneumonia requiring intravenous (IV) antibiotics for resolution. The pediatric ICU (PICU) team is considering a diagnosis of agammaglobulinemia. Which of the following statements by the nurse indicates a need for further teaching?
   A. "Children affected by agammaglobulinemia do not mount a sufficient vaccine response."
   B. "Treatment with intravenous immune globin (IVIG) will be needed lifelong."
   C. "Affected children have hypertrophic lymphoid structures such as tonsils and lymph nodes on exam."
   D. "Agammaglobulinemia is a defect in the body's ability produce mature and functioning B lymphocytes."

65. The nurse is taking care of an adolescent undergoing plasmapheresis for an autoimmune disorder. Two hours into the procedure, the patient becomes irritable and complains of abdominal pain. The nurse's immediate intervention is to:
   A. Administer ondansetron
   B. Treat hypocalcemia
   C. Administer intramuscular (IM) epinephrine
   D. Prepare for intubation

66. A 12-year-old presents to the ED for an examination after sustaining a direct blow to their abdomen with a soccer ball. The nurse suspects that the child may have injured their spleen. Which of these statements is true regarding assessment of the spleen in this situation? The spleen:
    A. Is likely to be normally palpated upon routine examination
    B. Located in the right upper quadrant and is seldom injured because of rib cage protection
    C. If enlarged, should be palpated to determine its exact size
    D. Should not be palpated because it can easily rupture

67. Which of the following suggests possible abdominal compartment syndrome (ACS) findings and should be reported to the provider for a child who is nonventilated?
    A. Intermittent intra-abdominal pressure measurement recordings of 5 mmHg and polyuria
    B. Sustained intra-abdominal pressure measurement of 14 mmHg and oliguria
    C. Intra-abdominal pressure measurement of 10 mmHg and urinary output of 1 mL/kg/hr
    D. Intermittent intra-abdominal pressure measurement of 10 mmHg and diminished abdominal sounds

68. A pediatric ICU (PICU) nurse is caring for a 3-year-old with a 6-day history of fever, bilateral conjunctivitis, and lymphadenopathy. Which if the following orders would the nurse question?
    A. Acetaminophen (Tylenol) 75 mg/kg/day
    B. Serial echocardiography
    C. Electrocardiography
    D. Intravenous immunoglobulin 2 g/kg

69. A nurse has just received report on their patients. Which patient should the nurse assess first? The patient with:
    A. Necrotizing enterocolitis (NEC) whose nasogastric/Replogle tube is draining green bile
    B. A gastrointestinal (GI) bleed who is receiving blood and has a hemoglobin of 11 g/dL and hematocrit of 30%
    C. Appendicitis, postoperative day 1 with a hard, rigid abdomen and temperature 38.3°C (101°F)
    D. A bowel infarction who has had diarrhea and a potassium level of 3 mEq/L

70. Which medication would the nurse expect to administer to a patient with gastrointestinal (GI) hemorrhage?
    A. Vasopressin (Pitressin)
    B. Digoxin (Lanoxin)
    C. Enoxaparin (Lovenox)
    D. Polyethylene glycol (Miralax)

71. Nurses are caring for four patients in the pediatric ICU (PICU). After reviewing each patient's laboratory results, which patient should a nurse call the provider about immediately? The patient who:
    A. Is nothing by mouth (NPO) with a blood glucose level of 80 mg/dL
    B. Is postoperative day 1 after abdominal surgery for a bowel perforation and has hemoglobin and hematocrit of 14.5/40
    C. Is 8 hours postoperative for necrotizing enterocolitis with white blood cell (WBC) count of 20,000/µL
    D. Is 4 hours postoperative for exploratory laparotomy with a serum potassium level of 3.6 mEq/L

72. The nurse is attempting to place a post-pyloric feeding tube. The tip of the tube is sitting just past the pyloric sphincter on abdominal x-ray. In order to get the tube to move further into the intestine, which of the following medications does the nurse expect to administer to increase intestinal motility?
    A. Famotidine (Pepcid)
    B. Sucralfate (Carafate)
    C. Omeprazole (Prilosec)
    D. Metoclopramide (Reglan)

73. Which symptom is most commonly associated with malabsorption syndromes?
    A. Frequent regurgitation
    B. Weight gain
    C. Watery diarrhea
    D. Negative Trousseau sign

74. A pediatric ICU (PICU) nurse is admitting a 12-year-old patient with a several-day history of fever, vomiting, diarrhea, and new rash. They have no significant past medical history but had suspected COVID-19 3 weeks ago. Their vital signs on admission are:

Temperature: 38.5°C (101.3°F)
Heart rate (HR): 115
Blood pressure (BP): 85/55
Respiratory rate (RR): 20
SpO_2: 88% on room air

The nurse places the patient on oxygen, obtains intravenous (IV) access, and administers a normal saline (NS) fluid bolus. Which of the following does the nurse anticipate next?
A. STAT chest x-ray, EKG, and complete blood count (CBC)
B. Epinephrine 0.05 mcg/kg/min IV
C. An additional 20 mL/kg NS bolus
D. Milrinone load followed by 0.25 mcg/kg/min IV

75. Which of the following patients with hypertension is most concerning and warrants immediate intervention with an intravenous (IV) antihypertensive medication?
A. A 12-year-old with papilledema and seizures
B. A 16-year-old with dyslipidemia who was unable to refill their benazepril (Lotensin) for 2 weeks
C. A 6-year-old with rheumatoid arthritis who presents with myalgias
D. A 10-year-old with renal vascular disease and headaches

76. A toddler presents with agitation, mydriasis, and dry and flushed skin. Their vital signs are:

Temperature: 38°C (100.4°F)
Heart rate (HR): 140
Blood pressure (BP): 100/60
Respiratory rate (RR): 30

Which of the following ingestions is most likely?
A. Organophosphate
B. Tricyclic antidepressants
C. Gabapentin
D. Hydromorphone

77. Which of the following pediatric ICU (PICU) patients are likely candidates for urgent renal replacement therapy? (Select all that apply.)
A. 12-month-old with a heart rate (HR) 145 bpm, blood pressure (BP) 110/70, and a pericardial effusion on x-ray
B. 6-year-old with a history of hemolytic uremic syndrome with new seizures
C. 14-year-old with polyuria and hyponatremia receiving replacement fluid
D. 2-year-old with a HR 100, respiratory rate (RR) 50, and SpO_2 90% on heated-high flow nasal cannula

78. Over the last 12 hours, a nurse caring for a patient with acute tubular necrosis (ATN) has observed the urine output remain <0.5 mL/kg/hr. Which of the following is mostly likely?
A. The patient is in the initial phase of injury.
B. The patient is oliguric phase of injury.
C. The patient is in the diuretic phase of injury.
D. The patient is in the recovery phase of injury.

79. A 5-year-old presented with a 2-day history of fever, abdominal and back pain, and new incontinence after successful potty training. Which of the following diagnosis is most likely?
A. Acute glomerulonephritis
B. Peritonitis
C. Pyelonephritis
D. Hemolytic uremic syndrome

80. A recent snowstorm prevented an adolescent pediatric ICU (PICU) patient from receiving their scheduled hemodialysis. In addition to complaints of feeling like their hands and feet are burning, an EKG showed peaked T waves and a widened QRS. Which of the following interventions do you anticipate?
    A. Monitor EKG, q2 hour neurovascular assessments, and orders for magnesium oxide.
    B. Restrict oral fluids and give hypertonic saline.
    C. Administer diuretics and calcium supplements.
    D. Administer calcium chloride, sodium bicarbonate, and insulin and glucose. Prepare for dialysis.

81. A 3-year-old is admitted to your pediatric ICU (PICU) with a 3-day history of abdominal pain and diarrhea, fever, and lethargy. Laboratory results reveal:

    Serum creatinine: 1.2 mg/dL
    Blood urea nitrogen (BUN): 40 mg/dL
    Hemoglobin: 12 g/dL
    Platelets: 150,000/uL

    Which of the following nursing interventions are appropriate in the care of this patient? (Select all that apply.)
    A. Place an indwelling urinary catheter and record urine output hourly.
    B. Administer 20 mL/kg normal saline.
    C. Administer 10 mL/kg packed red blood cells.
    D. Verify meningococcal vaccination prior to eculizumab administration.

82. A pediatric ICU (PICU) nurse is caring for a critically ill 16-year-old patient receiving hemodialysis with the following vital signs: temperature: 36°C (96.8°F), heart rate (HR): 100, blood pressure (BP): 90/60, respiratory rate (RR): 14. Which of the following are priority interventions in this patient's care?
    A. Perform hand hygiene before all patient contact, monitor for signs and symptoms of infection.
    B. Measure weight daily, monitor intake and output closely.
    C. Administer electrolyte replacements as ordered, monitor serum electrolytes daily.
    D. Give albumin, monitor vital signs following dose.

83. A patient with respiratory failure was intubated in the pediatric ICU (PICU) for 6 days. Now 3 days postextubation, the patient's mother is concerned they are not acting like themself. Which of the following statements by the nurse most accurately describes pediatric delirium?
    A. "The benzodiazepines your child received help prevent PICU delirium."
    B. "The most important thing is to catch delirium early."
    C. "The sleepiness and decreased attention are signs of exhaustion and will improve as they rest and recover."
    D. "Agitated behaviors and hallucinations are the most common delirium symptoms in patients admitted to the PICU for 6 or more days."

84. When assessing a wound, how should you measure the length?
    A. The largest dimension of the wound is the length.
    B. The dimension from head to toe is the length.
    C. The dimension from hip to hip is the length.
    D. The dimension should be described using coins as reference.

85. A nurse identifies a 2 cm-by-2 cm area of nonblanchable erythema on a patient's heel. The nurse knows that this pressure injury:
    A. Will likely heal on its own without intervention
    B. Is more likely to become a stage 3 or stage 4 injury than if located elsewhere on the body
    C. Was likely caused by a medical device
    D. Requires immediate surgical intervention

86. A nurse is caring for a 17-year-old immobile patient who prefers the supine position and is refusing to turn. Which of the following interventions is most appropriate?
    A. Obtain a specialty bed for pressure injury prevention.
    B. Obtain an order from the physician that the patient does not need to turn/reposition.
    C. Explain to the patient/family the importance of repositioning and identify strategies that will make repositioning tolerable.
    D. Reposition the patient anyway every 2 hours using pillows and blanket rolls.

87. A pediatric ICU (PICU) nurse is caring for a critically ill oncology patient. While providing hygiene in the afternoon, the nurse observes a deep red lesion on the sacrum that was not present upon the morning assessment. The nurse can anticipate:
    A. The patient's impending death
    B. The patient's injury will heal upon recovery from their critical illness
    C. An order for platelet transfusion
    D. An order for a wound culture to determine etiology

88. A 13-year-old with history of myelomeningocele and a chronic stage 4 pressure injury of the ischial tuberosity has heart rate of 126, temperature of 38.6°C (101.5°F), and appears uncomfortable. What intervention should the nurse plan to perform?
    A. Remove packing from wound and culture the drainage.
    B. Remove packing from the wound for wound assessment.
    C. Obtain consent for bone biopsy.
    D. Ready the patient for MRI.

89. The nurse is caring for a terminally ill patient whose goals of care have been identified as prioritizing comfort. When offering pain medication, the nurse knows to prioritize:
    A. Adhering to the schedule of routine bathing and repositioning
    B. Allowing the patient to have consolidated sleep
    C. The patient and family's values and preferences
    D. Stopping all pressure injury prevention interventions in the interest of comfort

90. The priority of treatment for a patient with rhabdomyolysis would be which of the following?
    A. Addiction counseling
    B. Fluid restriction
    C. Physical therapy (PT) to restore muscle function
    D. Aggressive intravenous fluid (IVF) administration

91. A child sustained a radial fracture after a fall and a cast was just applied. Two hours later the child states that "it really hurts, and my fingers feel tingly." Which intervention should be a priority?
    A. Elevate the extremity on a pillow.
    B. Immediately call the provider.
    C. Prepare for a fasciotomy.
    D. Perform more frequent neurovascular checks.

92. A 14-year-old patient has suspected compartment syndrome. What sustained compartment pressures are indicative of compartment syndrome and would require a fasciotomy?
    A. 10 mmHg
    B. 15 mmHg
    C. 30 mmHg
    D. 40 mmHg

93. A 4-year-old child was just admitted with a closed left femoral fracture. They are not splinted or in traction and experiencing severe intermittent pain. What might be the cause of that pain and needs to be treated?
    A. Infection
    B. Muscle spasm
    C. Edema
    D. Hypothermia

94. A child is ordered fentanyl intravenously (IV) after sustaining multiple fractures for pain. What is a possible side effect of IV fentanyl?
    A. Chest wall rigidity
    B. Tachypnea
    C. Hyperthyroidism
    D. Nasal congestion

95. A nurse is providing intracranial pressure education to a group of nurses on orientation and explains that when cerebral perfusion pressure (CPP) falls too low, the brain is not properly perfused and brain tissue dies. An orientee asks what normal cerebral perfusion pressure is. The nurse's response should be:
    A. 5 to 10 mmHg
    B. 20 to 30 mmHg
    C. 40 to 50 mmHg
    D. >100 mmHg

96. A patient with a cerebral hemorrhage is at risk for developing increased intracranial pressure (ICP). Which sign or symptom is the EARLIEST indicator the patient is having increased ICP?
    A. Decreased level of consciousness
    B. Bradycardia
    C. Unequal pupil size
    D. Decerebrate posturing

97. A nursing student is studying the Monro-Kellie doctrine. Which statement by the student indicates the need for further teaching?
    "A compensatory mechanism performed by the body to decrease ICP naturally is:
    A. leaking proteins into the brain barrier."
    B. shifting cerebrospinal fluid to other areas of the brain or spinal cord."
    C. vasoconstriction of cerebral vessels."
    D. decrease cerebrospinal fluid production."

98. A nurse is caring for an 8-year-old child that has a cervical spinal cord injury and is at risk of neurogenic shock. What hallmark signs and symptoms, if experienced by this patient, would indicate the child is experiencing neurogenic shock?
    A. Blood pressure (BP) 140/80, heart rate (HR) 120, temperature 38.5°C (101.3°F)
    B. BP 70/40, HR 45, temperature 35°C (95°F)
    C. Cool and clammy extremities, BP 110/50, temperature 37°C (98.6°F)
    D. Warm and dry extremities, BP 68/42, temperature 39°C (102.2°F)

99. A teenager is hospitalized with a known arteriovenous malformation (AVM). The patient complains of a headache and becomes disoriented. What is the most appropriate action by the nurse?
    A. Document the changes and monitor the patient closely.
    B. Administer acetaminophen (Tylenol) for the headache.
    C. Prepare to give aspirin or another thrombolytic agent as ordered.
    D. Prepare the patient for surgery.

100. What type of traumatic brain injury (TBI) is defined as a short period of observed or self-reported transient confusion, or impaired consciousness?
    A. Mild TBI
    B. Moderate TBI
    C. Severe TBI
    D. Vestibular TBI

101. Which of the following is considered a sign or symptom of traumatic brain injury (TBI)?
    A. Glasgow Coma Scale (GCS) = 15
    B. Nystagmus
    C. Decreased level of consciousness (LOC)
    D. Decreased appetite

102. A 3-year-old child is admitted directly to the pediatric ICU (PICU) from the trauma bay after a fall on the playground with a witnessed trauma to the head. Vital signs on arrival are the following: heart rate (HR) 145, respiratory rate (RR) 22, SpO_2 98%, and blood pressure (BP) 131/72. The child's neurologic exam on arrival included a Glasgow Coma Scale (GCS) of 15; pupils, equal, round, reactive to light and accommodation (PERRLA); and crying inconsolably in the mother's arms. On assessment 2 hours postadmission, the RN found the patient unarousable to painful stimulation, the right pupil 4 mm and nonreactive, and left pupil 3 mm and sluggish to light. The critical care RN should be most concerned for the following:
    A. Increased intracranial pressure (ICP)
    B. Elevated cerebral perfusion pressure (CPP)
    C. Brain herniation
    D. Seizures

103. The most severe form of encephalitis is caused by _____ and can be treated with _____ to improve prognosis.
    A. Herpes simplex virus; acyclovir
    B. Autoimmune causes; high-dose corticosteroids
    C. *Streptococcus pneumoniae*; vancomycin
    D. *Neisseria meningitidis*; ceftriaxone

104. Which of the following is not an example of parental education that may help prevent spinal cord injuries (SCIs) and traumatic brain injuries (TBIs)?
    A. Proper installation and use of car seats
    B. Helmet use for bikes, scooters, and motorized toys
    C. Safe sleep practices
    D. Pedestrian safety

105. The best imaging technique to rule out spinal cord injury (SCI) in pediatrics is:
    A. CT
    B. X-ray
    C. MRI
    D. Ultrasound

106. A child is admitted to the pediatric ICU (PICU) after being involved in a motor vehicle crash (MVC). The nurse notices the child's parents frequently arguing with each other at the bedside. Which of the following actions are most appropriate?
    A. The nurse tells the parents they are not allowed to visit at the same time if the arguing continues.
    B. The nurse notifies security and has them on standby when the parents are in the room together.
    C. The nurse assists the family to identify support people or resources to help them deal with the stress of their child's illness.
    D. The nurse acknowledges the parents' situation and empathizes with them as the nurse was recently divorced as well.

107. The nurse is discussing gender differences in suicide risk and suicide rates for children and adolescents with a history of major depressive disorder. Which of the following statements made by the nurse is most accurate?
    A. The risk of suicide attempts and completions is higher in males.
    B. The risk of suicide attempts and completions is higher in females.
    C. The risk of suicide attempts is higher in females, but the risk of suicide completions is higher in males.
    D. The risk of suicide attempts is higher in males, but the risk of suicide completions is higher in females.

108. A nurse is administering fluoxetine (Prozac) to a patient who is admitted to the pediatric ICU (PICU). The patient's mother asks if this medication has any warnings or precautions. Which of the following statements made by the nurse is most accurate?
    A. "This medication does not have a black box warning."
    B. "This medication has a black box warning but only for the elderly."
    C. "This medication has a black box warning indicating an increased risk for suicidality."
    D. "This medication has a black box warning indicating it can increase mortality in children."

109. A 12-year-old is admitted to the pediatric ICU (PICU). The nurse notices that they are wearing bilateral wrist bands. The nurse asks the child, "Why do you have wrist bands on your arms?" The patient responds: "I think they look cool." A few hours later, the nurse needs to start an intravenous (IV) on the patient. When looking for a site, the nurse pulls back one of the wrist bands and notice what appear to be cut marks on their wrists. Which of the following would be the most appropriate response by the nurse?
    A. Obtain a psychiatric consult.
    B. Ask the patient, "I noticed scars on your arms; can you tell me how you got them?"
    C. Ask the child if their parents know about this.
    D. Confront the patient and say, "I see you are self-harming and I find it very upsetting."

110. A 2-year-old girl is brought in with significant neglect and abuse. Which of the following statements by the mother is concerning for abuse?
    A. "I am so worried about my little baby girl."
    B. "Do you know when my child is going to be seen by the doctor?"
    C. "I have no idea what happened, it's all her fault anyway."
    D. "I love her so much; I hope everything will be OK."

111. Which of the following statements is accurate about posttraumatic stress disorder (PTSD)?
    A. It is usually diagnosed within 1 to 2 weeks following a stressful incident.
    B. Patients may develop it after a short pediatric ICU (PICU) admission.
    C. It is most common in older, male patients.
    D. It usually occurs after an unexpected, prolonged admission.

112. Which of the following is important for the nurse to recognize when caring for a child who is experiencing anxiety?
    A. Anxiety is easier to treat than overt aggression.
    B. Anxiety reactions are usually the same in the child as it is in the parent.
    C. Family members usually have no effect on the anxiety experienced by the patient.
    D. Parents and children usually have the same anxiety triggers.

113. Which of the following is not consistent with anaphylactic shock?
    A. Urticaria
    B. Swelling of the lips
    C. Elevated temperature
    D. Tachycardia

114. A 5-year-old admitted to the pediatric ICU (PICU) with an asthma exacerbation is requiring non-invasive ventilation via nasal mask and continuously inhaled albuterol. They are awake and alert with stable vital signs and improving air movement. A priority intervention for the critical care nurse would be:
    A. Apply padding over the nasal bridge and rotate their nasal mask with nasal prongs, if tolerated
    B. Administer 20 mL/kg bolus of 0.9% normal saline
    C. Prepare for intubation
    D. Administer antibiotics

115. A 3-year-old presents to the pediatric ICU (PICU) from home. They were born at 26 weeks' gestation and have a medical history of developmental delay, chronic lung disease, tracheostomy and ventilator dependence, gastrostomy tube, and a tunneled central venous catheter. The patient presents with fever, tachycardia, mottled skin, capillary refill time of 4 to 5 seconds, and rales on respiratory assessment. They received 40 mL/kg of Lactated Ringer's (LR) in the ED. The patient's current vital signs are

    39.4°C (102.9°F)
    heart rate (HR) 165
    respiratory rate (RR) 40
    blood pressure (BP) 68/40
    SpO_2 93%

    The critical care nurse should anticipate the following intervention as a priority:
    A. Obtaining blood and respiratory cultures
    B. Administration of 20 mL/kg of LR
    C. Intravenous (IV) cefepime STAT
    D. Initiation of a vasoactive infusion

116. The critical care nurse should anticipate the following vasoactive infusion as the first line for hypotension in septic shock:
    A. Epinephrine (Adrenalin)
    B. Dobutamine (Dobutrex)
    C. Vasopressin (Pitressin)
    D. Dopamine (Intropin)

117. A 15-year-old is admitted to the pediatric ICU (PICU) following an intentional ingestion of their parent's prescription alprazolam (Xanax). The critical care nurse anticipates the following treatment:
    A. Naloxone (Narcan)
    B. Cyproheptadine (Periactin)
    C. Diazepam (Valium)
    D. Flumazenil (Romazicon)

118. A 5-year-old weighing 19.5 kg presents to the ED from a birthday party where they told their mother they were having a hard time breathing. They have a history of asthma and use albuterol as needed for wheezing. Their mother states that she has administered four puffs of albuterol and the child appears to be struggling to breathe. They have some blotchy red spots on their arms and trunk and mild periorbital edema. They are audibly wheezing and tachypneic with a SpO$_2$ of 90% on room air. They are tachycardic and becoming increasingly agitated. The appropriate treatment includes:
    A. Nebulized albuterol
    B. 0.15 mg of intramuscular (IM) epinephrine via EpiPen®
    C. Noninvasive ventilatory support
    D. Oral corticosteroids

119. A child is admitted after drowning in the family swimming pool. The family is optimistic as within a few hours, the child opens their eyes. A day later the child no longer is responding to pain and is showing signs of increased intracranial pressure. The parent can't understand what happened. The nurse tries to explain that the worsening of condition is most likely due to:
    A. The development of an infection
    B. Cerebral edema post hypoxic event
    C. Development of a brain bleed
    D. Inability to ventilate the child

120. A 3-year-old presents to the ED obtunded, shallow breathing, with pinpoint pupils. In addition to interventions to support airway, breathing, and circulation, the nurse anticipates the following early action:
    A. Perform gastric decontamination with activated charcoal
    B. Obtain a history of the event and review of available medications and products in the home
    C. Obtain serial serum drug levels
    D. Perform ocular irrigation

121. A patient admitted to the pediatric ICU (PICU) develops a new fever and hypotension. They are postoperative day 4 following a posterior spinal fusion. They have a central line, the urinary catheter was removed on day 1 postoperative, and surgical wound dressings are clean, dry, and intact. Their pain has been well controlled with scheduled and as-needed intravenous hydromorphone and diazepam. Their fever and hypotension are most consistent with which hospital acquired condition?
    A. Catheter associated urinary tract infection (CAUTI)
    B. Surgical site infection
    C. Pressure injury
    D. Central line-associated bloodstream infection (CLABSI)

122. Which is the correct interpretation of the following arterial blood gas (ABG)?

    pH: 7.36
    PCO$_2$: 55 mmHg
    PO$_2$: 79 mmHg
    HCO$_3$: 28 mEq/L
    SaO$_2$: 95%
    A. Compensated respiratory acidosis
    B. Uncompensated respiratory acidosis
    C. Compensated metabolic acidosis
    D. Uncompensated metabolic acidosis

123. A 12-year old is receiving mechanical ventilation after an aortic valve repair. At 1430, additional sedation was required for postoperative chest tube manipulation. A scheduled arterial blood gas was obtained at 1545, with results as follows:

pH: 7.30
PCO_2: 62 mmHg
PO_2: 99mmHg
HCO_3: 23 mEq/L
SaO_2: 98%

Based on the results of this lab, what intervention would the nurse anticipate next?
A. Decrease FiO_2 on ventilator.
B. Increase respiratory rate on ventilator.
C. Decrease respiratory rate on ventilator.
D. Increase inspiratory time on ventilator.

124. A 3-month-old is admitted for management of acute fluid overload secondary to heart failure. The patient is being medically managed with the following: captopril, furosemide, and chlorothiazide. The patient experiences seizure-like activity and lab results show the following:

pH: 7.49
PCO_2: 35 mmHg
PO_2: 75 mmHg
HCO_3: 32 mEq/L
SaO_2: 96%

What is a possible cause of this patient's symptoms?
A. Hyperkalemia
B. Hypercalcemia
C. Diuretic use
D. Mineralocorticoid deficiency

125. A 7-year-old sustained a crush injury to the chest and abdomen after an all-terrain vehicle flipped on top of them. After a vigorous resuscitation, the team obtained return of spontaneous circulation. However, the patient continued to have extensive bleeding and dysrhythmias and experienced cardiac arrest twice in a 6-hour period. The family wishes to withdraw care and allow for natural death. Which of the following is the priority nursing action to provide care to the dying patient?
A. Ensure all dressings are clean, dry, and intact.
B. Assess and treat for signs of pain or discomfort.
C. Label all lines with date/time of expiration.
D. Assess for signs of altered skin integrity.

126. A 20-month-old presents to the ED with a 2-day history of vomiting and diarrhea. The patient is pale, minimally responsive to interventions, and cries upon placement of intravenous (IV) catheter but makes no tears. Vital signs are as follows:

Heart rate (HR): 160
Respiratory rate (RR): 40
Blood pressure (BP): 62/40
O_2 sat: 96%
Temperature: 36.7°C (98°F)

The nurse anticipates which of the following interventions?
A. Immediate transfer to the pediatric ICU (PICU)
B. Administration of a dextrose 10% bolus, 5 mL/kg
C. Administration of a 0.9% NaCl bolus, 20 mL/kg
D. Obtaining blood cultures and administering antibiotics

127. Which of the following is the primary treatment for graft-versus-host disease (GVHD)?
A. Steroids
B. Antibiotics
C. Immunosupressents
D. Antifungal

128. A 12-year-old patient with systemic lupus erythematosus underwent a kidney transplant secondary to refractory lupus nephritis. They are being admitted with headaches, hypertension, and decreased urine output. The nurse suspects which of the following?
A. Sepsis
B. Rejection of the organ
C. Lupus flare
D. Lymphoma

129. What is the gold standard for diagnosis of cardiac organ rejection?
A. Troponin level
B. Direct intracardiac pressure measurements
C. Echocardiogram
D. Tissue biopsy

130. A 3-year-old with a diagnosis of acute lymphoblastic leukemia is admitted with a presumed central line associated blood stream infection. The patient underwent surgical removal of the implanted port yesterday. Blood cultures were drawn and antibiotics were initiated. Today, the nurse records the following vital signs:

Heart rate (HR): 130
Respiratory rate (RR): 28
Blood pressure (BP): 99/74
O$_2$ sat: 98%
Temperature: 38.8°C (101.8°F)

The nurse anticipates administration of which of the following medications?
A. Acetaminophen (Tylenol)
B. Aspirin (Disprin)
C. Pentamidine (Nebupent)
D. Metoprolol (Lopressor)

131. A child has end-stage lung disease. They are currently being treated for aspiration pneumonia. The child is to receive nothing by mouth (NPO). They are receiving nasoduodenal feeds. The nurse notices the mother giving the child sips of water from her cup. Which of the following interventions would be most appropriate?
A. Do nothing; allow the mother to give the child fluids.
B. Gently but directly ask the mother why she is giving her child fluids.
C. Notify the provider that the mother is giving the child fluids during rounds.
D. Notify social service that the mother is noncompliant and putting her child at risk.

132. A child just diagnosed with chronic renal failure is being discharged to home. The child will go home on furosemide (Lasix) and it is vital the child receives this medication. The caregiver goes to the pharmacy to pick up the medication and returns without the medication. When the nurse inquires why they did not pick up the medication, the caregiver replies, "The hospital will not accept my insurance provider. I am sure my child will be fine without this medication." Which of the following is the most appropriate response by the discharging nurse?
A. "This is unacceptable, you need to go back down and get this medication, or your child may die."
B. "Let me call the social worker/case manager and see if they can assist you with this."
C. "Well, I guess it is all right that you go home without this medication, just be sure you go to your local pharmacy and pick it up later."
D. "Do you know anyone in your family that is on furosemide (Lasix) and could possibly share some of their medication with your child. It is vital that they get this medication!"

133. A 2-year-old child who suffered a traumatic brain injury (TBI) is being discharged home with a trach in place and continuous positive airway pressure (CPAP). The child's parents live in a camper in a year-round campground. They have a water and sewer hook-up, but electricity is not guaranteed. They do have a cell phone and a car. The father has a job. The next closest support person (maternal grandmother) lives 2 hours away and seems loving and attentive when visiting. Which of the patient characteristics are paramount in this case?
A. Resiliency
B. Resource availability
C. Participation in care
D. Predictability

134. A nurse who has a good awareness and anticipates changes in their patient, who is totally engaged with their patient, and who involves the patient/family in information, education, and changes in patient care would demonstrate what level of functioning when acting as a patient advocate?
    A. 1 (very low)
    B. 3 (moderate)
    C. 5 (very high)
    D. Unable to determine

135. Which of the following would contribute to a positive workplace environment?
    A. A business-oriented delivery of care model
    B. Caring for multiple complex patients while being short-staffed
    C. Presenting new innovative ideas to leadership that do not get implemented
    D. Nurses having a feeling of empowerment

136. A child is admitted to a nurse's unit and the family does not speak English. Which of the following is most appropriate when using an interpreter on the video language line on an iPad?
    A. Speak more slowly and louder than usual.
    B. Do not use any medical terms when explaining.
    C. Give the control of the conversations over to the interpreter.
    D. Speak to the family and make eye contact to ensure understanding.

137. A child with a tracheostomy and a gastrostomy tube is being discharged to home. They will need at-home ventilation and extensive care. In order to facilitate this discharge, the nurse should:
    A. Express their understanding of how overwhelming this situation will be for the family
    B. Notify the discharge planner of the child's home care and equipment needs
    C. Begin teaching the family of the anatomy and physiology of the airway
    D. Give the family numbers of at-home support groups

138. A nurse in the pediatric ICU (PICU) can manage a full patient assignment, is a unit preceptor, and participates in hospital interdisciplinary meetings. At what level of collaboration is this nurse functioning?
    A. Novice
    B. Advanced Beginner
    C. Competent
    D. Expert

139. An 18-year-old has terminal cancer. They verbalized to the nurse that after 7 years of treatment, they no longer want to continue with experimental treatments and they are ready to die. The patient has tried to talk to their parents about their feelings, but they refuse to talk to them about it and quickly change the subject. The patient is terminal, has become unconscious, and is having agonal respirations. The parents "want everything done" to save their child's life. Which of the following statements would be an example of a nurse acting as a moral agent for the patient?
    A. "Your child has verbalized that they no longer wish for further life-sustaining treatment to be done."
    B. "I totally understand; it is your child of course we will do everything to save their life."
    C. "What is going on? Why are you having trouble accepting your child's terminal diagnosis?"
    D. "Your child is not doing well; perhaps you should schedule a meeting with the treatment team to discuss the next course of action."

140. A 12-year-old child was in a house fire and suffered extensive burns to the lower extremities. As the wounds heal, the child expresses an interest in understanding their injuries. Which of the following statements by the nurse would demonstrate the example of participation in care and decision-making and leading to their own resiliency?
    A. "Today we are doing your dressing changes at 10 a.m. I expect you to start looking at your burns so you can help in dressing changes."
    B. "You are scheduled for a burn redress today at 10 a.m. I am going to ask your parent to help change the dressing today."
    C. "We are doing your burn redress today at 10 a.m. Would you like to take your sedation medication at 9 or 9:30 a.m.?"
    D. "You are scheduled for a burn redress today; what time this morning would you like to do it? Would you like to help me change your bandages today?"

141. A teenager with diabetes lives in a reportedly negligent household. They are frequently admitted with diabetic ketoacidosis (DKA). They purposely do not take their insulin so they can get a "vacation" from their home environment. Which statement by the nurse would be most appropriate?
   A. "What is going on at home should not interfere with you managing your insulin."
   B. "I think we should involve your parents more in your diabetic care so you take your insulin on time."
   C. "How are you doing managing your diabetes?"
   D. "Would you like to speak with our diabetic educator? This is your fifth admission for DKA."

142. A teenager with diabetes lives in a reportedly abusive household. They are frequently admitted with diabetic ketoacidosis (DKA). They purposely do not take their insulin so they can get a "vacation" from their home environment. The patient shares with the nurse that their family does not buy insulin because they have no money. What would be the best course of action?
   A. Involve the social worker to explore the family's resources and explore the teen's living environment.
   B. Immediately contact child protective services immediately as this is surely abuse.
   C. Schedule a family meeting involving the teen to determine if abuse is occurring in the home.
   D. Refer the teen to psychiatry as they obviously have a psychiatric issue.

143. Which of the following patient characteristics exemplifies the ability to maintain a constant steady state of functioning?
   A. Stability
   B. Resiliency
   C. Complexity
   D. Participation in care

144. A known diabetic patient comes in with diabetic ketoacidosis (DKA). They are homeless, have no insurance, and have no friends or family for support. Which of the following patient characteristics is this an example of?
   A. Participation on decision-making
   B. Resiliency
   C. Predictability
   D. Resource availability

145. A known diabetic patient comes in with diabetic ketoacidosis (DKA). They are homeless, have no insurance, and have no friends or family for support. Rate the patient's likely resiliency availability (likelihood of their resiliency and ability to return to a previous level of health and functioning).
   A. 1 (very low)
   B. 2 (moderate)
   C. 3 (very high)
   D. Unable to determine with the given information

146. A 19-year-old patient is admitted who is confused. They are in heart failure and need to be intubated, and their kidneys are failing and need dialysis. Which of the following would you say this patient does not have the ability to do?
   A. Be resilient
   B. Participate in decision-making
   C. Not exhibit being vulnerable
   D. Utilize resources

147. An 18-month-old special needs child is being discharged home with a trach in place and is on pressure ventilation, completely dependent on the ventilator for respiratory support. The child's parents live in a camper in a year-round campground. They have a water and sewer hook-up, but electricity is not guaranteed. They do have a cell phone and a car. The father has a job. The next closest support person (maternal grandmother) lives in another state hours away. What level of resource availability does this family have?
   A. Minimal
   B. Moderate
   C. High
   D. Cannot be determined

148. An 8-year-old patient is admitted to the ICU with myocarditis. They deteriorate rapidly and are placed on mechanical ventilation and vasopressors. After days, heart function remains poor and they are placed on veno-arterial extracorporeal membrane oxygenation (ECMO). They remain on ECMO for 30 days. They are unable to wean and transfer off. The patient is not a transplant or ventricular assist device candidate. The patient is in foster care and has no involved family. A discussion ensues as to whether to remove the patient from ECMO as many younger patients are in need of ECMO. While the treatment team proposes to do no harm, which ethical principle is presented in this case requires a care decision?
    A. Justice
    B. Futility
    C. Autonomy
    D. Beneficence

149. A child whose family recently immigrated to the United States is admitted to the pediatric ICU (PICU) with a head injury and increased intracranial pressure (ICP). Which of the following comments is most accurate in relation to providing culturally competent care?
    A. Culture does not affect children as they are too young to understand.
    B. Healthcare issues and concepts like ICP are universal and not affected by culture.
    C. It does not matter what the child thinks; the nurse needs to abide by the parent's wishes for care.
    D. Cultural factors can affect both the child's and family's response during hospitalization.

150. A child who has a fever is ordered acetaminophen (Tylenol). The nurse asks the child if they would prefer a chewable tablets or liquid. The child then turns to their mother and says, "Ok, but Mommy, which one do I like better?" This is an example of:
    A. Lack of cooperation
    B. Being shy
    C. Low level of decision-making
    D. Moderate level of decision-making

Practice Test: Answers

1. B) Apply pressure above the insertion site
The initial nursing action is to achieve hemostasis by applying direct pressure above the catheterization insertion site. Within 5 to 10 minutes, hemostasis should occur. Additional measures consist of notifying the physician, reinforcing the pressure dressing, and administering sedative medications as needed.

2. B) Infective endocarditis (IE)
A risk factor for IE is a prosthetic valve. The patient presented with the clinical findings of a new regurgitant murmur and nonspecific symptoms of infection such as prolonged low-grade fevers, malaise, weight loss, and myalgias, revealing IE as the most likely diagnosis. PE results from a thrombus that travels to the lung. Patients presenting with a PE event will have shortness of breath (SOB) and chest pain requiring emergency management. Patients with pericardial effusion may present with chest pain and SOB that is worse while laying flat. Constrictive pericarditis is a condition when the pericardium becomes stiffer and thickened, interfering with the heart's ability to pump blood out of the heart. Patients with constrictive pericarditis may present with SOB, chest pain, fatigue, and dizziness.

3. B) Hepatomegaly
Pulmonary stenosis is characterized as an acyanotic congenital heart defect with obstruction blood flow. Blood circulating on the right side of the heart meets an obstruction at pulmonic valve due to stenosis. When blood on the right side of the heart is obstructed, fluid backs up into the systemic circulation. This can lead to signs of congestive heart failure, which present as hepatomegaly, neck vein distention, peripheral edema, and ascites. Obstruction on the left side of the heart, such as in aortic stenosis, will cause blood to back up into the pulmonary circulation leading to pulmonary edema, orthopnea, dyspnea on exertion, and shortness of breath.

4. B) The elevated CVP measurement may result from pulmonary hypertension.
A CVP catheter is generally indicated to measure preload/venous return, end diastolic right ventricle function, and blood sampling for mixed venous O_2 saturations. Normal values are 0 to 5 mmHg. In this case, the CVP reflects elevated right atrial pressure due to increased pulmonary artery pressure from pulmonary hypertension. A CAVC defect is characterized as an acyanotic congenital heart defect with increased pulmonary blood flow. Long-term complications of prolonged exposure to increased pulmonary blood flow can have detrimental effects on the pulmonary vasculature, which may result in pulmonary hypertension. A decreased CVP is noted in patients with low intravascular volume such as hemorrhage, dehydration, or shock following cardiopulmonary bypass surgery.

5. D) Weak pulses
Low cardiac output syndrome (LCOS) is defined by ineffective cardiac output that cannot meet the metabolic demands of body tissues due to myocardial dysfunction, increased pulmonary vascular resistance (PVR) and systemic vascular resistance (SVR), anaerobic metabolism, and lactic acidosis. LCOS patients' clinical findings include cool, mottled extremities, delayed capillary refill time, decreased pulses and narrowed pulse pressure, tachycardia, altered level of consciousness, and decreased blood pressure.

6. C) The increase in right ventricle outflow tract (RVOT) obstruction causes right to left shunting.
Patients with TOF are at risk for tet spells. In this scenario, the tet spell (hypercyanotic episode) is caused by the noxious stimuli of a venipuncture. The episodic event causes an increase in RVOT obstruction, which results in a right to left shunting across the ventricular septal defect (VSD) and decreased pulmonary blood flow. The patient will present with cyanosis and decreased oxygen saturations. Interventions such as 100% oxygen aim to decrease pulmonary vascular resistance (PVR) and **increase** pulmonary blood

flow. The knee-to-chest intervention aims to increase SVR and promote an increase in pulmonary blood flow. A tet spell is a medical emergency and that a patient should not frequently experience. Surgery should be scheduled following the first hypercyanotic spell.

7. D) Pericardiocentesis
The patient is presenting in obstructive shock from *cardiac tamponade*. An abrupt stop in chest tube output along with the clinical findings of tachycardia, weak pulses, and muffled heart sounds is concerning for tamponade physiology. The excessive pericardial fluid leads to increased intrapericardial pressure, which impairs the heart ability to fill and decreases cardiac output. Cardiac tamponade requires emergency treatment with pericardiocentesis to remove the pericardial fluid drainage that has collected around the heart. The patient's clinical findings do not suggest infection therefore antibiotic therapy would not be a suggested intervention at this time. Antithrombotic therapy is a treatment intervention utilized in patients presenting with pulmonary embolism (PE). The patient's assessment did not reveal common clinical findings of PE such as tachypnea, dyspnea, and hypoxia. Crystalloid fluid administration would further exacerbate the patient's symptoms.

8. A) Initiate a pharmacologic and nonpharmacologic pain management plan.
A thoracotomy incision is more painful compared to the median sternotomy incision (MSI). A thoracotomy requires an incision on the side of the chest between two ribs, where there is more muscle and nerves. A pain management plan with a combination of pharmacologic (e.g., morphine, acetaminophen [Tylenol]) and nonpharmacologic (e.g., music, pacifier) therapies is most appropriate for a post-thoracotomy patient with the objective clinical findings of inconsolability along with tachycardia, and tachypnea. A BP of 80/38 is within normal limits for a neonate and does not need to be treated with a crystalloid fluid bolus. The patient has an increased RR of 66 due to pain; suctioning the patient would only further the patient's agitation. The patient is still in the recovery period postsurgical intervention; resumption of feeding should be paused till the patient has recovered for a few hours.

9. B) Furosemide (Lasix)
This infant presents with signs and symptoms of congestive heart failure due to pulmonary over circulation. Diuretic therapy should be initiated, and furosemide (Lasix) is the only diuretic medication listed.

10. A) Cool and sedate the patient.
This patient is at high risk for junctional ectopic tachycardia (JET). Having an increased temperature, long bypass run, and surgery in the area of conduction, and being on dopamine and epinephrine, which can increase the heart rate and potentiate the shift into JET, leading to decreased cardiac output. Turning down the environmental temperature and giving acetaminophen and fentanyl can keep the heart rate down and lessen the risk. There is no indication for attaching the pacemaker at this time. The patient will most likely have LCOS but closer to the 6-to-12-hour post-op time period. All post-op heart patients should receive an EKG within a few hours of returning from surgery; however, this is not an "initial" intervention.

11. B) Near infrared spectroscopy
Near infrared spectroscopy is a noninvasive monitoring technology that measures regional oxygen saturation and is used following cardiac surgery to trend changes in cardiac output. Pulse oximetry and transcutaneous oxygen monitors assess oxygenation and bispectral index monitoring is used to measure level of consciousness.

12. B) Failure to capture
Capture is evident when a pacer spike is followed by a contraction, either a P wave or a QRS, depending on the mode. "Failure to capture" occurs when more energy is needed for the pacemaker to take over the conduction of the heart. This appears as a pacemaker spike without the correlating expected response of a P or QRS. "Failure to sense" happens when the heart is beating but the pacemaker is not aware of the heart's activity. This will be apparent when a random pacer spike is on the monitor that does not correlate with a P or QRS following the spike. "Failure to pace" occurs when no pacing spikes are seen when they should have occurred often due to oversensing or pacer lead malfunction. "Failure to contract" is not a pacemaker term, though the heart muscle not contracting following an electrical impulse is akin to pulseless electrical activity (PEA).

13. D) Loss of atrial kick
A patient that is in a junctional rhythm is missing the P wave, which means that the atria aren't depolarizing and "kicking" 20% to 30% of blood volume into the ventricles. This leads to decreased cardiac

output due to hypotension. Slower heart rate is true, as a junctional rhythm is usually slower, but the loss of the atrial kick is more significant to decreased cardiac output. Poor contractility may not be a factor in junctional rhythm. Faster heart rate is not correct as a junctional rhythm arises from the atrioventricular (AV) node and is usually slower.

14. C) Vagal maneuvers
Vagal maneuvers include ice to the face (to elicit the diving reflex), suctioning, or doing a rectal temperature. In older kids, having them hold their breath and bear down, blow through a straw, or take a syringe and have them try to blow the plunger off may work to resolve supraventricular tachycardia (SVT). The nurse can assume this is SVT as the heart rate is >220 beats/min in an infant and the symptoms are consistent per the parent report. Vagal maneuvers are benign and, since this patient is hemodynamically stable (defined by the blood pressure being within normal limits), are an appropriate intervention. A 12 lead EKG would be required if the SVT persists despite the vagal maneuver. The next step would be to obtain IV access as adenosine would be the next treatment as long as the patient remains hemodynamically stable. Administering acetaminophen could be considered but not the initial intervention for this patient.

15. A) Call a code.
This patient needs help as soon as possible. Most likely the shunt is occluded or stenotic and the patient needs to go to the cath lab emergently. Getting people to the bedside to start this process is fastest by calling a code. Administering sedation may be useful to try to get some flow into the pulmonary vasculature and starting an IV to quickly give heparin to hopefully open the occluded shunt would be good to do, after calling for help. Applying oxygen via the BVM would be what the bedside nurse would do after calling a code. But until more people get to the bedside, the patient could fully arrest, and the nurse needs to be present.

16. D) Calcium
The heart requires calcium for contractility. Administering calcium gluconate or calcium chloride can increase blood pressure. Ionized calcium (iCal) levels should be maintained above 1 to 1.2 millimoles per liter. Postoperative heart patients use up calcium at a higher rate due to the dilution effects from cardiopulmonary bypass, fluid administration during surgery, as well as children and infants having less iCal reserves. Potassium replacement will help when K+ is low and premature ventricular contractions (PVCs) are noted. Sodium and glucose replacements are administered for patients at risk of seizures or neurological issues.

17. A) Get warm blankets for the patient.
The patient's heart rate is low because the temperature is low. Once the patient is warmed up, the heart rate will increase to a level better able to support cardiac output. The frontline practitioner should be notified but after the initial intervention is done and a repeated temperature. A blood gas may show some acidosis due to hypothermia, but this should not be an initial intervention. Checking a rectal/core temperature would be acceptable but knowing that the heart rate is low and the axillary temperature is low should be enough information to recognize that the patient is cold.

18. D) Chest tube cell count/triglyceride
The chest tube is most likely draining chylous fluid from the thoracic duct inadvertently being nicked in the operating room (OR) from the left thoracotomy. This is a known risk of this procedure, which can lead to chylous pleural effusions. The left pleural chest tubes are left in place until the patient drinks fat containing products to assess for this complication. A blood culture/CBC or chest tube culture is not correct because there are no signs of infection. An ABG/iCal is not the correct answer because it will not confirm the diagnosis of a possible chylous drainage. A chest x-ray may be useful, but as long as the chest tube is in place, this fluid will easily drain from this location.

19. A) Cool, mottled extremities, delayed capillary refill time, and decreased pulses
LCOS physical exam findings include cool, mottled extremities, delayed capillary refill time, decreased pulses and narrowed pulse pressure, tachycardia, altered level of consciousness, and decreased blood pressure (late sign).

20. A) Transition off iNO to sildenafil.
iNO has a few seconds half-life and must be watched closely. Some patients are not able to wean off iNO and therefore cannot leave the ICU. The family will have to learn how to care for a tracheostomy and ventilator and G-tube care, and when a family is excited to bring a patient home, this happens quickly.

Patients can be home on a milrinone infusion; therefore, this does not preclude a patient leaving the ICU or hospital.

21. D) Synchronized cardioversion.
In recognizing this rhythm as supraventricular tachycardia (SVT), the nurse note that this infant is hemodynamically **unstable**. The initial treatment for hemodynamically unstable SVT is immediate synchronized cardioversion.

22. C) Administer epinephrine.
This patient appears to be in sinus bradycardia except the observation that they have no pulse. This is pulseless electrical activity (PEA). The immediate treatment for PEA is to begin compressions and administer Epinephrine.

23. B) Magnesium sulfate
This is a strip of Torsade's de Pointes. The treatment for it is magnesium sulfate. The other options, norepinephrine, lidocaine, and atropine, are not indicated.

24. C) Administer an antiarrhythmic, such as amiodarone.
This rhythm strip shows junctional ectopic tachycardia (JET). Administering an antiarrhythmic, such as amiodarone, will slow the junctional rate and improve cardiac perfusion. Increasing the epinephrine infusion will not correct the arrhythmia. While JET generally resolves spontaneously in the weeks after surgery, this patient requires immediate intervention now. Ventricular pacing will not correct this arrhythmia.

25. C) Cool, mottled skin and oliguria
Cool, mottled skin and oliguria are signs and symptoms of cardiogenic shock. The other assessment findings are not consistent with cardiogenic shock.

26. B) Bronchiolitis
Bronchiolitis typically presents after 3 to 7 days of upper respiratory infection (URI) symptoms that progresses cough, rhinorrhea, respiratory distress, low-grade fever. *Tachypnea is the most consistent clinical manifestation.* Pneumonia presents with fine crackles, dullness, or diminished breath sounds. The hallmark sign of laryngotracheobronchitis is stridor and a barky hoarse cough, which is not present in this patient. Bronchitis presents with a dry, brassy cough, coarse breath sounds, or rhonchi on exam.

27. C) Respiratory syncytial virus (RSV)
RSV is the most common cause of bronchiolitis. Hib is the most common cause of acute epiglottitis. *Staphylococcus aureus* is a common organism associated with bacterial tracheitis. Parainfluenza is a common organism associated with bronchitis.

28. A) Nasal suctioning, high flow nasal cannula, nebulized 3% saline
The nurse can attempt to suction this patient, but it appears this infant's status has deteriorated. Infants at this age are obligate nose breathers to keeping the nares patent is very important. One of the common findings in bronchiolitis is nasal congestion. Albuterol, a bronchodilator is not routinely recommended and is rarely helpful in the management of bronchiolitis. The infant most probably will need high flow nasal cannula. Nebulized 3% saline will assist in thinning the infant's secretion. Nebulized racemic epinephrine is most often used for upper airway obstruction like stridor and croup.

29. A) Acute respiratory distress syndrome (ARDS)
Shock is among the top causes of ARDS; patients with ARDS develop hypoxia, hypocarbia, and tachypnea as a means to increase minute ventilation. Air leak syndrome can develop after the use of positive pressure ventilation and in this patient the nurse would anticipate the risk for pneumothoraces. A PE occurs when a blood clot gets stuck in an artery in the lung, blocking blood flow to part of the lung. While possible, it is not likely in this case. In this short period of time from ED to PICU, it is unlikely a pneumonia has developed. Respiratory symptoms have worsened from the shock.

30. D) Packed red blood cell (PRBC) transfusion
The goal in acute respiratory distress syndrome (ARDS) is to maintain the patient's hemoglobin (Hgb) above 7, so a value of 6.4 indicates a need for PRBC transfusion. Oxyhemoglobin is formed during

physiological respiration when oxygen binds to the heme component of the protein hemoglobin in red blood cells (RBCs). Without an adequate number of circulating RBCs the oxygen can't adequately be delivered. The platelet level of 147,000 is grossly normal and doesn't indicate a need for transfusion. There is no information given that the patient is hypotensive or requires additional fluid boluses, so normal saline and albumin bolus can be eliminated as incorrect.

31. A) Spare trach (same size and one size smaller), spare trach ties, lubricant, normal saline, suction equipment, manual resuscitator bag, and oxygen
A larger size trach would not be part of the emergency equipment the nurse would have available, as upsizing a trach would be something planned and managed by an ear, nose, and throat provider, not something that is done in an emergency. The nurse must have a trach one size smaller than the patient's current size in the event that the nurse is unable to replace the dislodged tracheostomy tube.

32. C) Begin discussing the upcoming transplant in advance and support explanations with diagrams, pictures, and models.
When time permits, school-aged children can be prepared weeks in advance of an upcoming procedure. The use of age-appropriate models and pictures can augment explanations. Toddlers and preschool children should be prepared closer to the procedure. Children should always be given choices when possible, but the decision to transplant may not be within the patient's decision-making capacity as it would for an older adolescent patient. Minimizing parental separation and supporting parental anxiety are helpful but not the best strategy to prepare this patient for the upcoming transplant.

33. C) Allow the child to assume a position of comfort and immediately notify anesthesiology and otolaryngology.
This patient is demonstrating signs and symptoms of acute epiglottitis, which is a life-threatening emergency. The patient should be kept calm and transported immediately to the operating room for laryngoscopy and intubation. Obtaining an x-ray would delay care. Distressing or anxiety-inducing procedures such as placing an IV or attempting to visualize the airway should be avoided.

34. A) Chest wiggle
Patients on high frequency oscillatory ventilation should have good chest wiggle. Chest wiggle should be noted from clavicle to the mid-thigh on both sides. Any change in quality or laterality of the chest wiggle could indicate a problem such as pneumothorax, mainstem intubation, long compliance change, or need for airway suctioning. The frequently used pneumonic "DOPE" is helpful when troubleshooting an acute change in an intubated patient. "D" stands for displacement of the ETT; "O" for obstruction; "P" for pneumothorax"; and "E" for equipment failure. While maintaining a patent ETT is important for all intubated patients as an obstruction impedes ventilation, ETT size is not typically a factor. Ventilator circuit connections should always be checked when an intubated patient has an acute change in condition and other causes are ruled out. Train of four test for adequate paralysis would only be performed after assessing chest wiggle and ruling out other complications. Patient appears adequately sedated, but sedated should always be reassessed.

35. A) Prepare for emergent needle decompression of the right chest.
Patients on the high frequency oscillatory ventilator are at higher risk for developing a pneumothorax. Breath sounds cannot be auscultated in patients on this type of ventilator, so assessment of the presence and quality of chest wiggle is imperative. A sudden decrease in chest wiggle on one side of the chest accompanied by an acute decrease in saturations and compromised hemodynamics indicate the presence of a pneumothorax and urgent intervention is necessary. The physician should be immediately notified, and the nurse should prepare for needle decompression; needle decompression is typically performed at the second intercostal space midclavicular line. Sedating the patient may further compromise hemodynamics in this patient. Turning the patient with the right side facing down will likely further compromise the patient's saturations and overall hemodynamics. Deflating the cuff on the patient's ETT may compromise airway pressure; a small leak around the cuff may be intentionally allowed for CO_2 elimination. However, the maintenance of mean airway pressure must be monitored.

36. A) Ketamine (Ketalar)
Ketamine is an anesthetic medication that is also recognized as a bronchodilator and has been shown to do this by blocking N-methyl-D-aspartatereceptors to prevent bronchoconstriction and decreasing nitric oxide production in pulmonary tissues to reduce bronchospasm. Vasopressin causes vasoconstriction and

increasing blood pressure. Propofol is an anesthetic medication but has not shown a role in the treatment of asthma. Morphine is not known to have bronchodilatory effects.

37.   D) Increased susceptibility to infections
In long-term therapy, patients receiving corticosteroids may be more susceptible to infections due to the alteration of cytokine production, which leads to immune system suppression and a decreased inflammatory response. Hypertension (not hypotension) can be a side effect related to fluid retention and/or excretion of potassium, calcium, and phosphate. Hypoglycemia is not a typical problem, while hyperglycemia occurs related to development of insulin resistance by the liver. Patients receiving steroids may sometimes develop increased appetite related to changes in metabolism.

38.   A) "This medication does not require any additional monitoring or follow-up."
Anticoagulants require routine monitoring to ensure safe therapeutic care. Parents of children receiving oral anticoagulants should be aware of the risk of bleeding with activities and the importance of communicating acute illness to prescribers so dosing can be adjusted. Children should be encouraged to wear Medi-Alert ID bracelets so other caregivers are aware.

39.   C) Increase the tidal volume on the ventilator.
You should increase the tidal volume. When it comes to alveolar ventilation, increasing tidal volume can be a more efficient way than increasing respiratory rate, it is now believed. Maintaining current ventilator settings, when proven ineffective, is not appropriate as a first choice. Putting a patient on a bicarbonate drip is not an effective way to treat respiratory acidosis. Decreasing the respiratory rate will cause a further retention of CO_2.

40.   C) Pulmonary hypertensive crisis
Pulmonary hypertensive crisis is the most likely cause of the patient's hypoxia given the acute nature of the desaturations associated with the patient's agitation and the fact that the patient has not had their sildenafil in 5 days. While mucus plugging may explain the patient's acute episode at home, the recurrent episodes and history of not having sildenafil is more indicative of uncontrolled pulmonary hypertension. The mother reconnected the patient to the ventilator after suctioning and bagging and the patient improved, which does not indicate a ventilator malfunction. There is no history of fever or change in secretions so no evidence of tracheitis.

41.   C) Decrease the rate.
The child is in respiratory alkalosis, which is probably due to increased respiratory rate (ventilation). The rate of the ventilator should be turned down, and additional sedations/analgesia should be administered if needed. Increasing the rate will blow off more CO_2, making the alkalosis worse. Increasing FiO_2 will not fix this situation. Increasing PEEP does hold the alveoli open but does not help in this case.

42.   C) Resting pulmonary artery pressure of >25 mmHg
Pulmonary hypertension is defined as a resting pulmonary artery pressure of >25 mmHg.

43.   D) Hemothorax
The patient had known trauma and developed respiratory distress, hemoptysis, tachycardia, and hypotension, which are all indicative of hemothorax. Rib fractures present with point tenderness and localized ecchymosis but would not impact hemodynamics; tension pneumothorax is possible in this scenario, but the hemoptysis is more indicative of hemothorax. Finally, posttraumatic atelectasis presents with dyspnea, cyanosis, cough, wheezing, rhonchi, and rales but would not cause hemoptysis and does not impact hemodynamics.

44.   A) Esophageal rupture
Esophageal rupture is a potential complication of foreign body aspiration, and signs and symptoms include chest and back pain, subcutaneous emphysema, hematemesis, and pneumomediastinum. There is no report of trauma, so traumatic rupture of the diaphragm is unlikely in this patient and there is no report of abdominal tenderness or rigidity in this patient. Tracheobronchial trauma is unlikely as there is no report compression or blunt trauma to the neck; while the patient does have subcutaneous emphysema and pneumomediastinum, in this patient with known foreign body aspiration esophageal rupture is the more likely cause. There is no evidence of hemodynamic compromise or tracheal deviation so tension pneumothorax is not likely.

45. B) Rib fractures
Rib fractures are causing this patient's symptoms given the history of known trauma, point tenderness, and worsening pain with movement. There is no report of respiratory distress, hemodynamic compromise, or tracheal deviation, so tension pneumothorax is not likely. There is no report of back pain, so spinal fractures are not the cause of the symptoms. The patient has no respiratory distress, hemoptysis, tachycardia, or hypotension, which are all indicative of hemothorax.

46. D) Cosmetic concerns
Cosmetic concerns are the most common reason for surgical correction. Respiratory and cardiac compromise are uncommon in patients with pectus excavatum. Pectus does not delay growth.

47. C) Atelectasis
Atelectasis is a known potential complication of a VATS procedure and is evidenced by his decreased breath sounds, increased oxygen requirement, and consolidation on CXR. The patient has no history of fever so pneumonia is unlikely; they are hemodynamically stable so tension pneumothorax can be ruled out. The diminished breath sounds at the base, as opposed to the apex of the lung, eliminate pneumothorax as the cause.

48. B) Tracheomalacia
The common presenting signs and symptoms of tracheomalacia are stridor and increased work of breathing. Choanal atresia has varying presenting signs and symptoms; however, stridor and suprasternal retractions are part of the common presentation. Pulmonary interstitial emphysema typically presents as a gradual deterioration including hypoxemia, hypercarbia, and acidosis. Pulmonary embolism typically presents as hypoxemia, tachypnea, dyspnea, or chest pain. Risk factors include fractures of the lower extremities, trauma, central venous lines, chemotherapy, infection, heart disease, oral contraceptive use, cancer, and immobility, and it is uncommon in an otherwise healthy neonate.

49. D) Turn the ventilator settings back to the previous settings.
This patient displayed classic signs of failure to wean from mechanical ventilation. There could be several potential causes. In the scenario described above several adjustments were made all at once, making it less likely for the patient to tolerate such a drastic change. The most important next intervention would be to return the ventilator settings to their previous settings to avoid further decline and monitor the patient. The sedation may need to be increased as well; however, the scenario does not describe the patient as more awake or interfering with the ventilator. Obtaining a CXR may be helpful to determine if the patient has become derecruited during the attempted wean but is not the most important step. Increasing the FiO_2 will not likely be helpful as the patient is not displaying oxygen desaturation, the FiO_2 was not weaned, and overutilization of oxygen could cause oxygen toxicity.

50. C) Increased renal potassium excretion
Aldosterone helps control the balance of water and salts in the kidney by keeping sodium in and releasing potassium from the body. The principal effect of holding onto sodium is to hold onto water. This does not increase or decrease serum sodium levels. Potassium excretion is not decreased, it is increased.

51. A) Decreased $PaCO_2$ and increased PaO_2
If the PIP is increased on the ventilator, it will cause the child to excrete more CO_2, thereby decreasing $PaCO_2$ and, as a result, increasing PaO_2.

52. D) 35 mg/dL
The most concerning of these results is the blood sugar of 35 mg/dL. That would require an immediate intervention by the nurse to prevent a severe hypoglycemic response.

53. C) Adrenocorticotropic hormone (ACTH)
Given the choices here, the anterior pituitary produces ACTH so that would be affected as well as sex hormones such as estrogen, progesterone, and testosterone. The adrenal glands produce cortisol, and the hypothalamus produces ADH. Glucagon is made by the alpha cell in the pancreas. It is stored in the liver and muscles.

54. D) Maple syrup urine disease
A sweet sugar-like smell is indicative of maple syrup urine disease, which is an inborn error of metabolism. This smell would not be present in any of the other disease processes noted here.

55. A) Respiratory acidosis
This patient is in respiratory distress and failure despite being intubated and placed on a ventilator. This is worsening respiratory acidosis due to the low pH, high CO_2, and low HCO_2. The base deficit indicates the worsening of the state and probably accumulation of lactic acid in acute respiratory distress syndrome (ARDS).

56. B) Diabetes insipidus (DI)
The scenario, especially with the high sodium and high urine output, is indicative of DI. The glucose level is normal, so it is not diabetes mellitus. In SIADH, the sodium level is low and urine output is low to none. Cushing syndrome presents with severe fatigue, headache, new or worsened high blood pressure, muscle weakness, depression, anxiety and irritability, and loss of emotional control, as well as cognitive difficulties.

57. A) Glucose consumption that exceeds glucose production
Glucose consumption that exceeds glucose production can cause acute hypoglycemia. Insulinoma is a tumor in the pancreas. Using oral antihyperglycemic agents should not cause acute hypoglycemia. Gastroenteritis would only cause a decrease in glucose if the child has profuse diarrhea and becomes extremely dehydrated. Due to the body's homeostatic mechanisms, this should not occur.

58. B) Continue with the current insulin infusion and add dextrose to the intravenous fluid (IVF).
It is important when caring for a patient with diabetic ketoacidosis (DKA) not to drop the blood sugar too quickly. Dropping from 1,120 to 580 is a significant drop and can lead to cerebral edema. Blood glucose should not drop faster than 50 to 100 mg/dL/hr. Because of this, dextrose should be added to the IVF, or a 2-bag system should be in place (one with NSS and the other with D10W). The nurse would not hold the insulin as this patient is still in DKA. This patient does not need a NSS bolus. Giving a large amount of IVF as a bolus would increase in intracranial pressure (ICP) and worsen the situation.

59. D) Cerebral edema
Although rare, 1% to 3% of children will develop cerebral edema. This is especially so if the blood glucose level drops too quickly. When recognized, cerebral edema can be treated with mannitol or hypertonic saline. There is no indication of sepsis or seizure activity. Because glucose and electrolytes are returning to normal, hyperkalemia is not likely, nor are these symptoms of hyperkalemia.

60. B) White blood cell (WBC) count of 256,000/μL
A child presenting with a high white count like this (hyperleukocytosis) is a classic presenting sign of leukemia. A high reticulocyte count is seen with hemolytic anemias. A low factor VIII level is seen in hemophilia. Pancytopenia is expected with this diagnosis; no Hgb and HCT within normal range would be inconsistent.

61. D) Immune-mediated complexes cause platelet activation resulting in thrombus formation and thrombocytopenia
Heparin-induced thrombocytopenia is caused by the formation of antibodies against heparin complexes bound to platelet factor 4 (PF4). These immune-mediated complexes cause platelet activation resulting in thrombus formation and thrombocytopenia. An autoimmune response where platelets are inappropriately identified as foreign and targeted for phagocytosis in the spleen is seen in immune thrombocytopenia (ITP). Heparin doesn't cause systemic microhemorrhages or megakaryocyte suppression in the bone marrow.

62. A) Splenic sequestration
The child is presenting with classic signs of splenic sequestration, which is life threatening if circulating blood volume isn't restored in a reasonable amount of time. Acute chest syndrome presents more consistently with fevers and increased work of breathing (WOB). Aplastic crisis is associated with infections causing bone marrow suppression. Although splenic sequestration is a type of vaso-occlusive crisis, the life-threatening physiology presented in the case differs from a vaso-occlusive pain crisis.

63. D) Low grade glioma
Low grade gliomas are benign brain tumors that are slow growing and unlikely to spread or cause spinal cord compression. Neuroblastoma, rhabdomyosarcoma, Ewing sarcoma, and soft tissue sarcomas account for over 50% of tumors in children presenting with spinal cord compression.

64. C) "Affected children have hypertrophic lymphoid structures such as tonsils and lymph nodes on exam."
Agammaglobulinemia is a defect in the body's ability to produce mature and functioning B-lymphocytes, which then impairs plasma cell and gamma globulin production. Children affected by agammaglobulinemia have hypotrophic or absent tonsils and adenoids due to the diminished production and maturation of B lymphocytes. Children with agammaglobulinemia do mount an immune response to vaccines; however, it's deficient and short-term with titers decreased or absent 2 to 4 months after immunization. Lifelong treatment with IVIG is the current standard therapy. The risks of curative therapies such as haematopoietic stem cell transplantation (HSCT) are thought to outweigh the benefits in this population.

65. B) Treat hypocalcemia
Hypocalcemia is a most common complication of plasmapheresis in pediatrics. It manifests in a variety of ways including numbness, tingling in hands/feet, abdominal pain, and mental status changes. Acute hypotension can result necessitating immediate treatment once hypocalcemia is recognized. Treating the hypocalcemia will be more effective at alleviating the nausea/abdominal pain than ondansetron. IM epinephrine is indicated for anaphylaxis. Cardiopulmonary compromise can be prevented when electrolyte abnormalities are promptly corrected, so the need for intubation and mechanical ventilation at this time is low.

66. D) Should not be palpated because it can easily rupture
An enlarged spleen should not be palpated as it can easily be ruptured. Only approximately 10% of normal, healthy children have a palpable spleen. Normal-sized spleen is contained within the rib cage and usually cannot be palpated. The spleen is a fist-sized organ located in the upper left side of the abdomen (as opposed to the right) with the spleen being the most commonly injured intra-abdominal organ in children. Rupture and hemorrhage could be life-threatening.

67. B) Sustained intra-abdominal pressure measurement of 14 mmHg and oliguria
A sustained intra-abdominal pressure that falls between 12 and 15 mmHg is identified as a Grade I for ACS and the associated diminished urine would be congruent with ACS symptoms. ACS is defined as a sustained rise of the intra-abdominal pressure together with newly developed organ dysfunction. Normal intra-abdominal pressure in a well-child is 0 mmHg. Expected intra-abdominal pressures in critically ill children ranges from 4 to 10 mmHg and in a child with positive pressure ventilation it is 1 to 8 mmHg, but this recording is intermittent, below 10, and not a sustained pressure. Intra-abdominal pressure measurement of 10 mmHg and urinary output of 1 mL/kg/hr is concerning but the urine output is normal. Intermittent intra-abdominal pressure measurement of 10 mmHg with diminished bowel sounds is concerning but does not yet meet the criteria of ACS.

68. A) Acetaminophen (Tylenol) 75 mg/kg/day
This patient has signs and symptoms of Kawasaki disease (KD). Patients may also present with a strawberry tongue and generalized rash. Management of KD includes high-dose acetylsalicylic acid and intravenous immunoglobulin, EKGs, and serial EKGs to diagnose coronary aneurysms and monitor ventricular function.

69. C) Appendicitis, postoperative day 1 with a hard, rigid abdomen and temperature 38.3°C (101°F)
A hard, rigid abdomen and increased temperature are signs of peritonitis (infection) which can be a complication of abdominal surgery. Peritonitis is a priority and requires immediate attention by the nurse. It is expected for a patient with NEC to have green bile drainage. A blood transfusion is appropriate treatment for a patient with a GI bleed with low hemoglobin and hematocrit, so this patient is stable and is not the priority. The patient with a bowel infarction has a low potassium level and does not need to be assessed first.

70. A) Vasopressin (Pitressin)
Vasopressin is a vasoconstrictor and decreases blood flow. It is used to treat acute GI hemorrhage. Digoxin, enoxaparin, and polyethylene glycol are not used to treat GI hemorrhage.

71. C) Is 8 hours postoperative for necrotizing enterocolitis with white blood cell (WBC) count of 20,000/µL
This patient has elevated WBC, which may indicate infection and peritonitis. All other laboratory results are considered normal.

72. D) Metoclopramide (Reglan)
Metoclopramide (Reglan) increases intestinal motility and should enable the tip of the tube to migrate farther into the duodenum. Erythromycin may also be used for this. Famotidine is an histamine H2-receptor antagonist (H2RA) and omeprazole is a proton pump inhibitor (PPI). They both decrease gastric acid production. Sucralfate coats the stomach. The other medications have no effect on intestinal motility or forward movement of the tube.

73. C) Watery diarrhea
Diarrhea (frequently watery) is the most common symptom associated with malabsorption. Frequent regurgitation may be indicative of gastrointestinal reflux disease. Weight loss is a finding usually associated with malabsorption disorders. A positive Trousseau sign may be found. This finding is usually associated with hypocalcemia often seen in malabsorption syndromes and disorders.

74. C) An additional 20 mL/kg NS bolus
Multisystem inflammatory syndrome in children (MIS-C) is a rare complication of COVID-19 in children. Children who present in shock with MIS-C should be managed according to shock guidelines and receive 10 to 20 mL/kg fluid boluses up to 40 to 60 mL/kg followed by the initiation of vasoactive medications, commonly epinephrine or norepinephrine. Chest x-ray, EKG, CBC, and milrinone may be later interventions.

75. D) A 10-year-old with renal vascular disease and headaches
Patients who present with acute, severe hypertension, defined as systolic and diastolic blood pressures >90th percentile, and life-threatening symptoms such as headache or chest pain require urgent treatment with an intravenous beta-blocker, calcium channel blocker, or vasodilator. Seizures should be managed first with a benzodiazepine and receive neuroimaging to rule out other causes.

76. B) Tricyclic antidepressants
This patient is demonstrating classic symptoms of an anticholinergic ingestion (recalled with the mnemonic "red as a beet, dry as a bone, blind as a bat, mad as a hatter, hot as a hare, full as a flask"). Common anticholinergic drugs include antihistamines, atropine, carbamazepine, sleep aids, and tricyclic antidepressants. Organophosphates are cholinergic drugs, gabapentin is a sedative, and hydromorphone is an opioid.

77. A) 12-month-old with a heart rate (HR) 145 bpm, blood pressure (BP) 110/70, and a pericardial effusion on x-ray; B) 6-year-old with a history of hemolytic uremic syndrome with new seizures; and C) 14-year-old with polyuria and hyponatremia receiving replacement fluid
Renal replacement therapies should be considered for critically ill children with acute kidney injury (AKI) experiencing severe symptoms of fluid overload such as pericardial infusion or worsening respiratory status requiring escalating respiratory support. Severe metabolic acidosis and electrolyte abnormalities or symptoms of uremia are also indications for dialysis. Polyuria and hyponatremia are signs of the diuretic phase of acute tubular necrosis.

78. B) The patient is oliguric phase of injury.
The oliguric phase of ATN occurs over several days and is characterized by oliguria. The initial phase is the time when the initial insult occurs. During the diuretic phase, urine output will increase to large volumes of unconcentrated urine. The recovery phase is the period when renal recovery occurs. Renal function will improve but polyuria may persist.

79. C) Pyelonephritis
Pyelonephritis is an upper urinary tract infection that presents with fever, abdominal pain, back pain, dysuria, or new-onset incontinence. Symptoms of peritonitis include cloudy peritoneal fluid, abdominal pain, and fever. Sudden onset of hematuria with proteinuria are typical symptoms of acute glomerulonephritis. Hemolytic uremic syndrome presents as a triad of features: thrombocytopenia, anemia, and acute kidney injury (AKI).

80. D) Administer calcium chloride, sodium bicarbonate, and insulin and glucose. Prepare for dialysis.
Signs of hyperkalemia include paresthesia and EKG changes. Symptomatic hyperkalemia should be treated with medications: calcium chloride, sodium bicarbonate, and insulin and glucose. Dialysis should be resumed as soon as possible. Neurovascular assessments and magnesium oxide is the treatment for hypomagnesemia. Hypermagnesemia is managed with diuretics and calcium supplements and hyponatremia is managed with fluid restriction and hypertonic saline.

81. A) Place an indwelling urinary catheter and record urine output hourly; B) Administer 20 mL/kg normal saline.
Nursing interventions for patients in acute kidney injury (AKI) include close monitoring of urine output with an indwelling urinary catheter and administration of isotonic crystalloid to manage hypovolemia. The hemoglobin and platelet results are within normal limits and this patient does not require a blood transfusion or administration of the monoclonal antibody eculizumab, a therapy given to hemolytic uremic syndrome patients with central nervous system (CNS) involvement.

82. D) Give albumin, monitor vital signs following dose.
Hypotension is a common complication of dialysis. Patients who become hypotensive during dialysis should receive albumin or fluid to support BP. All other interventions are appropriate but not the priority in the care of this patient.

83. B) "The most important thing is to catch delirium early."
Pediatric delirium is common in critically ill patients. Early identification of delirium and recognizing causes of delirium is most important in preventing long-term sequelae. A risk factor for the development of delirium is the use of sedatives, such as benzodiazepines. Signs of hypoactive delirium include sleepiness and decreased attention. Hyperactive delirium is characterized by agitation, restlessness, and hallucinations. Mixed hyperactive-hypoactive delirium, not hyperactive delirium, is the most common type of pediatric delirium.

84. B) The dimension from head to toe is the length.
The dimension going from "head to toe" is the length. The dimension from "hip to hip" is the width. Using the largest dimension or using coins as reference does not determine the width.

85. B) Is more likely to become a stage 3 or stage 4 injury than if located elsewhere on the body
This is a stage 1 pressure injury. Pressure injuries in areas with less adipose tissue are more likely to become advanced (stage 3 or 4 injuries) than those areas with more fat padding. The injury needs intervention to prevent worsening. There is not an indication that this was caused by a medical device and surgery is not indicated.

86. C) Explain to the patient/family the importance of repositioning and identify strategies that will make repositioning tolerable.
No specialty bed replaces the need for routine repositioning. It is important to ensure the patient/family's values and preferences are honored and informed. Forcing them to turn q2 hours any way does not build a therapeutic relationship or include them in decision-making about their care.

87. A) The patient's impending death
A Kennedy terminal ulcer (KTU) presents 2 hours to 2 weeks before the patient's death and progresses rapidly. It will not heal upon recovery from illness. Platelet transfusion and wound culture are not indicated.

88. B) Remove packing from the wound for wound assessment.
If a patient has a change in status, assessment is appropriate. Cultures would be obtained after careful consideration and only after wound cleansing. Bone biopsy is the gold standard for identifying osteomyelitis, but it is invasive; ruling out other sources of infection prior to an invasive procedure is necessary. An MRI would help identify osteomyelitis, but assessment is the appropriate first step.

89. C) The patient and family's values and preferences
It may not be appropriate to adhere to the schedule at life's end. Priorities should be set together with the patient and family. Continue what interventions the family prioritizes. Allowing for consolidated sleep is important but should not deter comfort. The nurse should always pay attention to the skin and not stop pressure injury prevention just because the patient is on "comfort care." Attention should still be given to maintain skin integrity.

90. D) Aggressive intravenous fluid (IVF) administration
Aggressive administration of IVFs is most important to increase renal blood flow, decrease the concentration of nephrotoxic pigments, and to prevent subsequent kidney dysfunction or damage. You would not want to restrict fluids. Addiction counseling would not be indicated. PT should not be initiated and in fact has not been shown to be helpful with this condition.

91. B) Immediately call the provider.
Compartment syndrome occurs when edema causes increased pressure in the muscle compartment. This can lead to decreased blood flow and potential muscle and nerve damage. This is a medical emergency. The provider should be called immediately so that the cast can be removed to assess the extremity. A fasciotomy is indicated when there is still increased pressure after the cast is removed. Neurovascular checks should be done more frequently but after the cast is removed as that is the constricting source at this point. Elevation of the extremity on a pillow should have been done after casting to help decrease edema.

92. C) 30 mmHg
Sustained compartment pressures of 30 mmHg are suggestive of compartment syndrome. This level of pressure would require and immediate surgical fasciotomy to release this pressure.

93. B) Muscle spasm
Muscle spasm frequently accompanies a femoral fracture. When the femoral bone is broken it caused trauma and injury to the surrounding tissue and muscle. The muscle may spasm and cause the bone to shift causing severe, intermittent pain. This should be treated with a muscle relaxant (methocarbamol [Robaxin], cyclobenzaprine [Flexeril], or diazepam [Valium]). It would be too soon for an infection to be present on admission. Edema on the first day should not significant enough to cause severe pain. Hypothermia would not be a cause of the pain. They are in the hospital and should be normothermic.

94. A) Chest wall rigidity
If fentanyl is pushed too quickly, it can cause acute chest wall rigidity. Management would then include ventilatory support and using a reversal agent with either naloxone or a short-acting neuromuscular blocking agent. Fentanyl might cause respiratory depression or arrest, not tachypnea. It does not affect the thyroid gland in any meaningful way. Nasal congestion is not a side effect of giving IV fentanyl.

95. C) 40 to 50 mmHg
Forty to 50 mmHg is a normal CPP. Five to 10 mmHg is the normal range for intracranial pressure. Twenty to 30 mmHg is too low of a range for CPP, and sustained low CPP values could result in neuronal cell death. >100 mmHg is too high of a range and could lead to a stroke if the blood pressure is also elevated.

96. A) Decreased level of consciousness
Mental status changes are the earliest indicators that a patient is experiencing increased ICP. All the other symptoms are later signs of increasing ICP.

97. A) leaking proteins into the brain barrier."
Leaking proteins into the brain barrier is not a compensatory mechanism and will increase ICP. Leaking protein leads to more swelling of brain tissue as water is attracted to protein. Shifting cerebrospinal fluid to other areas of the brain or spinal cord, vasoconstriction of cerebral vessels, and decrease cerebrospinal fluid production are all compensatory mechanisms to lower ICP.

98. B) BP 70/40, HR 45, temperature 35°C (95°F)
Hallmark signs and symptoms of neurogenic shock are hypotension, bradycardia, hypothermia, and warm/dry extremities.

99. D) Prepare the patient for surgery.
A ruptured AVM is a surgical emergency, and symptoms of a rupture include headache, change in level of consciousness, nausea and vomiting, and neurologic deficits that mimic a brain bleed. Administering aspirin to impact coagulation will only make bleeding worse. Administering acetaminophen (Tylenol) and continuing to monitor the patient are inappropriate interventions in a medical emergency.

100. A) Mild TBI
Mild TBI involves <30 minutes loss of conscious and <24-hour period of posttraumatic amnesia. In moderate TBI, a patient reports a >30 minute loss of consciousness. Severe TBI is characterized by >24 hours of loss of consciousness and requires prompt recognition and treatment and is associated with intracranial abnormalities such as bleeding and cerebral swelling. Vestibular TBI is a type of concussion characterized by difficulty with balance, motion, and vision.

101. C) Decreased level of consciousness (LOC)
Change or decrease in mental status often occur directly following a TBI. LOC should be monitored frequently by the critical care nurse following severe TBI. A GCS of 15 is normal. Nystagmus and decreased appetite are common symptoms following TBI.

102. A) Increased intracranial pressure (ICP)
Increased ICP answer due to patient having a witnessed mild traumatic brain injury (mTBI) and stable vital signs and neurologic exam 2 hours prior. It is associated with a decreased CPP. Increased ICP can lead to brain herniation if not emergently managed. While seizure activity can occur with most TBI, it is not the best answer here.

103. A) Herpes simplex virus; acyclovir
Steroids are not routinely recommended. *Streptococcus pneumoniae* is not the most severe form of encephalitis and is a type of meningitis. *Neisseria meningitidis* is incorrect as it is a type of meningitis.

104. C) Safe sleep practices
Proper use of car seats, helmet use, and pedestrian safety are preventative care for SCIs and TBIs. Safe sleep practices do not relate to TBI and SCI. It is important education for sudden infant death syndrome (SIDS) prevention.

105. C) MRI
SCI without radiographic abnormality is predominant in pediatrics. MRI can usually identify this pathology, where other imaging (like x-ray and CT) cannot. MRI is also helpful in identifying ligamentous injury in the pediatric population and being able to clear a C-spine to remove a C-collar. Ultrasound is not recommended for the diagnosis of SCI.

106. C) The nurse assists the family to identify support people or resources to help them deal with the stress of their child's illness.
The best course of action is to assist the family to find support individuals. They may be displacing anger on each other in this case. The nurse cannot deny their ability to visit their child. Having security on stand-by is not the best course of action to build a therapeutic relationship. The nurse sharing their personal situation of recently being divorced is not professional and should not be done.

107. C) The risk of suicide attempts is higher in females, but the risk of suicide completions is higher in males.
While females are more likely to attempt suicide, males are more likely to complete suicide.

108. C) "This medication has a black box warning indicating an increased risk for suicidality."
Fluoxetine (Prozac) has the back box warning indicated for all antidepressants, which includes the increased risk for suicidality. The other statements are inaccurate.

109. B) Ask the patient, "I noticed scars on your arms; can you tell me how you got them?"
The correct response is to acknowledge the scars, open the lines of communication, and explore how she got them. The nurse should not immediately get a psych consult. If the nurse asks the patient if their parents know, it may destroy the patient's trust in the nurse. A nurse should never directly confront a patient and share their own personal feelings about the situation.

110. C) "I have no idea what happened, it's all her fault anyway."
Blaming the child is an indication the mother might be responsible for the neglect. Being worried and saying she loves her child would be perceived as very caring. Asking, not demanding, when the child will be seen by the doctor is not indicative of being an abuser.

111. D) It usually occurs after an unexpected, prolonged admission.
Most children who go on to develop PTSD have a sudden, unexpected admission. They usually are in the PICU longer than 30 days. It is more common in younger, female patients.

112. A) Anxiety is easier to treat than overt aggression.
It is much easier to treat anxiety before it escalates into aggression. Anxiety is usually different in parents and children, and one can provoke a reaction in the other. Parents and children usually have different anxiety triggers.

113. C) Elevated temperature
Urticaria, angioedema, tachycardia, wheezing, agitation, and diaphoresis are all typical presentations of anaphylactic shock. Elevated temperature is most often seen with infection and may be part of the symptomology of septic shock.

114. A) Apply padding over the nasal bridge and rotate their nasal mask with nasal prongs, if tolerated
Device-related pressure injuries account for up to 30% of hospital-acquired pressure injuries. Padding and device rotation are integral parts of pressure injury prevention. The patient is otherwise improving, with no current indication for normal saline bolus, intubation, or antibiotics.

115. D) Initiation of a vasoactive infusion
The patient is presenting with signs of uncompensated shock. Based on their risk factors (central venous catheter, chronic ventilation), they are likely in septic shock. Early treatment would include obtaining blood and respiratory cultures and administration of antibiotics; however, treating their hypotension is the priority. The respiratory assessment is concerning for fluid overload and would suggest additional fluid administration could be harmful. The most appropriate action is to prepare a vasoactive infusion to improve the patient's blood pressure.

116. A) Epinephrine (Adrenalin)
Epinephrine and norepinephrine are recommended as first line agents in septic shock. Dobutamine provides inotropy and afterload reduction via vasodilation and is most appropriate for patients without acute hypotension. Dopamine is no longer widely used in septic shock as evidence has shown improved mortality with epinephrine; however, it may be used if epinephrine or norepinephrine is unavailable. Vasopressin is recommended as a second line infusion in septic shock.

117. D) Flumazenil (Romazicon)
The antidote for benzodiazepine toxicity is flumazenil. Naloxone is the antidote for opioid toxicity, while cyproheptadine may be used with serotonergic overdose, such as methylphenidate. Diazepam is another benzodiazepine.

118. B) 0.15 mg of intramuscular (IM) epinephrine via EpiPen®
Despite the child's history of asthma, the patient's symptoms are most consistent with anaphylaxis. The first-line treatment for anaphylaxis is IM epinephrine injection. Nebulized albuterol and oral steroids would be part of a treatment plan for asthma exacerbation. Noninvasive ventilatory support is not currently indicated. If respiratory failure occurred due to airway swelling endotracheal intubation would be a more appropriate intervention.

119. B) Cerebral edema post hypoxic event
Cerebral edema can occur 24 to 48 hours post-event, particularly in those who were submersed for a longer period of time. This is not likely the development of an infection or brain bleed. This change in neuro status has nothing to do with the ability to ventilate their child.

120. B) Obtain a history of the event and review of available medications and products in the home
Understanding the events leading up the event, if there was any observed ingestion, and what is available in the home is an integral part of early care with suspected poisoning. This allows targeted and prompt treatment. If this information is not available then symptomology can be used to guide treatment, but delays in appropriate treatment may occur while the team treats for several possible causes. Gastric decontamination may be used following some acute ingestions including salicylates or hypoglycemics but is not likely indicated in this case based on the presenting symptoms. This is true for ocular decontamination as well. Serial serum drug level may be useful in ingestions such as acetaminophen (Tylenol) but are unlikely to be part of early interventions as serial labs occur over time.

121. D) Central line-associated bloodstream infection (CLABSI)
Fever with hypotension is most consistent with bacteremia from a central line. The patient's pain medications are being administered as intermittent doses, which results in several central line entries per day, increasing her risk for CLABSI. CAUTI often presents with fever; hypotension is atypical. A surgical site infection could lead to bacteremia; however, the clean, dry, and intact dressings do not suggest infection. A pressure injury does not typically cause fever and hypotension.

122. A) Compensated respiratory acidosis
The pH is trended toward acidosis but within normal range, which indicates the body is compensating to maintain the physiologic pH range. The CO_2 is 10 units above normal, which will precipitate acidosis. The HCO_3 is slightly elevated in an attempt to raise the pH and avoid acidosis. Because the CO_2 is the primary

and most pronounced derangement, it can be concluded this is a compensated primary respiratory acidosis. Uncompensated states are when the pH is out of the normal range of 7.35 to 7.45.

123. B) Increase respiratory rate on ventilator.
The patient's blood gas demonstrates respiratory acidosis and hypercarbia. This is likely secondary to the sedation that was administered 1 hour prior causing respiratory suppression. Increasing the respiratory rate will result in clearance of retained CO_2. The PO_2 is within the normal range of 75 to 100 mmHg, a decrease is not required. Decreasing the respiratory rate would worsen CO_2 retention. Increasing the expiratory time could aid in removal of CO_2.

124. C) Diuretic use
Contraction alkalosis can occur with diuretic use secondary to loss of extracellular fluid volume and an increase in serum HCO_3 levels. Low levels of potassium and calcium can result in metabolic alkalosis. Mineralocorticoid deficiency is associated with metabolic acidosis.

125. B) Assess and treat for signs of pain or discomfort.
Pain control and comfort optimization are key components of care for the dying patient. This has been expressed by patients and families alike. The other options address high quality risk reduction for all patients. While they are not incorrect actions for this patient, they are not priority actions.

126. C) Administration of a 0.9% NaCl bolus, 20 mL/kg
The primary intervention in hypovolemic shock is to replace the intravascular fluid volume. Transfer to PICU is likely, but not before fluid resuscitation. Dextrose is not indicated in fluid resuscitation for hypovolemia. The patient is showing no infectious signs indicating need for blood cultures.

127. A) Steroids
High-dose steroids function as an immunosuppressant to stop the grafted cells from attacking the host cells. GVHD is not infectious and does not require antibiotics. Immunosupressents, such as tacrolimus, are part of the standard posttransplant regimen but not indicated for GVHD. Antifungals, such as pentamidine, are used prophylactically to prevent pneumocystis carinii pneumonia.

128. B) Rejection of the organ
Organ rejection often presents with signs of dysfunction in that organ/organ system. Decreased urine output and hypertension are indicative of renal concerns. While risk for infection remains a concern for all transplant patients, there are no infectious signs in this scenario. Lymphoma generally presents with lymphadenopathy, weight loss, and fatigue.

129. D) Tissue biopsy
Tissue biopsy is the gold standard for histological analysis to determine the type of rejection. Troponin levels are indicative of cardiac damage but are nonspecific. Intracardiac pressure measurements can be helpful in determining function but do not always correlate to rejection. An echocardiogram is an effective diagnostic tool for function and structural analysis, but does not aid in detection of rejection.

130. A) Acetaminophen (Tylenol)
Fever reduction is important to decrease metabolic demand and improve comfort. Use of aspirin is not recommended in pediatric patients because of the risk of Reye syndrome. Pentamidine is a prophylactic drug administered to posttransplant patients to protect against pneumonia. Metoprolol is a beta-blocker that would slow the heart rate but not address the fever.

131. B) Gently but directly ask the mother why she is giving her child fluids.
This action can cause additional aspiration. The nurse should explain to the mother and educate her. The nurse should not ignore the mother's actions. The nurse may want to make the provider aware but during rounds in front of the entire team may not be the best time. The nurse would not notify social services for this and judge her as noncompliant without having a conversation with the mother. It may just be a knowledge deficit or the mother thinking they are attending to the child's needs. The child could be asking the mother for water.

132. B) "Let me call the social worker/case manager and see if they can assist you with this."
The nurse should involve the social worker/case manager/discharge planner to get involved to be sure the child leaves the hospital with the appropriate medication. The other responses are not acceptable or helpful.

133. B) Resource availability
The biggest area of concern in this patient is the extent of family resources, the first of that being a stable home with a guaranteed electric source. While there is a grandmother involved, she lives 2 hours away. Resiliency of the child would be to return to their prior level of functioning. While that is important, the primary area of concern here is a reliable home with running water, sanitation, and dependable and guaranteed electricity. At age 2, participation in care may be minimal. The predictability of the child and how likely they are expected to follow a certain course of events or their illness trajectory is not the most important concern upon discharge.

134. C) 5 (very high)
This example would demonstrate a nurse functioning at a very high competency of providing patient care.

135. D) Nurses having a feeling of empowerment
Nurses feeling empowered and having their voice heard help them be happier, content, and feeling included. A business-as-usual approach, nurses being short-staffed, stressed, and overwhelmed does not contribute to a positive and health work environment. Nurses who produce and present new innovative ideas to leadership that go nowhere or are ignored causes frustration and dissatisfaction with the work environment.

136. D) Speak to the family and make eye contact to ensure understanding.
Even though the nurse may be using a language translation service like a video language line on an iPad, the nurse should look directly at the family to make sure they are understanding what is being said as well as allowing time for questions. The interpreter should not be in control of the conversation. They are interpreting what the nurse has to say. The nurse does not need to speak more slowly or loudly. If medical terms are needed to explain the situation, the nurse can use them. They should not be avoided. The interpreter will be able to interpret those terms.

137. B) Notify the discharge planner of the child's home care and equipment needs
To begin preparation for discharge, the nurse should involve the discharge planner early so that home care nursing, supplies, ventilator, and other items are in place for this family. They should not wait until the moment before discharge. This discharge requires much coordination. While the nurse may convey their support to the family, they should not say that the care will be overwhelming. Even if that might be true, the nurse should support the family and not create undue anxiety. The nurse may begin teaching at a level the family understands. Anatomy and physiology may be taught where appropriate. However, that is not the priority at this time. Support groups may be important later on, but right now the priority is getting the family set up for discharge with supplies, equipment, and home nursing.

138. C) Competent
The nurse described in this scenario is at the level of competent. A novice level would be primarily focused on learning. An advanced beginner would be refining their skills and not yet be at the level of being a preceptor. The expert level would being clinically competent, engaged in committees, and participating in evidence-based practice projects and perhaps advanced education and certifications.

139. A) "Your child has verbalized that they no longer wish for further life-sustaining treatment to be done."
Conveying the patient's wishes is the best example of speaking or interacting or someone's behalf representing their beliefs, concerns, and desires for care (moral agent) trying to resolve ethical and/or clinical concerns within or outside the clinical setting. This includes providing accurate education so one can provide truly informed consent and accurate decision-making. Sympathizing with the family is ok but example B is reversing what the adolescent wants. Confronting the parents is not appropriate. Scheduling a team meeting to discuss the next course of action when there likely is no next course of action and, most importantly going against the wishes of the patient, who is a legal adult, is not acting as a moral agent.

140. D) "You are scheduled for a burn redress today; what time this morning would you like to do it? Would you like to help me change your bandages today?"
The nurse should give the patient the ability to make decisions and offer the ability to participate in their care. The nurse setting the time and expectations does not allow any patient decision-making. Involving

the parents and not the child does not give the patient the ability to participate. Pain medication may be indicated but if the child is sedated, they cannot participate.

141. C) "How are you doing managing your diabetes?"
Asking an open-ended question to explore how the patient feels about managing their diabetes is the best way to explore understanding and identify any barriers. Involving the parents would not help this situation nor would referring them to a diabetic educator. There may be something more going on in this situation. Telling the patient that their home life should not interfere with their insulin management is too confrontational and will not establish a caring and trusting relationship.

142. A) Involve the social worker to explore the family's resources and explore the teen's living environment.
If there are financial issues that prevent the family from obtaining the insulin, these can be remedied. It also would be good to verify if the child is telling the truth about the home living environment. If abuse is suspected, child protective services should be contacted but involving the social worker first would be the first step. A family meeting might not be helpful to determine if abuse is indeed happening. If it is true, the teen would be reluctant to talk about it in front of the family. This is not a psychiatric issue at this point.

143. A) Stability
Stability is when the patient stays in a steady state. This is when the patient stays stable over a period of time. A patient who is resilient may suffer an insult but has the ability to bounce back and return to their previous level of health and physical functioning. A complex patient has not only multiple physical symptoms but also a complex social since they have no family or person to contribute to decision-making. A patient who is able to take an active role in treatment has participation in care.

144. D) Resource availability
This is an example of resource availability. A patient who has a known physical problem and has no social support, friends or family, or resources available to them exemplifies a patient circumstance with very limited resources to help them maintain a stable state of health.

145. A) 1 (very low)
In this situation the person has very few (if any) resources. Their capacity to return to a previous level of health and functioning using their own compensatory/coping mechanisms is very unlikely. This is the type of patient that will be admitted numerous times for their condition. These patient characteristics are sometimes interrelated. Having limited resource availability will lead to low stability and resiliency. This may be of no fault of their own, just due to their circumstances.

146. B) Participate in decision-making
This patient, due to their confusion, may not fully be able to understand what is happening to them and be able to make a fully informed decision. It is best if they have designated a medical power of attorney that this person be involved in the decision-making for this patient when possible.

147. B) Moderate
This scenario represents a family with moderate available resources. They do have limited knowledge, the father has a job, they have a home even though it is a camper, and they have electric water and sewer, but the electric is not dependable. In this situation, a social worker needs to get involved. The fire department can be contacted to be sure this family has a portable generator for the ventilator should they electric supply be disrupted. Also, a phone call can be made to the local utility company to be sure not to turn off the electric to this home site if the bill is not paid due to medical necessity. The family needs to be hooked up with additional social services. A minimal level of resource would be no home, family, or social support. High availability would have many more resources and a house with reliable electricity and utilities. There is enough information given to determine their level of resource availability.

148. B) Futility
This is an example of futility. Despite best efforts, the patient's condition has not improved. Without a heart transplant, for which this patient is not a candidate, the patient will die. Treatment is futile at this time.

149. D) Cultural factors can affect both the child's and family's response during hospitalization.
When providing culturally competent care with respect to diversity, it is important to understand that culture can affect not only the child's but the family's response to the situation and hospitalization. It is not true that a child of any culture is too young to understand. Nurses must also value what a child thinks and

how they react in relation to the parent's wishes. Nurses may need to advocate for the child, considering their parent's wishes.

150. D) Moderate level of decision-making

This is an example of moderate decision-making. The child is simply seeking advice. They have made the decision to take the medicine, so they are cooperative, just seeking guidance and support. They are talking so they are not shy. A low level of decision-making would be not being able to make a decision at all.

Index

Index